Third Edition

Evaluating Research in Communicative Disorders

Third Edition

Evaluating Research in Communicative Disorders

Nicholas Schiavetti
State University of New York at Geneseo

Dale Evan Metz
State University of New York at Geneseo

Allyn and Bacon
Boston • London • Toronto • Sydney • Tokyo • Singapore

Executive Editor: Steve Dragin
Editorial Assistant: Christine Svitila
Senior Marketing Manager: Kathy Hunter
Editorial-Production Administrator: Donna Simons
Editorial-Production Service: Shepherd, Inc.
Composition and Prepress Buyer: Linda Cox
Manufacturing Buyer: Suzanne Lareau
Cover Administrator: Suzanne Harbison

Library of Congress Cataloging-in-Publication Data

Schiavetti, Nicholas
  Evaluating research in communicative disorders / Nicholas
Schiavetti, Dale Evan Metz.— 3rd ed.
    p. cm.
  Rev. ed. of: Evaluating research in speech pathology and audiology /
Ira M. Ventry, Nicholas Schiavetti. 2nd ed. c1986.
  Includes bibliographical references and indexes.
  ISBN 0–205–19396–X
1. Speech disorders—Research—Evaluation.   2. Audiology—
Research—Evaluation.   I. Metz, Dale Evan.   II. Ventry, Ira M.
Evaluating research in speech pathology and audiology.   III. Title.
  [DNLM: 1. Communicative Disorders.   2. Evaluation Studies.
3. Research.   4. Research Design.   WM 475 S329e 1996]
RC423.V45   1996
616.85'5'0072—dc20
DNLM/DLC
for Library of Congress   96–23757
                                                                              CIP

Printed in the United States of America

10 9 8 7 6 5   01 00 99 98

Dedicated to the Memory of

Ira M. Ventry
1932–1983

"Technical progress evolves through applied scientific research and propagation of the knowledge acquired. It is not enough to pursue the knowledge of wine in the laboratory alone, it must be spread through the wineries in order for this knowledge to become part of daily practice. Moreover, the faster scientific progress advances, the greater risk there is of widening the gap between what we know and what we do. It is necessary to narrow this gap and speed up evolution."

—Emile Peynaud, *Knowing and Making Wine,*
New York: John Wiley & Sons, 1984, p. vii.

Contents

Preface

The third edition of this book remains faithful to the basic purpose of the first two editions, but many differences will be evident in reorganization, updating of material, changes in perspective, and addition of new content.

The main audience for the first edition of this book proved to be master's degree students preparing for a clinical career in communicative disorders. The original intent was to help such students prepare for a clinical career that would be guided by a reasonable assessment of developments in the field as reported in the research literature published in the professional journals. We also hoped to introduce those master's degree students who planned to pursue doctoral study to some of the basic concepts and terminology that they would encounter in the more rigorous research training that doctoral programs provide for potential producers of research.

The vast majority of professionals in communicative disorders are not *producers* of research but most of them are *consumers* of research in their professional activities. Therefore, this is *not* a book that describes *how to do* research. It *is* a book about how to *read, understand,* and *evaluate* research that someone else has done. It should be apparent, however, that the ability to read, understand, and evaluate the research done by others is a basic prerequisite to doing good research. It is sometimes difficult to write about research for the consumer without discussing some of the considerations that face the producer of research, and we tried to limit our treatment of these considerations.

Many revisions have been incorporated into the third edition in accordance with our experiences in teaching and conducting research over the past decade. The text has also been revised in places where reviewers, colleagues, and students have suggested improvements. Several of these changes are evident in the reorganization of Part I of the book. The material on research strategies and design has been expanded, while the material on internal and external validity has been refocused on treatment efficacy research. The small section on measurement in previous editions has been expanded into a chapter: Unfortunately, measurement needs at least a full book to do complete justice to the topic, but we lack space. We hope that these changes will be as well received as were those incorporated into the second edition. Many of the examples have been changed, particularly excerpts in Part II and articles in Part III of the book. Some examples were replaced by newer examples that illustrate points more clearly, and some new examples were added to illustrate points that were not made in the first two editions. A new example is not necessarily better than an old one, however, so many of the examples are old friends that have returned to illustrate points that have remained important over the years.

The third edition, like Gaul and the first two editions, is divided into three parts. Part I includes basic information on research strategies and design in communicative disorders, measurement issues, evaluation criteria, treatment efficacy research, and organization and analysis of data. Part II reflects the four typical parts of a research article: introduction, method, results, and conclusions. The excerpted examples in Part II are intended to illustrate the points made in Part I. Part III contains three complete research articles reprinted with evaluation checklists to guide students in evaluating the important features of research discussed in Parts I and II.

We gratefully acknowledge permission granted by the American Speech-Language-Hearing Association and by the many authors and coauthors to reprint selections from the journal articles. We are especially indebted to Pamela Souza, Christopher Turner, Vicki Hammen, Kathryn Yorkston, Fred Minifie, Janna Oetting, and Mabel Rice for allowing us to reprint their articles *in toto*.

The senior author of the first edition of this book was Ira Ventry who died in 1983. Although there have been many revisions made in the second and third editions, his influence remains obvious to those who knew him or his work. We thank Nona Ventry for graciously affording us access to Ira's notes and files, which were helpful in preparing the revisions for the second and third editions.

We wish to thank the many colleagues and students who have offered suggestions for the three editions of this book. In addition, we extend our appreciation to the following reviewers: Raymond Daniloff, University of North Texas; E. Charles Healey, University of Nebraska; Virgina Walker, Florida State University; and Charles Woodford, West Virginia University.

Six people deserve special thanks. Our department chair, Linda House, has provided a working environment that fosters creativity, independence, and accomplishment: We couldn't ask for a better boss. Kris Farnsworth and Steve Dragin have proven to be conscientious, patient, and understanding editors: We couldn't ask anyone to take better care of our work. Ray O'Connell has been the guardian angel of this book for the better part of two decades: No one understands better than he does why it is still being read. Finally, we thank our wives, Carolyn Schiavetti and Wendy Metz, for the love, encouragement, forbearance, and support that we needed to complete this task in time for the favorite holiday.

Nicholas Schiavetti
Dale Evan Metz
Geneseo, New York

Third Edition

Evaluating Research in Communicative Disorders

Basic Considerations in Evaluating Research

Overview

The six chapters of Part I introduce basic principles for evaluating communicative disorders research. Part I lays the foundation for evaluation of the excerpts from research articles that are presented in Part II and the complete articles found in Part III.

Chapter 1 discusses the relationship between clinical and research enterprises and presents a rationale for the improvement of clinical practice through the application of research findings in applied settings. As Kent (1983, p. 76) has said:

> *A profession that provides its own research base is much more in charge of its own destiny than a profession that doesn't. . . . As clinical practice changes, it will change in large part in response to new knowledge gained through research.*

Common ground in clinical and research activities and in basic and applied research is considered in Chapter 1 and emphasis is placed on the critical evaluation of research as an important activity for all professionals in the field: clinicians and researchers, consumers and producers of research. As Kent (1983, p. 76) further stated:

> *It is tempting to cast a discussion of research into a simple framework in which master's graduates are viewed as users of research and Ph.D. graduates are seen as the producers of research. However, this simplistic framework has important exceptions, and failure to recognize these exceptions may lead us into a faulty first step.*

The tension between basic research and practical application is not unique to our field. Gershenfeld (1995, p. 50) clearly expressed it in his essay "Why I Am/Am Not a Physicist":

> *There is a vigorous battle being fought between the defenders of curiosity-driven basic research and the proponents of applied development to solve practical*

1

problems. I would like to suggest that this polarization risks satisfying neither camp, because it misses the deeper and much more interesting interrelationship between research and application. Neither curiosity nor practice arises in a vacuum [emphasis ours].

Chapter 1 outlines some important principles of scientific method, empirical and rational knowledge, and theory construction in behavioral science. Finally, the editorial process that determines whether or not an article sees the light of day is considered.

The primary focus of Chapter 2 is research strategies in communicative disorders. Commonalities and differences among various experimental and descriptive research strategies are discussed and examples are presented of various approaches. Relationships among independent and dependent variables are discussed and different strategies for examining different kinds of variables are explored. Chapter 3 discusses research design in communicative disorders and examines some basic principles of many group and single-subject designs commonly encountered in the research literature. Measurement issues in communicative disorders are the topic of Chapter 4. Measurement is defined, different levels of measurement are specified, and some general and specific factors that affect the quality of measurements, especially reliability and validity, are discussed.

Chapter 5 considers the important topic of evaluating treatment efficacy research, which, perhaps more than any other area, exemplifies the linkage of research and clinical enterprise. Using the framework of Campbell and Stanley (1966) for the evaluation of research designs in educational psychology, this chapter discusses the important criteria of internal and external validity and factors that may jeopardize them. Some specific treatment efficacy research designs are reviewed relative to these factors and some matters concerning meta-analysis and research ethics are also considered.

Chapter 6 concludes Part I with an overview of important principles in the organization and analysis of data for consumers of research. The purpose of this chapter is to familiarize readers with some terminology, concepts, and statistical methods, without a lengthy discussion of calculation procedures. The material in this chapter, along with the examples in Part II, is intended to assist students in the reading of the results section of a research article. It is beyond the scope of this book to teach statistics *per se* and it is assumed that graduate students in communicative disorders will have at least a one-semester introductory course in statistics. Chapters 6 and 9 review the major terms and concepts of a semester's survey of statistics and provide relevant examples from the communicative disorders literature.

Part II will follow with excerpts from the communicative disorders research literature that provide specific examples of the concepts discussed in Part I.

References

Campbell, D. T., & Stanley, J. C., (1996). *Experimental and quasi-experimental designs for research.* Chicago: Rand McNally.

Gershenfeld, N. (1995). Why I am/am not a physicist. *Physics Today,* 48(7), 50–51.

Kent, R. D. (1983). How can we improve the role of research and educate speech-language patholo-gists and audiologists to be competent users of research? In N. S. Rees & T. L. Snope (Eds.), *Proceedings of the 1983 National Conference on Undergraduate, Graduate, and Continuing Education* (pp. 76–86). St. Paul, MN: American Speech-Language-Hearing Association.

Chapter *1*

Introduction: The Consumer of Research in Communicative Disorders

Beliefs are tentative, not dogmatic;
they are based on evidence, not on authority.
—BERTRAND RUSSELL (1945)
HISTORY OF WESTERN PHILOSOPHY

The purpose of this book is to help practitioners and students in communicative disorders become critical readers of the research literature in the field. Here and throughout, the word *critical* is used to mean "involving skillful judgment as to truth, merit, etc. . . . as in critical analysis" (*American College Dictionary,* 1965). Our intended meaning of the word critical is consistent with Minifie, Hixon, and Williams (1973, p. 9) who stated that "simply understanding journal reports of research is not sufficient, we must be able to evaluate them critically." The book, then, facilitates the practitioner's use of the research literature to improve, modify, and update clinical practice through reasoned assessment and evaluation of the literature relevant to clinical practice. Our goal stems from the basic premise that sound clinical practice should be based, in large part, on the relevant basic and applied research rather than on pronouncements by authorities, intuition, or dogma. As Siegel (1993, p. 36) states:

> *Clinicians need to have enough familiarity with research to judge whether the claims are reasonable and to determine just how closely the proposed clinical procedures adhere to the research methods and the underlying theory. Informed clinicians need not be sophisticated researchers, but they should have had first-hand experience with research during their graduate education to help them*

3

understand the limitations and the possibilities of research and the decisions that face researchers at so many turns in the conduct of a study.

The whole point of the text is to assist the clinician and student to arrive at reasoned decisions about the adequacy of the research reported in our journals and to make independent judgments about the relevance of the research to their clinical activities. In the process, we hope to dispel some of the more common myths about the research article, myths such as "You must be a statistician to read the literature" or "If it is in print, it must be good" or "The more difficult to read, the more scholarly an article must be."

In addition to our goal of helping clinicians develop the critical skills required in reading research, we have two additional goals: we hope the book serves as a bridge between clinician and researcher; and we view the text as a foundation, as a *first* course for the student who plans a career in research or for practitioners interested in conducting research within a clinic or school setting. It must be emphasized, however, that this is not a book on how to do research; it is a book on how to *read* research. It will become apparent, however, that intelligent evaluation of research has much in common with the intelligent conduct of research.

The Clinical Enterprise in Communicative Disorders

Most persons in the discipline of communicative disorders are clinicians and most students currently training will become involved in clinical practice. The American Speech-Language-Hearing Association's (ASHA) 1994 membership database indicates that 76.4 percent of ASHA members provides direct clinical service as their primary employment function. Three percent of the members' primary employment function is supervision of clinical activity. The sum of these two percentages indicates that approximately 80 percent of ASHA members are engaged primarily in direct clinical service. This percentage is in sharp contrast to the 0.7 percent of ASHA members who report research as their primary employment activity. It is further interesting to note that the percentage of members who reported research as a primary employment activity in 1994 is down 0.3 percent from the percentage reported by Punch (1983) a little more than ten years ago.

It can be argued, then, that the clinical enterprise constitutes the heart of the communicative disorders profession. That this is the case is reflected in various certification and accreditation activities of ASHA. These include the certification of clinical competence of the individual clinician and accreditation of both clinical service programs and academic programs and the activities of the Ethical Practice Board. The publication program of ASHA also recognizes the clinical focus of the profession through three important journals, the *American Journal of Speech Language Pathology: A Journal of Clinical Practice,* the *American Journal of Audiology: A Journal of Clinical Practice,* and *Language, Speech, and Hearing Services in Schools.*

In addition, the house organ, *Asha,* contains many articles relevant to the practitioner. In sum, then, the work activities of communicative disorders specialists, the accreditation and certification activities of ASHA, as well as its publication program, attest to the primacy of the clinical enterprise.

How does the clinical enterprise grow? How is it modified to reflect changing client needs and to take into account new and important information emerging from the laboratory? Many forces act on the profession to change its shape and alter its course. Federal and state legislation have an important impact on the development and growth of a profession. Technological advances play a significant role in affecting clinical practice. Advances in theory create new models of diagnosis and treatment. Even economic conditions can play a crucial part in determining the future of a clinical profession. Most relevant for our purposes, however, is that clinical practice also changes or should change as the empirical foundation, on which the practice rests, develops and expands.

How is the student or practitioner exposed to such knowledge—to this information base? It happens in a variety of ways. Professional conventions at the national, regional, and state level play an important part in helping the clinician to keep abreast of significant new developments. Interaction with colleagues is also of value. However, three of the most important ways of maintaining contact with new developments are through formal course work taken in an academic program, reading texts, and ongoing exposure to the periodical literature, that is, the journals relevant to the profession of communicative disorders.

The student's knowledge about clinical practice and the scientific basis of that practice come primarily through exposure to academic course work offered in the formal setting of a college or university. The student, in a very real sense, sees the profession through the eyes of the professor. Theory is presented, principles are expounded, practice is described, and clinical performance is evaluated under the close supervision of an academic staff member. The student depends, to a very large extent, on the knowledge, wisdom, and experience of the mentor. Ideally, the mentor provides the framework and the tools that enable the students to arrive at independent decisions once they become practicing clinicians. How successful the process is depends not only on the skills and the talents of the professor but also on those of the students.

In addition to the interaction that takes place within the confines of academe, the student and the practitioner look toward textbooks for new learning and new information. Textbooks obviously can contribute substantially to our knowledge and provide an excellent impetus to professional growth—but a text is basically a secondary source. That is, the author of a text has distilled, synthesized, organized, and clarified for the reader that theory and research the author believes are important and essential. The reader of the text, again, sees the world of communicative disorders through the eyes of the writer. The reference lists and the bibliographies in textbooks identify many, if not all, of the *primary* sources used by the author. On occasion, the reader may check on a primary source but more often than not, relies on the author's interpretation of the source rather than evaluating both the original source *and* the author's interpretation of the original data.

It is not easy to assess the adequacy of a textbook. Logical organization, clear and precise writing, comprehensive coverage, the extent and thoroughness of the bibliography, and the frequency with which the text is referred to in other texts or articles are some of the factors that need to be considered in the evaluation of a textbook. Book reviews are also helpful. *Contemporary Psychology,* a journal devoted exclusively to book reviews, is an excellent source of reviews of texts and books in psychology and related disciplines. Books on normal and disordered aspects of communication are often reviewed here. *Asha* has a section devoted to reviews of books in communicative disorders, but these reviews are frequently less critical and less scholarly than those appearing in *Contemporary Psychology*. Also, the coverage of new books is more limited than it should be. It should come as no surprise that textbooks contain errors, have misprints, promote the author's biases, and, at times, are simply poorly written. Given sufficient problems, a poor text will disappear from the marketplace. Perhaps that is the final judgment of the adequacy of the text.

Although the textbook can make a valuable contribution to the growth and development of clinical practice, the original research, the primary source for change in scholarly practice, makes an equally important contribution. For example, many of the tests that are used in communicative disorders are first described in the periodical literature. Follow-up studies and continued evaluation of the tests are reported in subsequent years. The test, if it withstands careful scrutiny, is gradually incorporated into clinical use and eventually becomes a routine part of a test battery. The emphasis on acoustic immittance measurement and its widespread adoption in the audiology clinic is an excellent example of the way in which a "new" test becomes part of the clinical test battery (see Jerger, 1975). Similar examples can be cited from communicative disorders literature. Diagnostic techniques and therapy approaches, the tools of the trade, often first see the light of day in the periodical literature.

At some point, sooner or later, the clinician must make a decision on whether to incorporate the test, the therapy approach, the rating scale into his or her clinical practice. The student clinician may have little choice; the student's supervisor or professor, presumably after a careful evaluation of the available data, recommends the procedure and the student accepts the recommendation, at least for the present. The professional, on the other hand, will probably no longer seek the professor's advice. Rather, the clinician may turn to colleagues in the clinic, texts, or information obtained at professional meetings. The professional may also go to the primary sources, the journal articles themselves, to help arrive at a decision based on a careful evaluation of the relevant research. It is to this evaluative process, this critical review, that we address ourselves in this text.

It is interesting to note, and also somewhat surprising, that there is little available to guide the practitioner or student in this evaluation process. There are a number of texts in the behavioral sciences that deal with research methodology and there is certainly no dearth of books on statistics. There are far fewer texts and articles on evaluation of research, and in communicative disorders, this literature is nearly nonexistent. As an example, Auer's (1959) text, *An Introduction to Research in Speech* first appeared almost forty years ago and is only one of a few books of its kind remotely related to our interests here. The Auer text, however, deals primarily with the conduct of research; considerable space is devoted to research methodology in general speech, rhetoric, and the like. Fewer than five pages of the book are devoted to the evaluation of experimental research (see pp. 39–40 and 201–203). Also, the relevance of Auer's book to today's communicative disorder specialist is limited in view of the dramatic changes that have taken place in the profession in the last forty years.

The periodical literature on the evaluation of research in communicative disorders is equally limited. There are only a few current articles relevant to the research evaluation process. For example, Armson and Kalinowski (1994) describe the difficulties in interpreting results of research designed to compare the fluent speech of persons who stutter to the speech of persons who are normally fluent; Young (1993) discusses the limitations of statistical significance testing and how to supplement such tests with measures that examine variance; and Cordes (1994) discusses procedures for improving reliability estimates using Generalizability Theory. The point is that remarkably little has been written about research design and methodology in communicative disorders *per se* and that there is very little information available regarding the evaluation of research in communicative disorders.

There is, however, an often overlooked source of evaluation material that does appear in the periodicals. That source is the "Letters to the Editor" section found in many journals. In many research-oriented journals, the letter to the editor is usually a critique of a published article and, in most instances, the researcher is given the opportunity to respond to the criticisms. These letters make interesting and educational reading. A case in point is the criticism by Cannito (1992) of an article entitled "Consistency of fundamental frequency and perturbation in repeated phonations of sustained vowels, reading, and connected speech" by Fitch (1990). Cannito noted that there were two explicit references in the prose to "correlation" between original and replicate measurements, but there were no correlation coefficients reported. Cannito also criticized Fitch's use of an F-ratio as a consistency measure and further noted the ambiguous use of the terms *consistency, reliability,* and *correlation.* Interestingly, Fitch's response (Fitch, 1992, p. 1269) was that he agreed with Cannito's criticisms and explicitly stated that "the original manuscript contained test-retest correlations. The reviewers, however, recommended that the table [of correlation coefficients] be removed." Regarding the use of an F-ratio as a consistency measure, Fitch went on to state that "The consensus of the reviewers appeared to be that the basic statistical model published in the final manuscript was a sufficient measure of consistency." Was the Fitch study flawed fatally by using the F-ratio as a consistency measure? Was the ANOVA model that was published a sufficient measure of consistency? What does the term *consistency* connote and when should it be used? Should the correlation coefficients have been reported in the original 1990 document? The intelligent consumer of research must be able to answer these questions. These questions, and their answers, again reflect the essence of this book.

In summary, we see the communicative disorders profession as primarily a clinical enterprise. It is an enterprise that is changing, growing, and developing. For growth to be truly substantive, it must rest, we believe, on a scientific and research basis, a basis that must be understood and incorporated into clinical practice.

Scientific Method

Siegel and Ingham (1987, p. 100) argue that the discipline of communicative disorders is "bound together by our concern for disordered communication. As a science, however, we share models, methods, and concepts with a larger community." They go on to say that most people "in the field of communicative disorders belong to the community of behavioral science."

Behavioral science, which has been differentiated from physical and natural sciences in the past, is that branch of science that deals with the development of knowledge concerning human or animal behavior. In recent years, physical and natural sciences (e.g., physics and biology) have been combined with the traditional behavioral sciences (e.g., psychology and sociology) for interdisciplinary research on many aspects of behavior. Areas of study such as sociobiology, neuropsychology, psychoacoustics, and vocal physiology illustrate considerable overlap among the behavioral, physical, and natural sciences in the study of human or animal behavior. Similarly, many disciplines contribute to the scientific underpinnings of communicative disorders. Physics, biology, physiology, computer science, speech science, hearing science, psychology, and psycholinguistics contribute directly or indirectly to the discipline of communicative disorders. These disciplines provide the knowledge and tools required to attack and solve clinical problems in communicative disorders.

To understand the research enterprise (i.e., common knowledge gathering) in communicative disorders, it is necessary to understand the general framework of behavioral science within which these research activities operate. Science is a search for knowledge concerning general truths or the operation of general laws, and it depends on the use of a systematic method for the development of such knowledge. This systematic method is commonly called the *scientific method.* The scientific method includes the recognition of a problem that can be studied objectively, the collection of data through observation or experiment, and the drawing of conclusions based on an analysis of the data that have been gathered.

Scientific research may be directed toward the development of knowledge *per se,* in which case it is called *basic research,* or it may be undertaken to solve some problem of immediate social or economic consequence, in which case it is called *applied research.* In recent years, professionals in many disciplines have realized that basic and applied research are not entirely separate or opposed activities. A piece of research that was done for the sake of basic knowledge may turn out to have an important application; a piece of research done to solve an immediate problem may provide basic information concerning the nature of some phenomenon. In the past, there have been instances of acrimonious opposition between people identified with the so-called basic and applied schools, and such opposition has resulted in communication failures that have retarded rather than advanced the development of knowledge. Today, many people recognize the importance of both basic and applied research, as well as the need for clear communication between researchers with more basic orientations and professionals with more applied orientations.

Within the framework of behavioral science, two major types of research may be identified: *descriptive* and *experimental.* Descriptive research examines group differences, developmental trends, or relationships among variables through the use of laboratory measurements, various kinds of tests, and naturalistic observations. Experimental research examines causation through observation of the effects of the manipulation of certain variables on other variables under controlled conditions. These two types of research are different empirical approaches to the development of knowledge.

Empirical and Rational Knowledge

Scientific endeavor depends on a complex interplay of empirical *and* rational inquiry, so it is important to understand the relationship between these two modes of inquiry in behavioral science.

Empiricism is a philosophy that assumes that knowledge must be gained through experience. Empiricists generally rely on inductive reasoning, that is, they use evidence from particular cases to make inferences about general principles. To be accepted into the realm of knowledge, explanations of phenomena must be based on evidence gained from observations of phenomena, and critical evaluation of the accuracy of observations is necessary before the observations can be accepted as evidence. This critical, self-correcting activity of empiricism is the core of scientific endeavor and is a necessary requisite of sound behavioral science research.

Rationalism is a philosophy that assumes that knowledge must be gained through the exercise of logical thought. Rationalists generally rely on deductive reasoning, that is, the use of general principles to make inferences about specific cases. Rationalism is often referred to as a *schematic* or *formal* or *analytic* endeavor because it deals with abstract models, and the logical criticism of propositions is necessary for the acceptance of explanations into the realm of knowledge.

Various schools of thought within the behavioral sciences differ in the extent to which they rely on empirical and rational endeavors. In linguistics, for instance, Chomsky (1968) insists that rational consideration rather than empirical inquiry is necessary for the development of a theory of language. In psychology, Skinner (1953) has relied on empirical evidence for a functional analysis of behavior and eschewed the exclusively rational approach. Although these two examples illustrate the extreme ends of the continuum of rational and empirical thought, many positions regarding the integration of empirical evidence and rational inquiry exist along this continuum. Stevens (1968, p. 850) suggested the term *schemapiric* for the "proper and judicious joining of the schematic with the empirical," and concluded (p. 856):

> *Science presents itself as a two-faced, bipartite endeavor looking at once toward the formal, analytic, schematic features of model-building, and toward the concrete, empirical, experiential observations by which we test the usefulness of a particular representation. Schematics and empirics are both essential to science, and full understanding demands that we know which is which.*

Common Steps in Behavioral Science Research

Examination of articles in the behavioral science literature reveals some common steps taken in empirical research. These steps exemplify the nature of the scientific approach discussed more thoroughly in texts such as Kerlinger (1973) and Bordens and Abbott (1988). Consideration of this simplified outline may enable consumers to understand the general framework underlying empirical research and to realize that the different types of research to be discussed here are variations on a common theme of empirical inquiry.

The common steps in empirical research are:

Statement of a *problem* to be investigated.
Delineation of a *method* for investigation of the problem.
Presentation of the *results* of this investigation.
Drawing *conclusions* from the results about the problem.

We outline as follows how these steps are usually presented in a research article. Part II of this book considers each of these steps in greater detail and presents examples with critical comments.

Statement of the Problem

The researcher usually begins with the formulation of a general problem, a statement of purpose, a research question, or a hypothesis. In some cases, there may be a general statement followed by its breakdown into a number of specific subproblems or subpurposes. Whether researchers choose to present their topics with a statement of the problem, a purpose, a research question, or a hypothesis seems to be a matter of personal preference and, in fact, there is disagreement among researchers as to which of these linguistic vehicles is best for conveying the nature of the topic under investigation. We are not interested here in the polemics surrounding the choice of wording in presenting the topic to be investigated. We are more concerned that researchers provide a *clear and concise statement of what it is they are investigating.*

The problem statement should also contain some material on the meaningfulness or relevance of the topic under investigation by placing it in context. This is generally accomplished by establishing a *rationale* for the study through a review of the literature that has already been published on the particular topic to be investigated. This review may provide a historical background of the research to date and perhaps provide a summary or organization of the existing data so that the reader has an overview of what is known, what is not known, and what is equivocal concerning this general topic. Eventually, the review should culminate in a statement of the need for the particular study and a statement of the significance of the particular study.

Method of Investigation

After stating the research problem and providing its rationale by placing it in perspective relative to the existing literature, the researcher outlines a *strategy* for investigating the problem. This is accomplished through the description of the method of investigation. It is common to find the Method section of an article divided into three subsections: (1) subjects, (2) materials, and (3) procedures. Although there are variations on these subsections, the important questions we are concerned with are: *How was the study carried out? Did the method provide valid and reliable results?*

Subjects

In this section of the research article, the researcher describes the people (or animals) that were studied. A careful description is generally provided of the relevant characteristics of the subjects (e.g., number of subjects, age, gender, intelligence, type of speech or hearing disorder, etc.). The important point is how well the general population under consideration (e.g., stutterers or presbycusics) is defined and how well the sample of subjects represents the population the researcher wishes to study.

Materials

In this section, the researcher describes the various tests, instruments, apparatus, or training materials used and may also describe the situation or environment in which the study took place. Information about the calibration, reliability, and validity of tests or instruments used is also presented here.

Procedure

In this section, the researcher describes how the *materials* were used to study the *subjects.*

Results of Investigation

Here, the researcher presents the results of the collection of data by means of the method of investigation just described. Tables and figures are often used to summarize and organize the data. Tables and figures are usually easier to understand than a simple listing of all the individual or raw data. It is important for a researcher to present a specific breakdown of the results as they relate to the specific subcomponents of the problem presented at the beginning of the article.

Conclusions

After presenting the results, the researcher draws conclusions from them that reflect on the original statement of the problem. The conclusions are often cast in the form of a discussion of the results in relation to previous research, theoretical implications, practical implications, and suggestions for further research.

This simplified discussion of the manner in which the common steps in empirical research are reported in a journal article may give beginning readers the impression that research is a drab activity that follows a single pattern. It is difficult to understand the excitement and creativity inherent in the design and execution of an empirical study unless the student experiences it directly. In fact all researchers may not necessarily follow the orderly steps outlined above in doing their research; adjustments may be made to meet the needs of a researcher in a particular situation. Skinner (1959, p. 363) has captured some of the flavor of scientific creativity and excitement in his famous statement:

> *Here was a first principle not formally recognized by scientific methodologists: when you run onto something interesting, drop everything else and study it.*

The common steps just outlined, then, are meant to illustrate the major components of the scientific method as reflected in the structure of most journal articles that report empirical research and should not be construed as an inviolate set of rules for defining *the* scientific method.

We also want to point out that readers are likely to encounter some articles that do not report original empirical research data, but, instead, review the existing literature on a particular topic in communicative disorders. These reviews are usually much more comprehensive and detailed than the literature review found in the introduction to a typical research article. They provide a historical perspective of trends in the development of thought about a particular topic and demonstrate how these trends may have shaped research approaches to these topics. Discussion of method and theory in historical research is beyond the scope of this book and readers are referred to Barzun and Graff (1970) for a general overview of historical research. A few brief points should be made about literature reviews as they relate to the commonalities of empirical research.

First, such reviews are important in synthesizing research developments to date, organizing our thinking regarding how past research has contributed to our present knowledge, and suggesting new avenues for exploration. Second, such devices are valuable in theory construction and in placing data into theoretical perspective. Third, such reviews are important sources of *critical* evaluation of the research literature. Finally, comprehensive reviews of the research literature also help to illuminate what Boring (1950) has referred to as the *zeitgeist* (German: "time spirit"), or the prevailing outlook that is characteristic of a particular period or generation. The zeitgeist influences research trends along particular lines and may proscribe other directions, but it may also shift to generate new research trends. Baken (1975), for example, has noted such a zeitgeist shift in his discussion of a renewed interest in physiological studies of stuttering behavior. Physiological studies of the 1930s had not proven to be particularly fruitful, partially because of technological difficulties that have now been overcome for the most part by advances in electronics. Of even more importance in the renewal of interest in physiological research, however, is what Baken called, "a retreat from the cortex." After reviewing the traditional stress on higher cortical functions in stuttering etiology as exemplified by cerebral dominance, semantic, Freudian psychodynamics, and non-Freudian psychological theories, Baken highlighted the new emphasis on peripheral physiological events in the "domain of quantifiable observations" that opened new areas of etiological research and has implications for biofeedback and behavior modification treatments. Lane and Tranel (1971) provided another example in their review of the Lombard sign. They pointed out that although this discovery has important implications for four areas of scientific investigation, researchers have failed to appreciate these ramifications and, therefore, have incorrectly relegated Lombard's work only to the area of audiometry. This constrained view of the importance of the Lombard sign has resulted in a narrow channel of research efforts concerning this phenomenon.

An example of a potential zeitgeist change is an article published by Hixon and Weismer (1995) where they reexamined published data from a complex study of speech breathing (Draper, Ladefoged, and Whitteridge, 1959) that has become known as the Edinburgh study. Hixon and Weismer (1995, p. 42) assert that:

> *The Edinburgh study has had a forceful, pervasive, and lasting impact on the speech sciences and is considered by many to be the definitive account of speech breathing function. Indeed, it is widely afforded the status of a classic.*

In a detailed critique, Hixon and Weismer (1995) pointed out several measurement and interpretive flaws in the Edinburgh study that serve to invalidate the study. In a sense, Hixon and Weismer's critique serves as a strong impetus to conduct new research in speech breathing processes. Hixon and Weismer (1995, p. 58), in fact, state:

> *There is still much to be learned about speech breathing and its role in human communication. Our hope for this article is that it will stimulate thinking and serve a useful tutorial purpose for those who will follow.*

The best way for students of communicative disorders to appreciate the common steps in empirical research that we have discussed thus far is to read journal articles that report empirical research. Sustained experience in the reading of empirical research will enable the student to eventually assimilate the concept or process of moving from the formulation of a problem that can be attacked empirically to the drawing of conclusions based on empirical evidence. Many students report that the reading of literature reviews is as important as the reading of original empirical articles in developing an appreciation of the common steps in empirical research.

Theory Construction in Behavioral Science

Empirical and rational inquiry leads to the development of theories that are statements formulated to explain phenomena. Kerlinger (1973, p. 9) stated that theory is the "ultimate aim of science" and defined a theory as:

> *a set of interrelated constructs (concepts), definitions, and propositions that presents a systematic view of phenomena by specifying relations among variables, with the purpose of explaining and predicting the phenomena .*

Rummel (1967) discussed the relationship of rational and empirical inquiry in theory construction and stated that empirical facts alone are meaningless unless they are linked through propositions that confer meaning on the facts. According to Rummel (1967, p. 454):

> *A scientific theory consists of two components:* analytic *and* empirical. *The analytic component is the linking of symbolic statements through chains of reasoning that obey logical or mathematical rules but that have little or no operational-empirical content. . . . this analytic component of theories can be the creation of the scientist's imagination, the distillation of a scholar's experience with the subject matter, or a tediously built structure slowly erected on a foundation of numerous experiments, investigations, and findings. The empirical component of theories is operational. It fastens the abstract analytic part of a theory to the facts.*

Theories generally fall into one of two broad categories (Sidman, 1960). First, they may be generalizations, developed after the facts are in, that try to synthesize the available empirical evidence into a coherent explanation of a phenomenon. Skinner (1972, p. 100) has called such a theory "a formal representation of the data reduced to a minimal number of terms." Second, theories may be tentative generalizations or conjectures that can be subjected to future empirical confirmation—as such, they are often called *hypotheses*. The first kind of theory looks back at available data and employs a formal logic to synthesize this empirical evidence; the second kind looks ahead to future empirical and rational inquiry for verification of the theory. Empirical and rational inquiry is necessary for verification of a theory or for its modification if observed facts do not fit the theory. A knowledgeable consumer of research should recognize the theoretical organization of empirical evidence and the empirical confirmation of theories as two activities that coalesce to form the "schemapiric view" in the behavioral sciences.

Bordens and Abbott (1988, p. 484) suggest that some theories have "stood the test of time, whereas others have fallen by the wayside." Many factors contribute to the longevity, or lack thereof, of any particular theory, and Bordens and Abbott (1988, pp 484–485) have listed five essential factors that can figure centrally in the life of theory. The first is the theory's ability to "account for most of the existing data within its domain." They explain that the amount of data accounted for is *most* not *all* because some of the data germane to the theory may be unreliable. Secondly, theories must have *explanatory relevance*. Explanatory relevance means that the "explanation for a phenomenon provided by a theory must offer good grounds for believing that the phenomenon would occur under the specified conditions" of the theory. The third condition is that of *testability*. Bordens and Abbott (1988 p. 484) state:

A theory is testable if it is capable of failing some empirical test. That is, the theory specifies outcomes under particular conditions, and if these outcomes do not occur, then the theory is rejected.

The theory's ability to predict novel events or new phenomena is the fourth characteristic of a sound theory. A theory should predict phenomena "beyond those for which the theory was originally designed." Such new phenomena were not taken into account when the theory was originally formulated. Lastly, the theory should be *parsimonious* (i.e., it should adopt the fewest and/or simplest set of assumptions in the interpretation of data).

There is controversy regarding the role of theory guiding research in the field of communicative disorders (Siegel and Ingham, 1987). For example, arguing strongly in favor of theory construction, Kent and Fair (1985, p. 26) stated that "science without theory may amount to little more than stamp collecting—systematic but without potential to advance knowledge." Similarly, Perkins (1986, p. 32) stated:

Theories are like maps. To do research without a theory is equivalent to traveling in a foreign territory without a map. Both tell you which way to turn. If the map is wrong, you soon discover you are lost and discard the map in favor of a better one. Likewise, theories are designed to be tested and discarded in favor of better ones that account for evidence more successfully.

In their response to Perkins (1986), Siegel and Ingham (1987) cite several examples of important and meaningful communicative disorders research efforts that were not motivated by theory. Siegel and Ingham (1987, p. 102) state:

Perkins (1986) is concerned that to do research unbounded by theory is like wandering in a wilderness without a map, but although that is a suggestive metaphor, it is not necessarily a useful one. In many areas of communication disorders we do not have a predetermined destination but are guided by the results of our research. We use as our map the questions that were raised as we were attempting to answer previous questions.

The arguments on both sides of the theory debate can be compelling, but in our view, the summary position of Siegel and Ingham (1987, pp. 103–104) is probably the most useful to the informed consumer of research:

Some research is clearly designed to test the current theories. Other research starts and ends with a particular phenomenon. A good theory will incorporate facts and data regardless of their lineage, and a good inductive program of research will take note of the conceptual integrations that theories provide; it cannot do otherwise.

The Nature of Research in Communicative Disorders

It is extremely difficult to paint a complete picture of the research enterprise in communicative disorders. No one has done it and we will not do it here. The data that would form the basis of such a picture are simply not available. A few generalizations should help, however, in understanding the broad scope of research activities that impinge, either directly or indirectly, on communicative disorders.

Although relatively few communicative disorders specialists are involved in full-time research, (ASHA Membership Database, 1994) the research enterprise in communicative disorders is much broader than would appear from surveys of the ASHA membership. One obvious reason is that not all people who are involved in communicative disorders research are members of ASHA. More important, though, is that many people are involved in research activities on less than a full-time basis. Perhaps the best example of such a person is the academician whose primary job responsibility is teaching. Such an individual is often involved in his or her own research or supervises doctoral dissertations or master's theses. The same person publishes the results of his or her research not only to advance knowledge but also to advance his or her own standing in the academic community because, unfortunately, the "publish-or-perish" phenomenon is still commonplace in university life. Other part-time researchers include doctoral students and clinicians working in a variety of clinical settings. Finally, much of the research appearing in the periodical literature is done by people working on the periphery of communicative disorders. These include individuals such as otolaryngologists, experimental psychologists, psycholinguists, and neurophysiologists. The numbers of published articles that relate directly or tangentially to the interests of professionals in communicative disorders attest to the numbers and different interests and backgrounds of individuals involved in the communicative disorders research enterprise.

The areas investigated are equally diverse, ranging, for example, from the study of the effects of noise on the hearing sensitivity of chinchillas to the study of hearing-aid evaluation procedures, from a study of infant respiration to a study of the most efficient way to teach esophageal speech to a laryngectomee, from the study of how children acquire language to the study of how aphasics relearn speech and language. The areas studied are almost as numerous as the people involved in their study.

The settings in which research is conducted are equally varied. Language acquisition of a normal child is studied in the naturalistic environment of the child's home; the efficiency of an auditory site-of-lesion test is evaluated in the audiology clinic. The chinchilla's hearing sensitivity is investigated within the confines of a laboratory; the effects of noise on human hearing sensitivity may be studied in a factory setting. Stuttering behavior may be investigated in a laboratory, clinic, or school. In broad terms, normal processes are usually but not always studied in a laboratory setting; the study of disordered communication is frequently but not always carried out in a clinical setting.

Finally, as we will see in Chapter 2, the research strategies in communicative disorders are also diverse, ranging from survey studies performed in the field to experimental research performed in the laboratory.

This section would be incomplete without some mention of the responsibilities incumbent on the researcher. In addition to doing "good" research, the researcher has two major responsibilities: to communicate and to be relevant. Jerger (1993, p. 47–48) has stated emphatically that a person conducting research must:

> be a leader, not a follower, in translating research findings into everyday clinical practice. . . . research is not complete until its implications have been translated into clinical practice.

Although few would dispute the need for communication scientists to communicate clearly about their research, the issue of relevance is another matter. Clinicians complain about the lack of relevance; yet, what is seemingly irrelevant today may have major clinical implications tomorrow. The examples in communicative disorders are almost too numerous to cite. The research done in the early 1950s on delayed auditory feedback, conducted originally to obtain a better understanding of normal speech and hearing processes, has found its way into stuttering treatment and the audiology clinic. The ear's ability to detect changes in intensity, first studied in the 1920s and 1930s, gave rise to the clinical techniques developed in the 1950s and 1960s for measuring differential sensitivity. The study of normal language acquisition and phonology provides a better understanding of the language problems of children seen in the clinic. The problem is not that our basic research is irrelevant to clinical practice but rather that the researcher may have failed to discuss the relevancy, or potential relevancy, of the research to the practitioner.

In addition to having a responsibility to communicate relevant findings, the researcher has other important ethical responsibilities—responsibilities that are inherent in the research process. Several professional associations have codes of ethics that specify the ethical constraints placed on investigators who do research with human subjects. For example, subjects must have the freedom to decline to participate in a research project or to withdraw from the project at any time. The welfare and dignity of subjects must be protected at all times. The investigator must protect the confidentiality of information obtained during the course of the study. The investigator must protect subjects from physical and mental discomfort, harm, and danger. Investigators must honor all agreements and commitments made to subjects. More complete descriptions of these ethical obligations can be found in such sources as *Ethical Principles in the Conduct of Research with Human Participants* (American Psychological Association [APA], (1992) and in Part III of the November 23, 1982, Federal Register.

The ethical responsibilities placed on the researcher are as stringent as those required of clinicians, especially when the researcher is using human subjects. In fact, researchers have both ethical *and* legal responsibilities to protect the rights of both human and nonhuman living subjects. Many institutions are required to have an Institutional Review Board that studies research proposals to ensure that the welfare of subjects is scrupulously maintained, especially if the institution is interested in obtaining governmental funds for the conduct of the research. Suffice it to say that researchers have important obligations to a varied constituency—to their audience, their subjects, their institutions, their profession, and themselves.

Consumers and Producers of Research

Kent (1985, p. 1) maintained that the field of communication disorders has had an "abiding conflict" between research and clinical practice. One need only read, for example, the exchanges between Jerger (1963) and Spriestersbach (see Jerger, 1964) and the flurry of ensuing position papers that were published during the 1970s and 1980s (e.g., Costello, 1979; Kent, 1983; Holley, 1983; Moll, 1983; Ringel, 1972) to confirm the long-standing and serious nature of this conflict. The essence of the conflict appears to be due to a conventional notion that research does little to inform clinical practice and an implicit idealized model of consumers and producers of research in communicative disorders. At a national conference on graduate education in communicative disorders, Kent (1983, p. 76) argued:

> It is tempting to cast a discussion of research into a simple framework in which master's graduates are viewed as users of research and Ph.D. graduates are seen as the producers of research.

Kent stated clearly that such a framework is too "simplistic," but the notion of such a conceptual framework was echoed at that same conference by Moll (1983, p. 32) who said:

> Although professional entry-level programs will not be designed to prepare persons for research careers, it is clear that graduates need to be consumers of research information if they are to keep current and be able to adapt new knowledge to their clinical practice.

In response to Moll's (1983) statements, Siegel and Spradlin (1985, p. 227) stated:

> To argue that clinicians are generally not researchers is not to suggest that they cannot be but only to recognize that despite a shared interest in disorders of communication, specialized education and training are required to do competent research. Realistically, it is rarely possible for this training to be incorporated into professional education, and the demands of most clinical positions make it difficult for research skills to be acquired on the job.

How can consumers and producers of research find common ground that will serve to ameliorate the abiding conflict to which Kent (1985) alluded? Although not all research findings may impact directly and immediately on the clinical enterprise, there are many research topics and paradigms that show great promise for both the researcher and the clinician. For example, Siegel (1993, p. 37) argued that treatment efficacy research "makes a natural bridge between the requirements of careful research and the needs of clinical practice." Similarly, Olswang (1993) suggested that clinical efficacy research can address both applied clinical questions and questions of a more theoretical nature. Specifically, Olswang (1993, p. 126) stated:

> *For those of us driven by both clinical practice and theory, we have found our playground. Efficacy research allows us to function within our split interests— addressing practice and the needs of the individual while investigating theory and the underlying mechanisms of communication. What we need is further research with this two-pronged approach, advancing our clinical and theoretical knowledge. Our profession and discipline indeed depend on both.*

There are potentially hundreds of legitimate research questions that fall under the general rubric of treatment efficacy research. Carefully controlled group studies could investigate the relative efficacy of two or more intervention paradigms designed to improve dysarthric speech, time series designs could be employed to investigate the immediate and long-term effectiveness of fluency-enhancing protocols, and single-subject designs could be used to investigate clinical strategies for increasing language output in children who are language delayed. It goes beyond the scope of this text to discuss all the potential treatment efficacy investigations, but the area is rich with research potential. Wertz (1993, p. 38) asks if the question "Does therapy work?" serves as a legitimate research question and proceeds to answer the question by responding:

> *It seems to me that the question is not only appropriate for research; it is essential for clinical practice. The rationale for not asking appears weak.*

The Editorial Process in the Publication of a Research Article

One common myth that needs to be dispelled early is that if an article appears in print, it must be worthwhile, valuable, and a significant contribution to the literature and to our knowledge. This is simply not the case. Inadequate research is reported, trivial problems are investigated, and articles vary tremendously in quality and value. Perhaps a brief description of the publication process will help the reader understand how an article gets published and how the quality of research can vary from one article to the next.

Although the editorial process differs from journal to journal, there are commonalities in the review process that cut across most journals. (For a description of the editorial process for articles published by the American Psychological Association, the reader should consult the Association's Publication Manual [American Psychological Association, 1994].) Let us use, as an example, a clinical research article submitted for publication to the *American Journal of Speech-Language Pathology: A Journal of Clinical Practice (AJSLP)*, one of the journals published by ASHA. At the time of writing, the journal was directed to professionals who provide services to persons with communication disorders. Manuscripts that deal with the nature, assessment, prevention and treatment of communicative disorders were invited. Note that the *Journal of Speech and Hearing Research (JSHR),* also published by ASHA, "invites papers concerned with theoretical issues and research in the communication sciences." Manuscripts submitted to *AJSLP* are considered on the basis of clinical significance, conformity to standards of evidence, and clarity of writing. The journal welcomes philosophical, conceptual, or synthesizing essays, as well as reports of clinical research. The details are contained in the Information for Authors section of each issue, a section that defines, in a general way, the scope and emphasis of the journal, thus helping potential contributors to decide whether *AJSLP* is the appropriate journal for their manuscript.

The editorial staff of *AJSLP* consists of an editor and several associate editors in areas such as fluency and fluency disorders, neurogenic communication disorders, dysphagia, voice disorders, and communication disorders in early childhood. In addition, there are more than one hundred editorial consultants, all of whom are knowledgeable in one or more areas of communicative disorders. Overall editorial policy is established by the editor and must be consistent with the general guidelines set by the Publication Board of ASHA.

On receipt of a manuscript, a decision is made into whose purview the manuscript falls. An associate editor is then assigned to oversee the review process and to serve as a reviewer. Next, the manuscript is forwarded by the associate editor to two editorial consultants who, after careful evaluation of the manuscript, recommend one of four alternatives: (1) accept for publication as is, (2) accept contingent on the author agreeing to make certain revisions recommended by the reviewers, (3) defer decision pending major revisions and another review by two different editorial consultants, and (4) reject outright. No matter which alternative is recommended, the final decision to accept or reject lies with the editor. If a decision to reject is reached, the evaluations by the reviewers are forwarded to the author, sometimes with a marked copy of the manuscript. The editorial consultants are not identified to the author and the editorial consultants do not know the name of the author or the author's institutional affiliation. That is, manuscripts are subjected to a "blind" review in which reviewers are ostensibly unaware of the identity of the author.

Although every effort is made to arrive at a publication decision quickly, the review process can be time consuming, especially if extensive revision is requested. The revisions may require considerable work on the part of the author, data may have to be reanalyzed or displayed differently, tables and figures may have to be added or deleted, and portions of the manuscript may have to be rewritten. Obviously, the more revisions required, the less likely is a manuscript to be accepted, particularly if a journal has a backlog of manuscripts already accepted for publication. All of this necessitates considerable correspondence between the author and the editor and, perhaps, even another review by two more editorial consultants. It is for these reasons that considerable time may elapse between the date the manuscript is received and the date it is finally accepted.

How do inadequate or marginal manuscripts end up being published? Despite the care that is taken to select knowledgeable and informed editorial consultants, not all editorial consultants have the same level of expertise, have comparable research or evaluative skills, are equally familiar with a given area, use the same standards in evaluating a manuscript, and give the same amount of time and energy to the evaluation process. One journal in the field of communicative disorders, the *Journal of Fluency Disorders*, periodically surveys the consulting editors regarding their interests and expertise in an attempt to provide competent and balanced manuscript reviews.

Finally, the research sophistication found among members of a profession or discipline can have a pronounced effect on the character and excellence of its journals. Equally important, however, is the great care of the journal staff to ensure a high degree of excellence in the review process. Despite everyone's devotion to quality, journal articles indeed differ in excellence, and educated consumers of research have the responsibility of being able to identify those differences.

Some Myths and a Caveat

One of our goals is to explode some of the myths surrounding research and the evaluation of research. We have noted already that the appearance of an article in a journal is no guarantee of the article's quality. There is good research and there is poor research, both of which may be published. The objective of the critical evaluation is to discern which is which. A stance of healthy skepticism is good for both the reader and, in the long run, for the researcher and the profession.

A major obstacle standing in the path of the consumer of research is the attitude that one must have a solid background in statistics before one can intelligently read the research literature. A similar attitude is that research and statistics are synonymous. Nothing could be further from the truth. For example, Plutchik (1974) stated that statistical analysis is not an end in itself and cannot ensure meaningful conclusions simply by its application to experimental data. This view continues to be held by current authors of research design textbooks such as DePoy and Gitlin (1994, p. 237) who point out that "conducting statistical analysis is just one action process in research." No matter how excellent and sophisticated the statistical treatment, a major weakness in any other part of the research study or article vitiates the value of the statistical analysis. A trivial problem is still trivial no matter how sophisticated the statistical analysis. A poorly conceived research design remains poorly conceived, despite a complex statistical approach. The inferences and generalizations drawn from the data may be appropriate and fair but the statistical analysis does not ensure this.

Statistical analysis is an essential tool for the researcher, but research and statistical treatment are not the same. A serious weakness in *any* part of a research article—introduction (rationale), method, data analysis, or discussion—weakens the whole.

Another myth, perhaps less widely held, is that the researcher is characteristically a recluse in a white coat isolated in the ivy-covered laboratory working on problems that have little relevance to human life, no less to the practicing clinician. Again, this is not true. Most researchers are concerned about people with communicative disorders, and it is this concern that continues to motivate their research. In fact, many of today's researchers have strong clinical backgrounds and extensive clinical experience. Many researchers, while perhaps not involved in research that has immediate application, are doing research that tomorrow may have considerable relevance to clinical practice. Researchers usually do not go out of their way to be obtuse or uncommunicative; some may not write well, but the poor writing is unintentional. A number of leading researchers have played important roles in the nonresearch professional aspects of communicative disorders. Some researchers are haughty and aloof; so, too, are some clinicians.

Now for the caveat. Although we are attempting to lead the interested clinician through the process of research evaluation, a fundamental prerequisite to intelligent consumership is the fund of substantive information possessed by the reader. To illustrate, let us take a research article on stuttering and, further, let us consider the introductory section devoted to developing the need for the study and the purpose of the study. How can one evaluate the author's rationale without some knowledge of the literature on stuttering? Have important citations been omitted because they are inconsistent with the author's purpose? Can the reader understand the theoretical framework within which the author is operating? Has the author misinterpreted or misunderstood previous research? The only way the reader can answer these questions is to have a strong background in the subject of stuttering. The identical problem exists for the editorial consultant; that is why journals have large rosters of reviewers. The information explosion in communicative disorders has made it almost impossible for one person to be truly knowledgeable in all substantive areas.

This is not a book on stuttering, aphasia, cleft palate, or audiometry; therefore, we have made the assumption that practitioners and students will approach a journal article with some background on the topic dealt with in the article. Although we have provided a framework for evaluation, the framework must rest on a substantive foundation which the reader must have.

Study Questions

1. Read the following article:

   Minifie, F. D. (1983). Research mentorship training in communication sciences and disorders. In N. S. Rees and T. L. Snope (Eds.), *Proceedings of the 1983 National Conference on Undergraduate, Graduate, and Continuing Education* (pp. 3–9). St. Paul, MN: American Speech-Language-Hearing Association.

   a. What are the major issues that Minifie raised regarding the need for research mentorships?

   b. What is his position on postdoctoral work in communication disorders?

2. Read the following articles:

   Dillon, H. (1993). Hearing aid evaluation: Predicting speech gain from insertion gain. *Journal of Speech and Hearing Research, 36,* 621–633.

   McHenry, M., Minton, J., Wilson, R., & Post, Y. (1994). Intelligibility and nonspeech orofacial strength and force control following traumatic brain injury. *Journal of Speech and Hearing Research, 37,* 1271–1283.

   Examine the overlap of physical and behavioral measurements in the investigation of speech and hearing phenomena in these two articles.

3. Read the following article:

   Stevens, S. S. (1968). Measurement, statistics, and the schemapiric view. *Science, 161,* 849–856.

   Summarize Stevens's viewpoint on the relationship between the schematic and empirical aspects of science. What is the meaning of Stevens's reference to the two faces of Janus?

4. Read the following articles:

   Hixon, T. J., & Weismer, G. (1995). Perspectives on the Edinburgh study of speech breathing. *Journal of Speech and Hearing Research, 38,* 42–60.

   Folkins, J. W., & Bleile, K. M. (1990). Taxonomies in biology, phonetics, phonology, and speech motor control. *Journal of Speech and Hearing Disorders, 55,* 596–611.

   Discuss the manner in which the authors deal with the relationship of empirical evidence to theory. Are theories cited that represent a synthesis of previous evidence? Are new theories advanced that need to be confirmed by future empirical evidence?

5. Read the following article:

   Perkins, W. H. (1990). What is stuttering? *Journal of Speech and Hearing Disorders, 55,* 370–382.

   What does Perkins say about the relationships among research, theory, and therapy?

References

American college dictionary. (1965). New York: Random House.

American Psychological Association. (1992). Ethical principles of psychologists and code of conduct. *American Psychologist, 47,* 1597–1611.

American Psychological Association. (1994). *Publication manual of the American Psychological Association* (4th ed.). Washington, DC: American Psychological Association.

American Speech-Language-Hearing Association. (1994). Membership database. Unpublished document.

Armson, J., & Kalinowski, J. (1994). Interpreting results of the fluent speech paradigm in stuttering research: Difficulties in separating cause from effect. *Journal of Speech and Hearing Research, 37,* 69–82.

Auer, J. J. (1959). *An introduction to research in speech.* New York: Harper and Row.

Baken, R. (1975). Overview of the conference. In L. M. Webster, & L. C. Furst (Eds.), *Vocal tract dynamics and disfluency* (pp. 1–9). New York: Speech and Hearing Institute.

Barzun, J., & Graff, H. F. (1970). *The modern researcher.* New York: Harcourt, Brace, & World.

Bordens, K. S., & Abbott, B. B. (1988). *Research design and methods: A process approach.* Mountain View, CA: Mayfield Publishing Company.

Boring, E. G. (1950). *A history of experimental psychology.* New York: Appleton-Century-Crofts.

Cannito, M. P. (1992). A questionable consistency: Response to Fitch. *Journal of Speech and Hearing Research, 35,* 1268–1269.

Chomsky, N. (1968). *Language and mind.* New York: Harcourt, Brace, & World.

Cordes, A. K. (1994). The reliability of observational data: I. Theories and methods for speech-language pathology. *Journal of Speech and Hearing Research, 37,* 264–278.

Costello, J. M. (1979). Clinicians and researchers: A necessary dichotomy? *Journal of the National Student Speech and Hearing Association. 7,* 6–26.

DePoy, E. & Gitlin, L. N. (1994). *Introduction to research: Multiple strategies for health and human services.* St. Louis: Mosby.

Draper, M., Ladefoged, P., & Whitteridge, D. (1959). Respiratory muscles in speech. *Journal of Speech and Hearing Research, 2,* 16–27.

Fitch, J. L. (1990). Consistency of fundamental frequency and perturbation in repeated phonations of sustained vowels, reading, and connected speech. *Journal of Speech and Hearing Research, 55,* 360–363.

Fitch, J. L. (1992). Response to Cannito. *Journal of Speech and Hearing Research. 35,* 1269.

Hixon, T. J. & Weismer, G. (1995). Perspectives on the Edinburgh study of speech breathing. *Journal of Speech and Hearing Research. 38,* 42–60.

Holley, S. C. (1983). Preparing for a changing society. In N. S. Rees & T. L. Snope (Eds.), *Proceedings*

of the 1983 National Conference on Undergraduate. Graduate. and Continuing Education
(pp. 58–62). St. Paul, MN: American Speech-
Language-Hearing Association.

Jerger, J. F. (1963). Viewpoint: Who is qualified to do
research? *Journal of Speech and Hearing
Research, 6,* 301.

Jerger, J. F. (1964). Viewpoint: More on "Who is qualified to do research?" *Journal of Speech and
Hearing Research, 7,* 4–6.

Jerger, J. F. (Ed.). (1975). *Handbook of clinical impedance audiometry.* Dobbs Ferry, NY: American
Electromedics Corporation.

Jerger, J. F. (1993). Research training and mentorship
in hearing disorders. In N. J. Minghetti, J. A.
Cooper, H. Goldstein, L. B. Olswang, & S. F.
Warren (Eds.), *Research Mentorship and Training
in Communication Sciences and Disorders.* (pp.
41–50). Rockville, MD: American Speech-
Language-Hearing Foundation.

Kent, R. D. (1983). How can we improve the role of
research and educate speech-language pathologists and audiologists to be competent users of
research? In N. S. Rees & T. L. Snope (Eds.),
*Proceedings of the 1983 National Conference on
Undergraduate, Graduate, and Continuing Education* (pp. 76–86). St. Paul, MN: American
Speech-Language Hearing Association.

Kent, R. D. (1985). Science and the clinician: The practice of science and the science of practice.
Seminars in Speech and Language, 6, 1–12.

Kent, R. D., & Fair, J. (1985). Clinical research: Who,
where, and how? *Seminars in Speech and
Language, 6,* 23–34.

Kerlinger, F. (1973). *Foundations of Behavioral
Research.* New York: Holt, Rinehart & Winston.

Lane, H., & Tranel, B. (1971). The Lombard sign and
the role of hearing in speech. *Journal of Speech
and Hearing Research. 14,* 677–709.

Minifie, F., Hixon, T. J., & Williams, F. (Eds.). (1973).
Normal aspects of speech, hearing, and language.
Englewood Cliffs, NJ: Prentice Hall.

Moll, K. (1983). Graduate education. In N. S. Rees &
T. L. Snope (Eds.). *Proceedings of the 1983*

National Conference on Undergraduate, Grad-
uate, and Continuing Education (pp. 25–37). St.
Paul, MN: American Speech-Language-Hearing
Association.

Olswang, L. B. (1993) Treatment efficacy research: A
paradigm for investigating clinical practice and theory. *Journal of Fluency Disorders, 18,* 125–134.

Perkins, W. H. (1986). Functions and malfunctions of
theories in therapies. *Asha. 28,* 31–33.

Plutchik, R. (1974). *Foundations of experimental
research* (2nd ed.). New York: Harper & Row.

Punch, J. (1983). Characteristics of ASHA members.
Asha. 25, 31.

Ringel, R. L. (1972). The clinician and the researcher:
An artificial dichotomy. *Asha, 14,* 351–353.

Rummel, R. J. (1967). Understanding factor analysis.
Journal of Conflict Resolution. 11, 444–480.

Russell, B. (1945). *History of western philosophy.* New
York: Simon & Schuster.

Sidman, M. (1960). *Tactics of scientific research.* New
York: Basic Books.

Siegel, G. M. (1993). Research: A natural bridge. *Asha,
35,* 36–37.

Siegel, G. M., & Ingham, R. J. (1987). Theory and science in communication disorders. *Journal of
Speech and Hearing Disorders, 52,* 99–104.

Siegel, G. M., & Spradlin, J. E. (1985). Therapy and
research. *Journal of Speech and Hearing
Disorders. 50,* 226–230.

Skinner, B. F. (1953). *Science and human behavior.*
New York: Macmillan.

Skinner, B. F. (1959). A case history in the scientific
method. In S. Koch (Ed.), *Psychology: A study of
a science* (Vol. 2, pp. 359–379). New York:
McGraw-Hill .

Skinner, B. F. (1972). *Cumulative record* (3rd ed.).
New York: Appleton-Century-Crofts.

Stevens, S. S. (1968). Measurement, statistics, and the
schemapiric view. *Science, 161,* 849–856.

Wertz, R. T. (1993). Adult-onset disorders. *Asha, 35,*
38–39.

Young, M. R. (1993). Supplemental tests of statistical
significance: Variation accounted for. *Journal of
Speech and Hearing Research, 36,* 644–656.

Chapter 2

Research Strategies in Communicative Disorders

This chapter reviews research strategies that are prevalent in the communicative disorders literature. Classification of research studies into mutually exclusive categories is difficult because of the variety of research strategies employed and the overlap among them. In addition, it is common for one journal article to report the results of large studies that include different research strategies used in the same investigation to study different aspects of the same research problem. Therefore, our categorization will be arbitrary as are those of other research textbooks. It is intended to illustrate common principles of empirical research in communicative disorders, some of the differences among various research strategies, and the appropriateness of certain strategies for the study of different problems.

Bordens and Abbott (1988) make a clear distinction between research strategy and research design. In their scheme, a research strategy is the general plan of attack, whereas the specific tactics used to carry out the strategy constitute the research design. Before choosing a specific research design, an investigator must first select an overall research strategy. This chapter will outline some of the more common research strategies used in communicative disorders research, and the next chapter will describe some specific research designs employed to carry out these major research strategies.

Variables in Empirical Research

Empirical research is concerned with the relationships among *variables*. Variables are measurable quantities that vary or change under different circumstances rather than remain constant. In geometry, for example, the radius and circumference of a circle are two variables: draw a large and a small circle and you can measure the different values of the radius and circumference of each circle. However, the formula that relates the radius and the circumference of a circle ($c = 2\pi r$) contains the term π (pi), which has a constant value of approximately 3.14159. Thus, π is a constant; it never varies regardless of the size of the circle. However, the radius and the circumference are variables, or measurable quantities that may differ from one circle to the next. In behavioral science, the variables studied are often common measurable quantities such as stimulus characteristics (tone intensity or frequency), environmental conditions (background noise level), speech behavior (rate of speech or number of nonfluencies), language performance (mean length of utterance or number of embedded clauses found in a language sample), or hearing ability (speech reception threshold). Kerlinger (1973) has outlined three classifications of variables that are important for understanding the ways in which behavioral research attempts to understand the relationships among important variables.

Independent and Dependent Variables

Kerlinger's most important notion is the distinction between *independent* and *dependent* variables. Indeed, this concept forms the core of the material in this chapter and underlies everything discussed in the rest of the book. According to Kerlinger (1973, p. 35):

> *The most important and useful way to categorize variables is as independent and dependent. This categorization is highly useful because of its general applicability, simplicity, and special importance in conceptualizing and designing research and in communicating the results of research. An* independent variable *is the* presumed *cause of the* dependent variable, *the* presumed *effect. The independent variable is the antecedent; the dependent is the consequent.*

Independent variables, then, can often be conceptualized as conditions that cause changes in behavior; dependent variables can be seen as the behavior that is changed. For example, delayed auditory feedback (independent variable) may cause a change in speech rate (dependent variable). Masking noise (independent variable) may cause a change in auditory threshold (dependent variable). Kerlinger cautions us, however, on the use of "the touchy word 'cause' and related words" in discussing independent and dependent variables. One problem is the level of causation that we talk about: the variable that we manipulate may cause a change in a variable that is unknown to us, and the change of the unknown variable is what causes the change we observe in our dependent variable.

Another problem facing researchers in discussing cause-and-effect relations among variables will be seen in our discussion in this chapter of the distinctions between experimental and descriptive research. Cause–effect relations are more logically inferred from the results of experiments than from the results of descriptive research because of the nature of the independent variables in these two kinds of research. In experimental research, the experimenter manipulates an independent variable (while holding other potential independent variables constant) to examine what effect the manipulation of the independent variable has on the dependent variable. In descriptive research, however, it is not possible for the researcher to manipulate the independent variable to see what effect that manipulation will have on the dependent variable. Independent variables in descriptive research usually include factors such as subject classification (e.g., normal vs. language-delayed children) that the researcher cannot manipulate. The descriptive researcher may be able to compare a group of normal children with a group of language-delayed children on some dependent variable, but he or she cannot directly manipulate the subject classification of the children to observe the effect of the manipulation on their behavior. (Some authors have called such descriptive research "experiments of nature" because nature has manipulated the independent variable in determining the children's subject classification.) Thus, direct cause–effect relations are difficult to infer from the results of descriptive research.

Kerlinger (1973) has also pointed out that the distinction between independent and dependent variables is really a distinction that is based on our *use* of variables rather than on some inherent property of a variable. We conceive of a certain variable as the antecedent that causes a change in another variable and, therefore, use that first variable as the independent variable and the second variable as the dependent variable. It is sometimes possible for researchers to conceive of a particular variable as being an independent variable in one situation and a dependent variable in another situation. For example, mean length of utterance is sometimes used (instead of chronological age) to classify children into groups that vary in degree of language development; mean length of utterance thereby becomes the measure of the values of the independent variable. In another study, however, a researcher may study the effect of manipulation of an independent variable on children's mean length of utterance; mean length of utterance thereby becomes the dependent variable. We must always look carefully at how a researcher employs the variables studied to determine the independent and dependent variables.

Kerlinger (1973) advocates thinking of independent and dependent variables in mathematical terms where X is an independent variable and Y is a dependent variable, and we may specify the relationship between X and Y as a mathematical *function.* Jaeger and Bacon (1962, p. 6) state that

> If two variables are related in such a way that the value of one is determined whenever the other is specified, the one is said to be a function of the other.

Thus, if we know the functional relationship of X and Y, we know how Y varies whenever X is varied. When we know the value of X, we can determine the value of Y from the functional relation of the two variables. In other words, if we know how the independent variable and the dependent variable are related and we know the value of the independent variable, we can determine the value of the dependent variable.

Functions can be demonstrated graphically by plotting the values of X and Y on the coordinate axes of a graph. Functions can also be demonstrated by writing an equation that shows how to calculate the value of Y for any value of X. The equation can be used to generate a line that connects all the plotted values of X and Y on the graph. The equation and the graph are just two different ways of displaying the same function—the equation with mathematical symbols and the graph with a line that connects the coordinate values of X and Y.

It is useful to exemplify this concept by examining the manner in which research results may often be presented in a graph. For example, the results of a research study examining the relationship of two variables might look like the hypothetical data shown in Figure 2.1. The values of the independent variable are indicated on the *abscissa* (horizon-

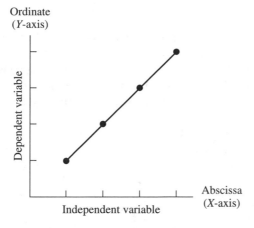

**FIGURE 2.1
Hypothetical Data Illustrating a
Dependent Variable That Increases
as a Function of Increases in the
Independent Variable**

tal or *X* axis), and the values of the dependent variable are indicated on the *ordinate* (vertical or *Y* axis). The values of the independent variable increase from left to right on the abscissa and the values of the dependent variable increase from bottom to top on the ordinate. The dots indicate coordinate points of values of the dependent variable (*Y*) that were found for each value of the independent variable (*X*), and the line drawn to connect these dots graphically shows the function relating the changes in the dependent variable to changes in the independent variable.

Figure 2.1 shows how the dependent variable varies as a function of changes in the independent variable in a graphic fashion. The function could also be shown with an equation relating the values of *Y* to the values of *X*. Because the function shown in Figure 2.1 is a straight line, a simple linear equation can be used to show the function

$$Y = a + bX$$

This equation states that values of the dependent variable (*Y*) can be calculated by taking the value of the independent variable (*X*) and multiplying it by a value (*b*) and adding to it another value (*a*). The *b* term is the slope of the line that indicates how fast *Y* increases as *X* is increased. The *a* term is the value of *Y* at the point where the line intercepts the *Y* axis when the value of *X* is zero and is called the *Y*-intercept. The formula can be used to calculate the value of *Y* for any value of *X* and can also be used to generate the line drawn through the data points. The values of *a* and *b* are calculated from the actual *X* and *Y* data. The particular function shown in Figure 2.1 shows that *Y* increases as a function of increases in *X*. There are many other possible functions that can be seen in actual research data. For example, *Y* may decrease as a function of increases in *X,* in which case, the line would slope downward to the right rather than upward as in Figure 2.1. Or the data points may not fall along a straight line; they may show a curvilinear relationship between *X* and *Y*. In any case, the function is a mathematical or graphic way of depicting the relationship between the independent variable and the dependent variable by demonstrating how the dependent variable changes as a function of changes in the independent variable.

Active and Attribute Variables

A second notion about classifying variables that Kerlinger (1973) discussed is the distinction between *active* and *attribute* variables. A variable that can be *manipulated* is an active variable. Thus, the independent variable in an experiment is an active variable because the experimenter can manipulate it or change its value. For example, an experimenter can change the intensity of a tone presented to a listener by manipulating the hearing-level dial on an audiometer.

There are many independent variables, however, that cannot be manipulated by an experimenter. Variables such as subject characteristics cannot be manipulated. An experimenter cannot change things such as a subject's age, gender, intelligence, type of speech disorder, degree of hearing loss, or history. Such variables have already existed for each subject—or have been "manipulated by nature." These variables are attributes of the subjects.

Some variables may be either active or attribute variables, depending on the circumstances of the research or on how the researcher uses the variable. Kerlinger (1973, pp. 38–39) uses the example of anxiety as a variable that may be either active or attribute. Anxiety may be thought of as an attribute of subjects—yet, anxiety could also be manipulated by inducing different degrees of anxiety in different subjects to see what effect the manipulation of anxiety has on some dependent variable. For example, anxiety could be raised in some subjects by telling them that the task they are about to undertake is a difficult one that will require great concentration, while telling other subjects not to worry about the task that they are about to complete because it is very easy.[1]

The important point is that the independent variable in an experiment is active—it can be manipulated in some way by an experimenter to see what effect it has on a dependent variable. However, the independent variable in descriptive research is an attribute—it cannot be manipulated by the researcher to see what effect it has on the dependent variable. In descriptive studies, the researcher must rely on comparisons of values of the dependent variable that correspond to some existing value of an attribute independent variable.

Continuous and Categorical Variables

A third notion about classifying variables discussed by Kerlinger (1973) is the distinction between *continuous* and *categorical* variables. A continuous variable is one that may be measured along some continuum or dimension that reflects at least the rank ordering of values of the variable and possibly reflects even more refined measurement of the actual numerical values of the variable. The intensity of a tone, for example, can be measured along a numerical continuum from low to high values of sound pressure level. Stuttering frequency can vary from zero nonfluencies to a high number of nonfluencies.

Categorical variables, however, cannot be measured along a continuum. Instead, different values of the variable can only be categorized or named. For example, tones could

---

[1]Kerlinger (1973, p. 39) however, says that: "Actually, we cannot assume that the measured (attribute) and the manipulated (active) 'anxieties' are the same. We may assume that both are 'anxiety' in a broad sense, but they are certainly not the same." Nevertheless, the example points out the principle that what may be an attribute variable in one situation may be an active variable in another.

be presented to a listener binaurally or monaurally. Subjects could be classified as "stutterers" or "nonstutterers" (although the degree of stuttering *severity* of the stutterers could be measured along some continuum from mild to severe). The ways in which we measure continuous and categorical variables differ—more will be said about this in Chapter 6 when we discuss data organization and analysis.

One immediate concern in this chapter is the way that continuous and categorical variables are displayed graphically. This is especially important in distinguishing between continuous and categorical independent variables. When graphing the change in a dependent variable as a function of changes in a continuous independent variable, it is common to use a line graph like the one in Figure 2.1. The line drawn through the data points in Figure 2.1 is an interpolation and intended to demonstrate what the values of the dependent variable ought to be for intermediate values of the independent variable that were not actually used. However, when graphing the changes in a dependent variable as a function of changes in a categorical independent variable, it is customary to use a bar graph in which the height of the bar that is aligned at each categorical value of the independent variable on the X axis is meant to indicate the value of the dependent variable on the Y axis for that categorical value of the independent variable. Several examples of both types of graphs are seen in this and later chapters, but it may be useful to illustrate briefly the way in which a categorical independent variable is presented in a bar graph.

Figure 2.2 shows the same hypothetical data that were illustrated in Figure 2.1, except that the four values of the independent variable are shown as four categories of a categorical variable rather than as four values on a continuous variable. The data in Figure 2.1 show a dependent variable that increases as the values of the independent variable increase along a continuum. The data in Figure 2.2 show the differences in the values of the dependent variable for four different categories of an independent variable. In general, throughout the rest of the book, we follow the convention of presenting data for a continuous independent variable with a line graph and data for a categorical independent variable with a bar graph.

Now that we have discussed the concept of variables in empirical research, we will examine some different research strategies in communicative disorders and consider their

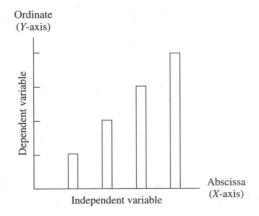

FIGURE 2.2
Hypothetical Data Illustrating Differences in the Values of the Dependent Variable for Four Different Categories of an Independent Variable

similarities and differences. We will outline various research strategies by presenting a description of the general purpose of each strategy, giving an example of their applications to problems in the field of communicative disorders, and discussing some advantages and disadvantages of each one.

Experimental Research

Experimental research is the appropriate method for investigating cause-and-effect relations among variables. With regard to the investigation of cause and effect, Underwood and Shaughnessy (1975, p. 15) have stated:

> *The critical strength of the experiment lies in the fact that when it is properly executed we learn about cause–effect relationships existing in nature. It is as near a foolproof technique for making these discoveries as has yet been devised. Those who have sought other approaches for determining cause–effect relationships in behavior have usually become discouraged.*

The ability to make conclusions about cause–effect relationships among variables, then, is a hallmark of experimental research.

There are numerous kinds of research problems in communicative disorders that have been studied through the use of experimental research. Experiments have been carried out to examine the effects of treatment on the behavior of persons with speech or hearing disorders. The experimental question in such cases would be "Does treatment cause a change in behavior?" In addition to such rather long-term treatment experiments, many experiments have examined more short-term cause–effect relationships in laboratories or clinics. For example, the research question "What effect does delayed auditory feedback have on speech behavior?" has been submitted to considerable experimental scrutiny over the years. Psychophysical experiments have been used to examine stimulus–response relationships to determine what effects certain changes in stimulus characteristics may have on people's responses. Psychophysical experiments of this nature have been especially common in audiology and underlie the development of most of the clinical tests used in audiometry. Questions such as "What effect does change in pure-tone frequency have on auditory threshold?" or "What effect does presentation level of phonemically balanced (PB) words have on speech intelligibility?" have been answered by psychophysical experiments.

In reality, there are so many potential uses of the experimental approach that it is difficult to classify all of its possible applications. As Kling and Riggs (1971, p. 3) have commented in attempting to define the experimental method in psychology;

> *contemporary methodology has become so highly specific that it is difficult to lay down general rules applicable to all experiments. However, a few characteristics of the experimental method may be mentioned.*

The four characteristics of experimental research that Kling and Riggs listed (1971, p. 3) are: (1) experimenters start with some purpose, question, or hypothesis that allows them to know when to observe certain specific aspects of behavior; (2) experimenters can control the occurrence of events and, thus, observe changes in behavior when they are best prepared to make the observations; (3) because of this, experimenters (or others) can repeat these observations under the same conditions; and (4) because experimenters can control the conditions of observation, they can systematically manipulate certain conditions to measure the effects of these manipulations on behavior.

The experimenter, then, can manipulate an independent variable to study its effect on the dependent variable. However, a change in an independent variable may be considered to cause a change in a dependent variable only if other potential independent variables have been controlled or held constant so that they will not be able to have a simultaneous effect on the dependent variable. Other potential independent variables are often called "extraneous" or "nuisance" variables because they may confuse the picture of a cause–effect relationship if left uncontrolled. Therefore, a major purpose of experimentation is to control potential extraneous variables while manipulating the independent variable of interest to the experimenter. We discuss several potential nuisance variables and how they may be controlled in Chapter 5. In this chapter, though, we are concerned mainly with the way in which the independent variable is manipulated as the basis for identifying different types of experiments.

Plutchik (1974) has outlined a classification of types of experiments that is based on the structure of the independent variables used. Plutchik's classification is useful as a first step toward understanding experimental research and appreciating the strategies that an experimenter might use to study the effects of manipulating an independent variable on some dependent variable. Not every experiment found in the literature falls into an exact niche in Plutchik's classification, but an understanding of the classification enables consumers of research to grasp the overall concept of how independent variables affect dependent variables and experimenters go about studying these effects. Plutchik's classification is based on the number of independent variables studied and the number of manipulated values of the independent variable. Although it may seem trivial at first merely to count variables and their values, it eventually becomes apparent that the number of independent variables and the number of values of an independent variable can be critical in enabling an experimenter to determine the nature of the functional relationship of an independent and a dependent variable.

Bivalent Experiments

The first type of experiment that Plutchik (1974) identified is the bivalent experiment in which the experimenter studies the effects of two values of one independent variable on the dependent variable. This type of experiment is called bivalent ("two values") because the independent variable is manipulated by the experimenter in a manner that allows for only two values of the independent variable to be presented to the subjects. In the case of a continuous independent variable, this means that the experimenter has selected only two of the many values that fall along the continuum of the independent variable to be the manipulated values of the independent variable. For example, an experimenter may wish to manipulate the intensity of tones presented to listeners and selects only two intensities to present to them: a "low" and a "high" intensity. In the case of a categorical independent variable, the researcher may select two of the many categories of the independent variable that are available. In some cases, the independent variable may be dichotomous and, there-fore, only classifiable into two categories. For example, the experimenter may wish to study the effects of binaural vs. monaural listening. In any case, regardless of the potential number of values of the independent variable at the researcher's disposal, only two are employed in the bivalent experiment.

The study by Adams and Moore (1972) of the effects of masking noise on stuttering behavior is an example of a bivalent experiment. In this experiment, stutterers spoke under two conditions: (1) in quiet and (2) when presented with a masking noise. The results of this bivalent experiment are illustrated in Figure 2.3, which shows that presentation of the masking noise caused a reduction in stuttering frequency relative to the quiet condition. A bar graph is used to display these results because the two conditions (quiet vs. noise) are categorical manipulations of the independent variable rather than manipulations that fall along a continuum of values of the independent variable.

In another example of a bivalent experiment, McClellan (1967) examined the effect of venting hearing-aid earmolds on speech discrimination in noise. Hearing-impaired sub-jects were given speech discrimination tests in a noisy background under two conditions: (1) while wearing hearing aid with an unvented earmold and (2) while wearing the same aid with a vented earmold. Figure 2.4 illustrates the results of this bivalent experiment. Inspection of Figure 2.4 reveals that the subjects showed better speech-discrimination scores when using the vented earmold than when using the unvented earmold. Again, the results of this bivalent experiment are presented with a bar graph because the independent variable was manipulated categorically (vented vs. unvented earmold) rather than along a continuum of values.

Many experiments examine the effect of the independent variable on more than one dependent variable. In the Adams and Moore (1972) experiment discussed previously, for example, the researchers actually studied more than just the effects of noise masking on stuttering frequency. They examined the effects of noise on four dependent variables: stut-tering frequency, palmar sweat anxiety, vocal intensity, and reading time in an attempt to explain the masking effect on stuttering in relation to potential changes in these other

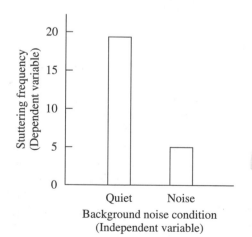

FIGURE 2.3
Results of a Bivalent Experiment
Showing the Effect of Masking Noise on
Stuttering Frequency

Drawn from the data of Adams and Moore, 1972.

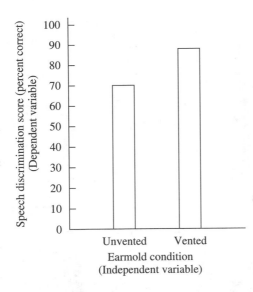

FIGURE 2.4
Results of a Bivalent Experiment
Showing the Effect of Earmold Venting
on Speech Discrimination in Noise

Drawn from the data of McClellan, 1967.

dependent variables. It is actually fairly common to examine the effects of an independent variable on several related dependent variables. The graphs in Figure 2.5 illustrate some results from an experiment by Sapienza and Stathopoulos (1994) on the effect of changing vocal intensity from a comfortable to a loud level on various respiratory and laryngeal variables. The figure demonstrates the effect of increasing intensity from comfortable to loud speech (bivalent independent variable) on six respiratory and laryngeal functions (dependent variables). Each of the six panels in the figure shows a different dependent variable plotted as a function of changing vocal intensity from the comfortable to the loud level. Many of the studies used throughout the rest of this chapter to illustrate various experimental and descriptive research strategies also used more than one dependent variable, but we will generally discuss only the single dependent variable that illustrates the point under consideration in each example.

Other examples of bivalent experiments might include studies of the effect of treatment vs. no treatment on the articulation performance of articulation-impaired children, studies of the effect of binaural vs. monaural stimulation on speech perception, studies of the effect of fluency reinforcement vs. no reinforcement on stuttering, or studies of the effect of delayed vs. normal feedback on speech rate. All of these examples represent problems for which bivalent experiments could be valuable in examining the effects of these independent variables on these dependent variables because the independent variables can be dichotomized to form two values for manipulation.

Categorical independent variables very often form dichotomies that require the use of bivalent experiments. For example, Sherman (1954) considered the merits of playing speech backward vs. forward to listeners for scaling of voice quality, the rationale being that variables, such as semantic content that could bias the ratings would be removed with backward playing of the tapes. Backward vs. forward tape playback is a true dichotomy because there are only these two ways of presenting the stimuli. A truly dichotomous independent variable like this requires a bivalent experiment.

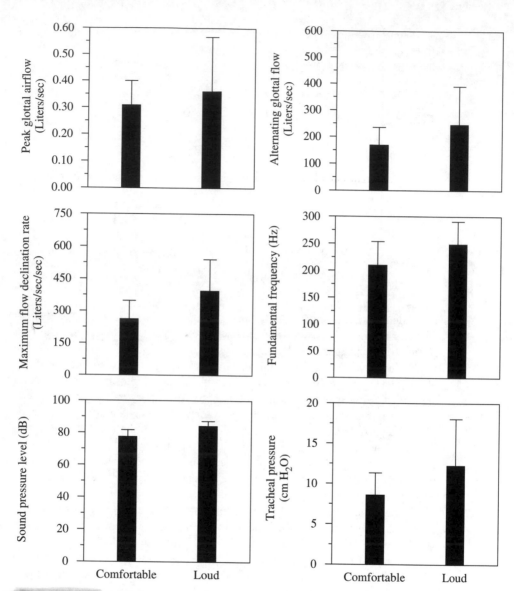

FIGURE 2.5   **Results of a Bivalent Experiment Showing the Effect of Changing Vocal Intensity from a Comfortable to a Loud Level on Six Dependent Variables**

From "Respiratory and Laryngeal Measures of Children and Women with Bilateral Vocal Cord Nodules," by C. M. Sapienza and E. Stathopoulos, 1994, *Journal of Speech and Hearing Research, 37,* p. 1236. Copyright 1994 by the American Speech-Language-Hearing Association. Reprinted with permission.

Some categorical independent variables comprise more than two categories. In that case, a researcher may select two of them to form a dichotomous independent variable, either because two of the categories are of more interest or because two of the categories seem to be opposed in a dichotomous fashion. For example, we could conceive of binaural vs. monaural stimulation as a dichotomous independent variable because stimuli can be presented to either one ear or both. However, we could also conceive of a more general categorical independent variable, mode of auditory stimulation, that includes values such as monaural left, monaural right, true binaural (dichotic), pseudobinaural (diotic), and so on. We could then select various apparent dichotomies from the available categories such as left-ear vs. right-ear monaural stimulation, monaural vs. binaural, dichotic vs. diotic, and so on to form the two values of a bivalent experiment. On the other hand, a researcher may decide to select more than two categories for manipulation and not do a simple bivalent experiment.

An experimenter may also take a continuous independent variable and use it to form a more or less artificial dichotomy in order to conduct a bivalent experiment. For example, the experimenter might study the effect of the presence vs. the absence of reinforcement on nonfluencies. Amount of reinforcement could be conceptualized as a continuous independent variable that could be artificially dichotomized into values of zero vs. a large amount, or "present" vs. "absent." In a sense, this is what happened in the Adams and Moore (1972) study of the effects of noise on stuttering. Noise intensity is a continuous independent variable that Adams and Moore artificially dichotomized into "quiet" and "noise" or presence vs. absence of noise.

Although bivalent experiments are valuable in examining the effects of categorical independent variables (especially those that reflect true dichotomies), Plutchik (1974) has indicated that they are limited in scope and may even lead to erroneous conclusions when the independent variable is continuous. Bivalent experiments are limited in scope because they do not always encompass as much of the potential range of values of the continuous independent variable as may be possible. In other words, presenting only two values of a continuous independent variable may not give as clear a picture of the function relating it to a dependent variable as presenting a larger number of values of the independent variable might. Bivalent experiments can lead to erroneous conclusions when the function being studied is not linear. Discussion of the next type of experiment in Plutchik's classification will help to clarify these two problems.

Multivalent Experiments

The second type of experiment that Plutchik (1974) identified is the multivalent experiment in which the experimenter studies the effects of several values of the independent variable on the dependent variable. This type of experiment is called multivalent ("many values") because the independent variable is manipulated in a manner that allows for at least three (and usually more) values of the independent variable to be presented to the subjects. When the independent variable is continuous, a multivalent experiment is more appropriate than a bivalent experiment for two reasons.

First, the multivalent experiment gives a broader picture of the relationship between the independent and dependent variables than the bivalent experiment does, because the experimenter samples the range of possible values of the independent variable more completely. If the dependent variable changes linearly as a function of changes in the independent variable (i.e., the graph slopes upward or downward in a straight-line fashion), then the bivalent experiment would show a pattern of results similar to the multivalent experiment. The results of the bivalent experiment, however, would be limited in scope, and the multivalent experiment would broaden the picture of the functional relationship between the independent and dependent variables.

A second and more serious problem occurs when the function takes the form of a curve rather than a straight line on the graph relating changes in the dependent variable to manipulations of the independent variable. At least three values of the independent variable must be used to identify a curvilinear function, because at least three coordinate points on a graph must be used to plot a curve. Because a bivalent experiment examines only two values of the independent variable, its resultant graph cannot reveal the shape of a curvilinear function. A multivalent experiment must be performed to reveal a curvilinear function. We now examine some examples from the research literature to demonstrate the appropriateness of multivalent experiments for studying the effects of a continuous independent variable on a dependent variable.

In the previous section, the study by Adams and Moore (1972) on the effects of noise on stuttering was presented as an example of a bivalent experiment. Although this study showed that stuttering frequency decreased from the quiet to the noise condition, it was somewhat limited in scope because it could not show how stuttering frequency changed as a function of increases in the intensity of noise. Adams and Hutchinson (1974) hypothesized, as a logical extension of the Adams and Moore study, that increases in the intensity of masking noise might cause decreases in stuttering frequency. To test this hypothesis, the authors conducted a multivalent experiment in which the masking noise was varied from quiet to 10, 50, and 90 dB above threshold. The results of this study are illustrated in Figure 2.6, which plots stuttering frequency as a function of masking noise intensity. Inspection of Figure 2.6 reveals systematic decreases in stuttering frequency from the quiet condition to the noise condition. Also, stuttering frequency decreased in a roughly linear fashion as masking noise was progressively increased in intensity from 10 to 90 dB above threshold. This multivalent experiment broadens the picture of the relation between stuttering and masking noise by showing the functional dependence of stuttering frequency on increases in the masking noise intensity.

An example of a multivalent experiment that demonstrates a curvilinear relationship is the commonly seen performance-intensity function. It demonstrates how word recognition varies as a function of the intensity at which words are presented to the listener. For normal-hearing persons listening to PB words, this curve rises rather sharply as presentation level is increased from 0 to about 50 dB sound pressure level (SPL) and then flattens out at a ceiling of about 95 to 100 percent correct as intensity is further increased to about 100 dB SPL. Figure 2.7 depicts a typical performance-intensity function for normal-hearing persons listening to PB words. The dependent variable is performance (percent of words correctly recognized), and the independent variable is the intensity of presentation

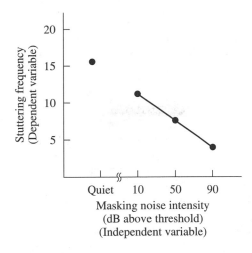

FIGURE 2.6
Results of a Multivalent Experiment Showing the Effect of Masking Noise Intensity on Stuttering Frequency

Drawn from the data of Adams and Hutchinson, 1974.

level of the words. As we can see in Figure 2.7, performance rises steeply from the lowest presentation level to about 50 dB SPL and then the curve flattens out from about 50 to 100 dB SPL.

Clearly, a multivalent experiment is necessary to discover the shape of this function. If a bivalent experiment were performed using the values of the independent variable indicated at points *A* and *B* on Figure 2.7, the function would seem to rise sharply, but there would be no indication of the curvilinearity of the relationship. If a bivalent experiment were performed using the values of the independent variable indicated at points *B* and *C* on Figure 2.7, the conclusion would be that presentation level had no effect on performance. Thus, a bivalent experiment would not be appropriate for examining the effect of presentation intensity level on word recognition because the dependent variable changes as a curvilinear function of changes in the independent variable.

In summary, a multivalent experiment is more appropriate than a bivalent experiment in the case of a continuously manipulable independent variable. Consumers of research should be cautious in drawing conclusions from bivalent experiments unless the independent variable can be dichotomized. When the independent variable can be manipulated along some continuum of values for presentation to the subjects, bivalent experiments suffer from two disadvantages. First, the picture of the functional relation of the dependent to the independent variable is limited in scope. Plutchik (1974) cautions that this limitation may force readers to overgeneralize to the effects of other possible values of the independent variable. Second, when the function is curvilinear, a bivalent experiment could lead to incorrect conclusions because at least three values of the independent variable (and preferably more) are necessary to determine the shape of the curve. These disadvantages can be overcome by conducting a multivalent experiment in which several values of the independent variable are manipulated or presented to the subjects. The multivalent experiment, then, is a much more comprehensive type of experiment for studying the functional dependence of one variable on another variable, especially when examining nonlinear functions.

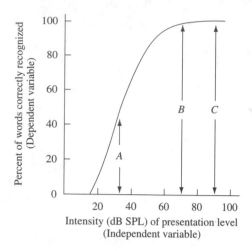

Percent of words correctly recognized (Dependent variable)

Intensity (dB SPL) of presentation level (Independent variable)

FIGURE 2.7
Results of a Multivalent Experiment Showing the Effect of Presentation-Intensity Level on Recognition of Monosyllabic PB Words. *A* and *B* or *B* and *C* Indicate Possible Outcomes of Bivalent Experiments.

Adapted from data of Hirsh et al., 1952.

Parametric Experiments

The third type of experiment Plutchik (1974) described is the *parametric* experiment in which the researcher studies the simultaneous effects of more than one independent variable on the dependent variable. It is called a parametric experiment because the second independent variable is referred to as the parameter.[2] The main effect of one independent variable on the dependent variable can be examined at the same time that the main effect of another independent variable on the dependent variable is studied. In addition, the *interaction* of the two independent variables in causing changes in the dependent variable can also be determined.

Why are parametric experiments important and what are their advantages over bivalent and multivalent experiments? First, parametric experiments can be more economical and efficient than bivalent or multivalent experiments because they examine effects of more independent variables in a single experiment. However, there is a rationale for parametric experiments that is even more compelling than conservation of time, effort, and money. The communication behaviors that we study in this complex world are multivariate in nature, and it is rare to encounter a single independent variable that can account for the entire causation of change in any dependent variable. In trying to explain the communication between a talker and a hearing-impaired listener, for example, it would be important to consider several variables that would affect the intelligibility of the speaker's message to the listener: acoustical characteristics of the talker's speech, the noise level in the background, distance between talker and listener, reverberation in the room, type and severity of the listener's hearing loss, amplification properties of the listener's hearing aid (e.g., gain, distortion), familiarity of the listener with the speaker and the topic, and so forth. Therefore, it is important in research concerning the nature and treatment of communicative disorders to design

---

[2]This is a special use of the term *parameter,* a word that has several uses. In mathematics, parameter means a variable quantity that may be arbitrarily held constant or changed to generate a family of curves. In statistics, parameter means a variable population characteristic; this statistical use of the word will be explained in more detail in Chapter 6.

experiments that examine the simultaneous effects of many relevant independent variables that may cause changes in the dependent variables of interest.

An example of a parametric experiment is the study by Erber (1971) of the simultaneous effects of distance (independent variable) and syllabic pattern of words (parameter) on visual recognition of speech through lipreading by deaf children (dependent variable). The results of this experiment are illustrated in Figure 2.8. Inspection of the figure reveals that recognition of words by lipreading decreased as the talker moved farther away from the receiver and that this function held true for three types of words differing in syllabic pattern. Also demonstrated was the fact that at any given distance, spondees were easiest to recognize by lipreading, trochees were somewhat more difficult, and monosyllables were most difficult. Therefore, there were two main effects operating on lipreading recognition: distance of talker from receiver and syllabic pattern of words spoken.

In a parametric experiment on speech recognition, Studebaker, Taylor, and Sherbecoe (1994) examined the simultaneous effects of signal-to-noise ratio and type of noise spectrum on speech recognition performance of adults with normal hearing. Figure 2.9 shows the main effects of the independent variable (signal-to-noise ratio) and the parameter (type of noise spectrum) on the dependent variable (speech recognition performance measured in percent correct). Inspection of Figure 2.9 reveals two things: (1) speech recognition performance increased as signal-to-noise ratio increased and (2) the slope of the functional

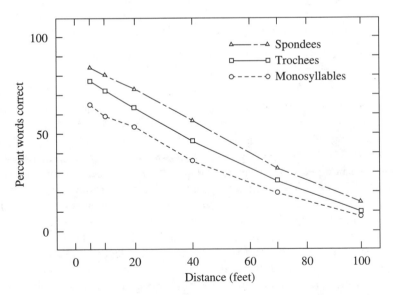

FIGURE 2.8   Results of a Parametric Experiment Showing the Main Effects of Distance of Talker from Receiver and Syllabic Pattern of Words on Recognition of Words by Lipreading

From "Effects of Distance on the Visual Perception of Speech," by N. P. Erber, 1971, *Journal of Speech and Hearing Research, 14,* p. 852. Copyright 1971 by the American Speech-Language-Hearing Association. Reprinted with permission.

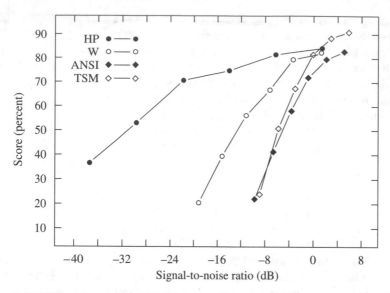

FIGURE 2.9   Results of a Parametric Experiment Showing the Main Effects of Signal-to-Noise Ratio and Type of Noise Spectrum on Speech Recognition Performance

From "The Effect of Noise Spectrum on Speech Recognition Performance–Intensity Functions," by G. A. Studebaker, R. Taylor, and R. L. Sherbecoe, 1994, *Journal of Speech and Hearing Research, 37,* p. 443. Copyright 1994 by the American Speech-Language-Hearing Association. Reprinted with permission.

relation of speech recognition performance and signal-to-noise ratio differed somewhat for each type of noise spectrum. Thus, the main effects of two independent variables on the dependent variable were explored.

Parametric experiments may employ more than one parameter, so it is not uncommon to encounter experiments that examine the simultaneous effects of three or four or five independent variables. It is much less common to find experiments that examine six or more independent variables, because they may become cumbersome and difficult to analyze and interpret, especially when considering the complexity of the potential interactions among so many independent variables. Figure 2.10 shows the results of a parametric experiment using three independent variables (i.e., one independent variable and two parameters). In this study Helfer (1994) examined the effects of (1) presentation mode (monaural, diotic, binaural), (2) listening condition (noise, reverberation, both), and (3) consonant position (initial, final) on the accuracy of consonant identification. Figure 2.10 shows that the combination of reverberation and noise reduced consonant identification more than either condition alone; that final consonants were affected more than initial consonants by reverberation and the combined condition, although not by noise; and that monaural, diotic, and binaural presentation modes did not differ markedly in this task.

So far, we have discussed only the *main effects* of the independent variable and the parameter on the dependent variable. The main effects of each of these independent vari-

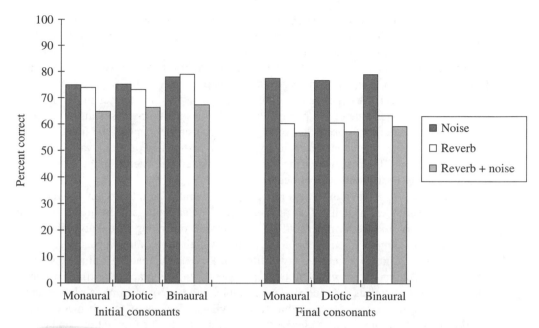

FIGURE 2.10 **Results of a Parametric Experiment Showing the Main Effects of Presentation Mode, Listening Condition, and Consonant Position on Consonant Identification**

From "Binaural Cues and Consonant Perception in Reverberation and Noise," by K. S. Helfer, 1994, *Journal of Speech and Hearing Research, 37,* p. 433. Copyright 1994 by the American Speech-Language-Hearing Association. Reprinted with permission.

ables and parameters could also be studied if the experimenter performed two different multivalent experiments to examine the effects of each of the independent variables on the dependent variables. For example, Erber (1971) could have studied the effect of distance on lipreading and then done a second experiment to study the effect of syllabic pattern on lipreading. Thus far, the experimenter has improved efficiency by studying the two main effects in the same experiment rather than performing a different experiment for each main effect. But the most important advantage of performing a parametric experiment rather than two multivalent (or bivalent if both independent variables are categorical) experiments is that the *interaction* of the two independent variables in causing changes in the dependent variable can be examined.

An interaction effect is a *joint* or *simultaneous* or *mutual* effect of the two (or more) independent variables on the dependent variable. We say that an interaction effect occurs when the independent variable affects the dependent variable in different ways for different levels of the parameter. An interaction effect can only be seen when two (or more) independent variables are studied *simultaneously* in a parametric experiment. An interaction effect cannot be seen when two separate multivalent experiments have been completed, even if the two independent variables employed in the two experiments would have interacted in a parametric experiment.

An interaction effect occurs when the function relating changes in the dependent variable to changes in the independent variable is not the same shape for all values of the parameter. For example, the dependent variable may *increase* as a function of increases in the independent variable for one value of the parameter, but the dependent variable might show *no change* as a function of increases in the independent variable for another value of the parameter. In fact, the dependent variable may increase with increases in the independent variable for one value of the parameter and *decrease* with increases in the independent variable for another value of the parameter. Whenever the shape of the function relating changes in the dependent variable to changes in the independent variable has a different form for different values of the parameter, an interaction between the independent variable and the parameter is said to occur.

An example of a parametric experiment that illustrates an interaction between two independent variables in their effect on the dependent variable is seen in the study by De Filippo, Sims, and Gottermeier (1995) on the effects of linking visual and kinesthetic imagery in lipreading instruction. Figure 2.11 shows their pretraining versus posttraining results for deaf adults who received two different kinds of lipreading training: viewing their own speech versus viewing the trainer's speech. In this graph, the time of testing (pre vs. post) is plotted as the independent variable, and type of training is plotted as the parameter. The figure reveals that subjects who viewed their own speech made greater pre–post gains than subjects who viewed the trainer's speech. The interaction can be visualized best by considering the crossing of the graphic lines. This crossing indicates that the self-viewing subjects scored slightly below the trainer-viewing subjects before train-

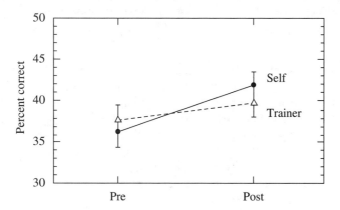

FIGURE 2.11   Results of a Parametric Experiment Showing the Main and Interaction Effects of Time of Test and Type of Training on Lipreading Performance

ing, but the self-viewing subjects scored above the trainer-viewing subjects after training. This reversing of the order of groups from before to after training is sometimes referred to as a *reversal-shift* interaction because of the shifting order of the group scores from one condition to another.

Another example of a parametric experiment with an interaction between two independent variables is seen in the study of Camarata, Nelson, and Camarata (1994) on imitative vs. conversational–interactive language interventions. They found that although imitation treatment was more effective than conversational–interactive treatment in producing elicited productions, the conversational–interactive treatment was more effective in producing spontaneous productions. This interaction of treatment type and production condition is illustrated in Figure 2.12, which shows fewer clinician presentations needed to generate elicited production for the imitation treatment but fewer clinician presentations needed to generate spontaneous production for the conversational treatment.

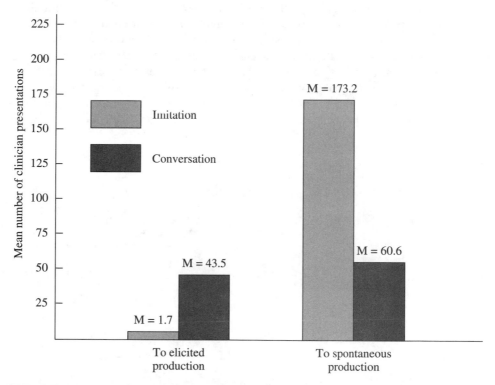

FIGURE 2.12   Results of a Parametric Experiment Showing the Main and Interaction Effects of Type of Treatment and Mode of Generalization on Number of Clinician Presentations Needed for Client to Produce a Target Utterance

From "Comparison of Conversational-Recasting and Imitative Procedures for Training Grammatical Structures in Children with Specific Language Impairment," by S. M. Camarata, K. E. Nelson, and M. N. Camarata, 1994, *Journal of Speech and Hearing Research, 37,* p. 1419. Copyright 1994 by the American Speech-Language-Hearing Association. Reprinted with permission.

In the previous two examples of interaction effects in parametric experiments, both independent variables were bivalent; that is, each independent variable had only two levels. Interaction effects are also encountered in parametric experiments using multivalent independent variables. Figure 2.13 shows the results of an experiment by Loven and Collins (1988) on the effects of signal-to-noise ratio (shown on the abscissa as the independent variable with six levels) and reverberation time (plotted as the parameter with three levels) on speech recognition. An interaction effect between the two variables was reported by the authors because speech recognition was not greatly affected by reverberation time at signal-to-noise ratios below O dB, but above O dB speech recognition at the 1.2 second reverberation time was deteriorated relative to the other two reverberation times. This interaction effect can be seen clearly in the figure: below O dB the three lines are close and overlapping; above O dB the three lines separate and the line showing the function for 1.2 seconds drops well below the other two lines.

An interaction occurs, then, when the function relating performance on the dependent variable to manipulation of the independent variable is not the same for all of the levels of the parameter. As a general rule of thumb, when the lines on a line graph are roughly parallel, there is no interaction between the independent variables, but when lines deviate grossly from parallelism, there is an interaction effect. Parallel lines on the graph indicate that the functions relating the changes in the dependent variable to manipulation of the independent variable are the same for each level of the parameter. Lines that are not parallel indicate that the functions relating the changes in the dependent variable to the manipulations of the independent variable are not the same for each level of the parameter.

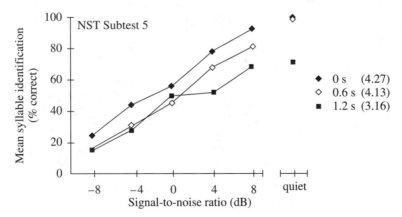

**FIGURE 2.13   Results of a Parametric Experiment Showing the
Main and Interaction Effects of Signal-to-Noise
Ratio and Reverberation Time on Syllable
Identification**

From "Reverberation, Masking, Filtering, and Level Effects on Speech Recognition Performance," by F. C. Loven and M. J. Collins, 1988, *Journal of Speech and Hearing Research, 31,* p. 689. Copyright 1988 by the American Speech-Language-Hearing Association. Reprinted with permission.

To summarize Plutchik's (1974) classification, experiments may be categorized as bivalent, multivalent, or parametric. Bivalent experiments examine the effects of two values of one independent variable on a dependent variable and are appropriate when the independent variable can be dichotomized. These experiments are inappropriate for studying independent variables that can be continuously manipulated, especially when examining nonlinear functions. Multivalent experiments examine the effects of several values of one independent variable on the dependent variable. They are more comprehensive and accurate than bivalent experiments in determining functional relationships when the independent variable is continuous. When there is the possibility of more than one independent variable having an effect on the dependent variable, the parametric experiment is appropriate for simultaneously manipulating an independent variable and a parameter to study their combined effects on the dependent variable. Any of these types of experiments could employ more than one dependent variable.

Descriptive Research

Descriptive research is used to examine group differences, developmental trends, or relationships among variables that can be measured by the researcher. Research of this type provides an empirical picture of what was observed at one time or of observed changes over a period of time, without manipulation of independent variables by the researcher. In descriptive research, researchers are essentially passive observers who try to be as unobtrusive as possible so that their presence (or the presence of their measuring instruments or techniques) causes minimal alteration of the naturalness of the phenomena under investigation. As pointed out earlier in this chapter, experimental research involves manipulation of an active independent variable to determine its effect on a dependent variable, whereas descriptive research involves the observation of relations between attribute independent variables and dependent variables. Descriptive research is an important endeavor in behavioral science and constitutes a large portion of the research found in the communicative disorders literature. There are, however, some common misunderstandings of descriptive research that should be discussed.

First, descriptive research results should not lead to the formulation of cause-and-effect statements. The description of differences between groups or of relationships among variables does not provide sufficient grounds for establishing *causal* relations. The discovery of cause and effect falls within the purview of experimental research, and the experimenter's ability to make things happen under controlled conditions is simply not possible in descriptive research. It is difficult, therefore, to draw conclusions from descriptive research about cause-effect relations because many factors beyond the control of the researcher may confound the results.

Second, statements such as the foregoing have led some people to disparage descriptive research as an inferior method. It is not an inferior method. There are situations in which descriptive research is more appropriate and situations in which experimental research is more appropriate. Descriptive research is more appropriate in a situation in which the researcher is interested in behaviors as they occur naturally without the interference of an experimenter. In other situations, when the researcher wishes to manipulate conditions to study cause–effect relations, experimental research is more appropriate.

There are, however, situations in which experimental research is desired, but ethical concerns such as the regard for protection of human subjects preclude the use of certain experimental techniques. For example, it would be unethical to conduct an experiment that would produce a conductive hearing loss in humans in order to study the effects of middle ear pathology on auditory perception or academic achievement. Therefore, researchers must rely on descriptive studies of children with and without middle ear pathology. Such descriptive research is not equal to experiments in determining cause–effect relationships, but it must be relied on as the best available compromise because of the ethical concern that forbids experimental studies of the effects of pathology on humans. The problems inherent in such a situation have led to much controversy concerning descriptive research such as investigations of the relations between middle ear pathology and auditory perception (Ventry, 1980). An exchange of letters in the *Journal of Speech and Hearing Disorders* between Ayukawa and Rudmin (1983) and Karsh and Brandes (1983) illustrates the dilemma facing researchers who must substitute a descriptive study for an experiment that is impossible to conduct.

Another example concerns research on the etiology of stuttering. It has been hypothesized that various conditions in the child's speaking environment may be responsible for the onset of stuttering. However, it would be unethical to manipulate systematically environmental conditions in an attempt to cause stuttering in children. Therefore, much research concerned with environmental factors related to the onset of stuttering has focused on descriptions of stuttering and nonstuttering children around the time of typical onset.

In summary, when observation of natural phenomena is necessary to solve a particular problem, descriptive research is appropriate. When the researcher wishes to examine cause-and-effect relations by manipulating variables, experimental research is appropriate. There may be situations in which experimental research is desirable but impossible. When descriptive research is substituted for experimental research in such a situation, the ensuing investigation is unable to determine the kind of direct cause-and-effect links that the experiment might have found.

Before discussing the different strategies used in descriptive research, it is worth commenting on the various terms that are used to describe independent and dependent variables in descriptive research. As stated previously, experimental independent variables are active and can be manipulated by the experimenter to examine their effects on dependent variables. The independent variables of descriptive research, however, are attribute variables that cannot be manipulated.

In certain kinds of descriptive research, subjects can be *classified* according to certain variables and comparisons can be made between the classifications with regard to some *criterion* variable. The terms *classification variable* and *criterion variable* are analogous, respectively, to the terms *independent variable* and *dependent variable*. For example, aphasics might be compared with persons without aphasia on some measure of linguistic performance. In such a case, the classification variable would be language status (aphasic vs. nonaphasic) and linguistic performance would be the criterion variable.

In certain other kinds of descriptive research, subjects of one classification are measured on a number of criterion variables to determine the relationships among these variables and the ability to predict one variable from another. In such a case, one of the variables can be designated the *predictor variable* and the other can be designated the *predicted variable*. Again, the terms *predictor variable* and *predicted variable* are analogous to the terms *independent variable* and *dependent variable*. The real difference between the two sets of terms lies in the ability of the researcher to manipulate the independent variable.

It might help consumers of research to differentiate experimental and descriptive research if they would examine the manipulability of the variables used in a research study. If the independent variable can be manipulated to determine its effect on the dependent variable, then the study is experimental. If the subjects are classified according to some nonmanipulable dimension and compared on some criterion, or if relationships are examined between nonmanipulable predict*or* and predict*ed* variables, then the research is descriptive. It should be pointed out to consumers that many authors use the terms independent and dependent variables for *both* experimental and descriptive research, so an analysis of the manipulability of variables is often necessary to determine whether a given research study is experimental or descriptive. As will be seen later, much research in communicative disorders is a *combination* of experimental and descriptive research.

Many different strategies for descriptive research can be found in the literature and those outlined as follows illustrate some of the common approaches found in communicative disorders. Four different strategies of descriptive research will be considered: (1) *comparative,* (2) *developmental,* (3) *correlational,* and (4) *survey* research.

Comparative Research

Comparative research is a strategy used to measure the behavior of two or more types of subjects at one point in time in order to draw conclusions about the similarities or differences between them.

For example, Shriner, Holloway, and Daniloff (1969) were interested in the syntactic performances of children with and without articulatory defects. They asked thirty children with severe articulation problems and thirty children with normal articulation to tell stories about pictures of children engaged in various activities, and they derived six measures of each child's syntactic use from their responses: length-complexity index (LCI), four subcategories of LCI, and mean length of response (MLR). Children with normal articulation performed better than did those with articulation defects on LCI, two subcategories of LCI that involve elaboration of noun phrases and verb phrases in sentences, and MLR.

The LCI scores of the two groups of children are illustrated in Figure 2.14. Inspection of Figure 2.14 shows that the children with normal articulation had higher LCI scores than did the children with impaired articulation. It also reveals that comparative research that examines dichotomous groups is analogous to a bivalent experiment, but it involves the selection of subjects from dichotomous classifications rather than manipulation of a dichotomous independent variable.

As pointed out earlier in the section on experimental research, many experiments have more than one dependent variable. The same is true for many descriptive studies. Figure 2.15 shows more results from the same example used to illustrate this point earlier. In this study by Sapienza and Stathopolous (1994), a comparison was made of the performance of children

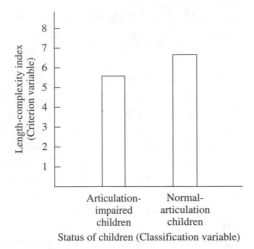

FIGURE 2.14

Results of a Bivalent Comparison of the Length-Complexity Index (LCI) Scores of Children with Normal and Impaired Articulation

Drawn from data of Shriner et al., 1969.

vs. adults on a number of respiratory and laryngeal functions; these bivalent descriptive comparisons are illustrated in the bar graphs of Figure 2.15. It is interesting to note the similarity of this figure to the example in Figure 2.5. Both figures show multiple dependent variables influenced by a single bivalent independent variable. In the experimental case the independent variable is an active variable manipulated by the experimenter by instructing speakers to talk at different loudness levels. In the descriptive case the independent variable is an attribute variable that cannot be manipulated by the experimenter: the speakers' ages. This example is an excellent illustration from the same study of two different types of independent variables that may influence the same dependent variables. The active variable may be studied experimentally, but the attribute variable may only be observed in a descriptive study.

Comparative research studies may also be found that are analogous to multivalent and parametric experiments. A comparative research study analogous to a multivalent experiment would involve comparison of three or more groups of subjects who could be classified along some continuum. For example, Brannon (1968) compared linguistic word-class usage in samples of the spoken language of normal-hearing, hearing-impaired, and deaf children. The children were classified along the continuum of hearing status from normal to hearing impaired to deaf, and linguistic word-class usage was the criterion variable on which they were compared.

To illustrate the analogy between this comparative study and a multivalent experiment, Brannon's data on the average number of words per subject found in the speech samples of the three groups are shown in Figure 2.16. The similarity between Figure 2.16 and Figure 2.6 illustrates the analogy between a multivalent comparison and a multivalent experiment. The graph relating the criterion variable to the classification variable can be evaluated in much the same manner as the graph relating the dependent variable to the independent variable in experimental research. The major difference between the multivalent comparison and the multivalent experiment concerns the ability to manipulate the independent variable in the experiment vs. the need to select already existing members of the classifications in the descriptive comparison. It would not have been possible to produce hearing impairment in the children and then study the effects of this impairment on word-class usage.

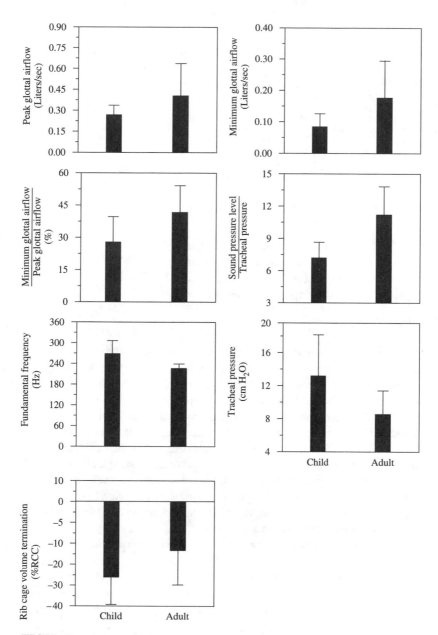

FIGURE 2.15   Results of a Bivalent Comparison of Children versus Adults on Seven Respiratory and Laryngeal Variables

From "Respiratory and Laryngeal Measures of Children and Women with Bilateral Vocal Fold Nodules," by C. M. Sapienza and E. Stathopoulos, 1994, *Journal of Speech and Hearing Research, 37,* p. 1235. Copyright 1994 by the American Speech-Language-Hearing Association. Reprinted with permission.

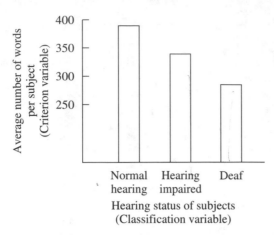

**FIGURE 2.16   Results of a Multivalent Comparison
of Number of Words per Subject
Produced by Three Groups of Subjects
Differing in Hearing Status**

Drawn from data of Brannon, 1968.

There is one minor difference between Brannon's (1968) results, as illustrated in Figure 2.16, and the results of Adams and Hutchinson (1974), illustrated in Figure 2.6. A bar graph was used instead of a line graph to illustrate Brannon's data. This was done because the three levels of the independent variable were three categorical values of hearing status rather than numbers on a numerical continuum to indicate degrees of hearing loss severity. The line graph was used for the Adams and Hutchinson data in Figure 2.6 because their independent variable was continuous rather than categorical. The categories in Brannon's data do, however, represent an approximation, at least, to a multivalent ordering of categories along a continuum of degree of hearing-loss severity. This graphical convention should not be construed as a reflection of a difference between experimental and descriptive independent variables but, rather, as reflecting a difference between categorical and continuous independent variables.

An interesting follow-up to the Brannon study by Elfenbein, Hardin-Jones, and Davis (1994) illustrates the attempt to quantify the continuum of hearing-impairment severity as an attribute independent variable in comparative research and relate it to a number of dependent variables to describe oral communication skills of children with hearing impairment. Elfenbein et al. (1994, p. 216) stated their purpose as follows:

> *The purpose of this study was twofold: (a) to describe the oral communication skills of children with mild to severe hearing losses, and (b) to determine where their skills lie along a continuum between children who are normally hearing and children who are deaf.*

Figure 2.17 shows the composite pure tone audiograms of the children who composed the three groups representing increasing degree of hearing impairment as the independent variable.

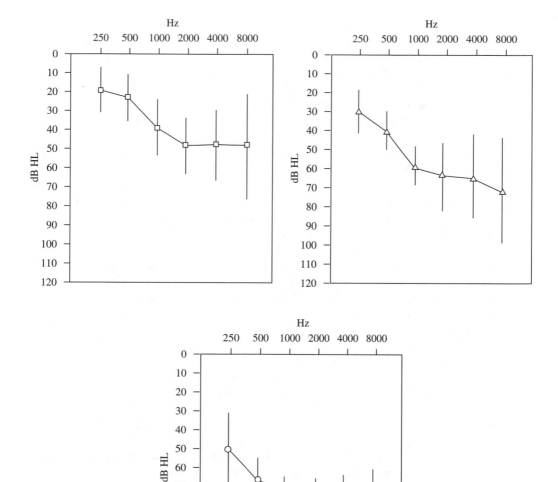

FIGURE 2.17   Composite Pure Tone Audiograms for the Better Ears of the Children in the Three Hearing Loss Groups. Mean and Standard Deviation Data are Shown for *(Top Left)* Group A (*N* = 16): *M* PTA = 31.56 dB HL, *(Top Right)* Group B (*N* = 15): *M* PTA = 51.93 dB HL, and *(Bottom)* Group C (*N* = 9): *M* PTA = 72.67 dB HL.

From "Oral Communication Skills of Children Who Are Hard of Hearing," by J. L. Elferbein, M. A. Hardin-Jones, and J. M. Davis, 1994, *Journal of Speech and Hearing Research, 37,* p. 218. Copyright 1994 by the American Speech-Language-Hearing Assocation. Reprinted with permission.

A comparative study that is analogous to a parametric experiment involves comparisons of groups that differ simultaneously with respect to two or more classification variables. For an excellent illustration of this point, let us return to the study by Elfenbein et al. (1994). In addition to the multivalent independent variable of degree of hearing impairment, the authors were interested in age as another independent variable (i.e., parameter) influencing oral communication skills (dependent variable). Table 2.1 shows their results for articulation test performance comparing children across the three hearing loss groups (A, B, and C) and the two ages (Younger, Older). Another good example of a parametric comparative study can be seen in the article by Geers and Moog (1992), which used a similar independent variable (degree of hearing impairment but over a much more severely impaired range) and incorporated type of communication mode used in their educational program (oral vs. total communication [TC]) as the parameter. Table 2.2 illustrates the composition of the groups of children arranged by pure tone average as an index of hearing-impairment severity and by communication mode indexed as oral, TC with hearing parents, or TC with deaf parents. Figure 2.18 shows their results for lipreading performance and indicates a main effect of hearing impairment, communication mode, and an interaction of the two variables. The main effects demonstrate that children with less severe hearing impairment had better lipreading scores than children with more severe hearing impairment, and children with oral communication mode had better lipreading than children with TC. The interaction effect is seen clearly as a wider gap between oral and TC students at the higher levels of hearing-impairment severity.

Another good example of a parametric comparative study can be seen in the results from Riddel, McCauley, Mulligan, and Tandan (1995) shown in Figure 2.19 on the intelligibility of speakers with amyotrophic lateral sclerosis (ALS). The two attribute independent variables are dysarthria and gender, and the figure illustrates more phonetic contrast errors for males than females and for those with dysarthria than for those without dysarthria.

Comparative research, then, involves the examination of differences and similarities among existing variables or subject classifications that are of interest to the researcher. This descriptive research strategy has the advantage of allowing researchers to study

TABLE 2.1   Articulation Test Performance of Children in Each Hearing-Loss and Age Group

| | Hearing Loss | | | | | | | |
| | Group A | | Group B | | Group C | | Total | |
Age Group	M	SD	M	SD	M	SD	M	SD
Younger	86.44	12.07	81.28	9.63	84.88	3.17	83.46	9.52
Older	90.63	5.78	94.07	4.48	83.60	10.50	89.28	8.25
Total	88.69	9.06	84.27	10.24	84.18	7.71	87.25	9.60

From "Oral Communication Skills of Children Who Are Hard of Hearing," by J. L. Elfenbein, M. A. Hardin-Jones, and J. M. Davis, 1994, *Journal of Speech and Hearing Research, 37,* p. 219. Copyright 1994 by the American Speech-Language-Hearing Association. Reprinted with permission.

TABLE 2.2   Number and Percentage of Subjects in Each Communication Mode and Hearing-Impairment Group

Communication Mode Group	Hearing-Impairment Group[a]							
	80–90 dB		91–100 dB		101–110 dB		>110 dB	
	n	*%*	*n*	*%*	*n*	*%*	*n*	*%*
ORAL (*n* = 100)	10	10	43	43	37	37	10	10
TC-HP (*n* = 63)	8	13	14	22	25	40	16	25
TC-DP (*n* = 64)	13	20	13	20	25	40	13	20

From "Speech Perception and Production Skills of Hearing-Impaired Children from Oral and Total Communication Education Settings," by A.E. Geers and J.S. Moog, 1992, *Journal of Speech and Hearing Research, 35,* p. 1388. Copyright 1992 by the American Speech-Language-Hearing Association. Reprinted with permission.

Note: ORAL = oral education program; TC-HP = total communication program—hearing parents; TC-DP = Total communication program—deaf parents.
[a]In dB HL (ANSI, 1969).

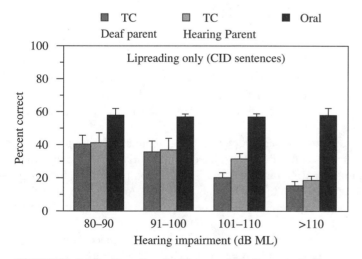

FIGURE 2.18   Results of a Parametric Comparison Showing Differences in Lipreading Scores for Children Classified According to Severity of Hearing Impairment and Communication Mode

From "Speech Perception and Production Skills of Hearing-Impaired Children From Oral and Total Communication Education Settings," by A. E. Geers and J. S. Moog, 1992, *Journal of Speech and Hearing Research, 35,* p. 1390. Copyright 1992 by the American Speech-Language-Hearing Association. Reprinted with permission.

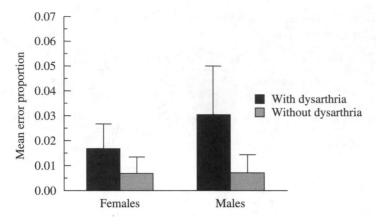

FIGURE 2.19   Results of a Parametric Comparison Showing Differences in Phonetic Contrast Error Proportions for Subjects Classified According to Gender and Dysarthria

From "Intelligibility and Phonetic Contrast Errors in Highly Intelligible Speakers with Amyotrophic Lateral Sclerosis," by J. Riddel, R. J. McCauley, M. Mulligan, and R. Tandan, 1995, *Journal of Speech and Hearing Research, 38,* p. 310. Copyright 1995 by the American Speech-Language-Hearing Association. Reprinted with permission.

variables that could not be manipulated experimentally. Sometimes these experiments are called "experiments of nature" because subjects belong to the classifications as a result of the vagaries of nature. These experiments may also be referred to as "natural-group" research studies for the same reason.

There are two disadvantages of comparative research that should be mentioned. First, it is difficult to draw conclusions about the causes of criterion-variable differences that may be found. This difficulty in attributing causation is due to the possibility that other variables may concurrently operate with the classification variable to influence the criterion variable. The lack of experimental control in the descriptive approach makes it difficult to preclude such a possibility.

Second, Young (1976, 1993, 1994)[3] criticized the use of group-difference data for generating knowledge about the performance of different groups of subjects on various criterion measures. He suggested correlational strategies and analysis of variation accounted for in dependent variables and group compositions as better strategies for assessing performance of subjects who differ in classification variables and has emphasized the difficulties of using descriptive comparisons for the development of conclusions about cause-and-effect relationships.

---

[3]Young uses the term *retrospective* to describe what we call comparative research, and our use of the term *retrospective* later in this chapter has a more restricted meaning than the one Young implied.

Developmental Research

A developmental research study is designed to measure changes over time in the behavior or characteristics of subjects, usually with reference to aging or maturation of the subjects. The independent variable in developmental research is maturation (e.g., physical or intellectual growth) and is usually indicated by measurements of chronological or mental age or by some index of maturation (e.g., mean length of response as an index of language maturity). Researchers, for example, have been interested in studying the form and function of emerging grammars as children develop language (Bloom, 1970) or in changes in hearing thresholds as adults progress through older age (Bergman, 1971). Three different developmental plans may be encountered in the literature: *cross-sectional, longitudinal,* and *semilongitudinal.*

A cross-sectional plan of observation involves the selection of subjects from various age groups and observing differences among the behaviors or characteristics of the different groups. For example, Lodge and Leach (1975) examined idiomatic comprehension of adults and six-, nine-, and twelve-year-old children. Sentences that could be interpreted idiomatically or literally were read to twenty subjects in each age group, and the subjects were asked to choose pictures closest in meaning to each sentence. More idiomatic comprehension was found for older subjects than younger ones, whereas all subjects performed at about the same level in literal comprehension. The authors concluded that literal meaning was acquired first by children and followed by acquisition of idiomatic meaning.

Figure 2.20 shows a portion of the data that Lodge and Leach (1975) presented in their article and is included here to illustrate how cross-sectional developmental data are often used to show changes in various dependent variables as a function of maturation as indexed by the ages of subjects in the different groups. The data in Figure 2.20 illustrate the conclusion that comprehension of literal meaning appeared to be acquired before comprehension of idiomatic meaning. The data for literal meaning showed that six-year-old children already comprehended more than 80 percent of literal items tested. Only a small increase in performance from children aged six to nine years occurred, with a similar performance revealed for the upper three age groups. The data for idiomatic comprehension, however, indicated a pronounced increase in performance as a function of the increased ages of the subject groups. These functions are shown in a similar format to the functions seen earlier in experimental and comparative research. In the developmental research, the independent variable is age acting as an index of maturation.

A weakness of cross-sectional research is that observations are made of differences *between* subjects of different ages in order to generalize about developmental changes that would occur *within* subjects as they mature. Direct observation of how subjects actually develop as they age and mature are made with a *longitudinal* plan of observation that involves following subjects as they mature or age and observing changes in their behavior. Longitudinal studies have the advantage of directly showing how subjects mature in their behavior while they are aging.

A good example of longitudinal research can be found in the study by Shriberg, Gruber, and Kwiatkowski (1994) that followed ten children with developmental phonological disorders for seven years. Figure 2.21 shows the averaged performance of the children at twelve age points (spaced about a half-year apart when the children were younger

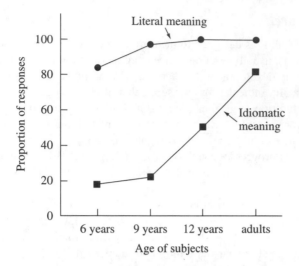

FIGURE 2.20   Illustration of the Results of a Cross-Sectional Developmental Study of Two Dependent Variables (Comprehension of Literal and of Idiomatic Meaning). Correct Literal and Idiomatic Responses Are Plotted as a Function of Age.

Adapted from the data of Lodge and Leach, 1975.

and about one year apart when the children were older) on five dependent variables that were observed over the seven-year span of the study. The figure depicts the developmental progress of the children's performance on these variables as they actually aged.

Despite their advantage of direct observation of actual development, longitudinal studies have the disadvantages of being expensive, time-consuming, and more subject to attrition than cross-sectional studies. Longitudinal studies may take years for data collection, resulting in high costs of data collection and loss of subjects or researchers from the study. As a result of their expense, attrition, and time consumption, longitudinal studies often include only small numbers of subjects, somewhat limiting generalization relative to cross-sectional studies. Although longitudinal studies are more desirable because they directly observe development, cross-sectional studies are often substituted for longitudinal plans because they are more cost-effective and practical.

A logical compromise to minimize the weaknesses and maximize the strengths of cross-sectional and longitudinal studies is a *semilongitudinal* plan of observation. This plan involves dividing the total age span to be studied into several overlapping age spans, selecting subjects whose ages are at the lower edge of each new age span and following them until they reach the upper age of the span. Wilder and Baken (1974), for example, were interested in observing respiratory parameters underlying infant crying behavior with a technique called impedance pneumography to record thoracic and abdominal movements. Ten infants entered the study at ages ranging from 2 to 161 days, and each was

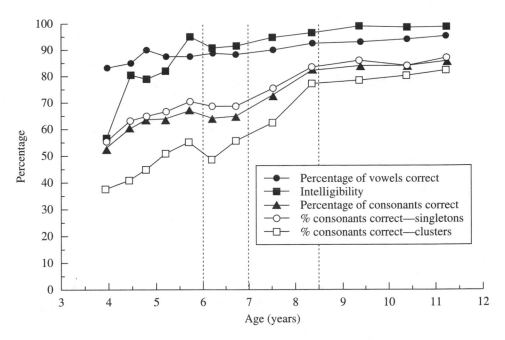

FIGURE 2.21   Results of a Longitudinal Developmental Study Showing Five Dependent Variables Plotted as a Function of Age

From "Developmental Phonological Disorders III: Long-Term Speech Sound Normalization," by L. D. Shriberg, F. A. Gruber, and J. Kwiatkowski, 1994, *Journal of Speech and Hearing Research, 37,* p. 1164. Copyright 1994 by the American Speech-Language-Hearing Association. Reprinted with permission.

observed over a period of four months. Rather than making one observation of infants of different ages or waiting for infants to be born and then following them for a year, a semi-longitudinal approach was adopted that allowed Wilder and Baken to make observations between *and* within subjects over a period of time in a more efficient manner.

In addition, it is not uncommon to see longitudinal and cross-sectional data put together for comparison to capitalize on the practical advantages of the cross-sectional plan and the scientific advantages of the longitudinal plan. Figure 2.22 shows such a comparison from the Shriberg et al. (1994) article of their longitudinal data for speech-delayed children with cross-sectional data for speech-normal developing age-mates on early-8, middle-8, and late-8 sounds. The six trends plotted in the graph illustrate the developmental progress on the three classes of sounds for the two groups of subjects.

As indicated in the previous comparison of longitudinal and cross-sectional data, developmental studies may be concerned with the comparison of developmental trends of normally developing and late developing populations on dependent variables that may be late in developing as a result of various disorders and conditions. Therefore, it is common for a developmental strategy to be combined with a comparative strategy in examining the developmental delay of one group of subjects compared to normative data for their peers. The longitudinal study of Ellis Weismer, Murray-Branch, and Miller (1994) illustrates this

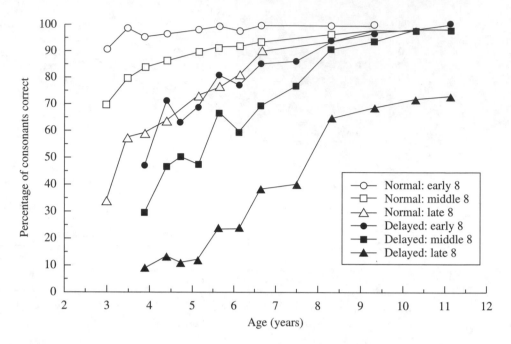

FIGURE 2.22   Longitudinal Data on Delayed Development (Filled Symbols) Compared with Cross-Sectional Data on Normal Development (Open Symbols) for Early, Middle, and Late Groups of Speech Sounds

From "Developmental Phonological Disorders III: Long-Term Speech Sound Normalization," by L. D. Shriberg, F. A. Gruber, and J. Kwiatkowski, 1994, *Journal of Speech and Hearing Research, 37,* p. 1167. Copyright 1994 by the American Speech-Language-Hearing Association. Reprinted with permission.

combined strategy in the study of language development in late talkers vs. typically developing talkers. Children were observed at three-month intervals for a year starting at about thirteen to fourteen months of age. Figure 2.23 shows their data on the number of different words produced at each observational visit over the course of the study for the late and typically developing talkers. This figure provides a ready picture of the developmental trends of the two subject groups.

Correlational Research

A correlational research strategy is used to study the relationships among two or more variables by examining the degree to which changes in one variable correspond with or can be predicted from variations in another. Details of the statistical procedure called *correlation and regression analysis* will be discussed in Chapter 6, but the logical framework of correlational research should be considered as a descriptive research strategy. Correlational research may range from a simple problem in which only two variables are studied to complex research in which the interrelation of a large number of variables is considered.

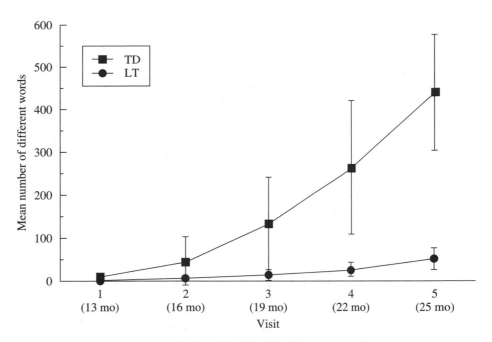

FIGURE 2.23   **Results of a Longitudinal Developmental Study Comparing Vocabulary Size of a Group of Typically Developing (TD) Children to a Group of Late Talkers (LT) at Various Ages**

From "A Perspective Longitudinal Study of Language Development in Late Talkers," by Ellis Weismer, J. Murray-Branch, and J. F. Miller, 1994, *Journal of Speech and Hearing Research, 37,* p. 858. Copyright 1994 by the American Speech-Language-Hearing Association. Reprinted with permission.

There are two basic questions asked in correlational research. First, how closely related are the variables? This question is answered by examining the performance of a group of subjects on the variables. The appropriate correlation coefficient is computed to indicate the strength of the relationship with regard to how much variation the two share. The correlation also indicates the direction of the relationship. A positive correlation indicates that increases in one variable are associated with increases in the other, whereas a negative correlation indicates that increases in one variable are associated with decreases in the other. A zero correlation indicates that the two variables are unrelated.

The concept of the correlation between variables can also be depicted visually on a graph called the *scatterplot* or *scattergram,* which will be discussed in more detail in Chapters 6 and 9. The scattergram will be mentioned here only to illustrate correlational research. Briefly, the scattergram shows the pairs of scores on the two variables that were attained by each subject. The graph is a plot of the functional relationship between the two variables and is similar to the functions plotted for the data of experimental, comparative, and developmental research.

The second question that can be asked in correlational research is how well performance on one variable can be predicted from knowledge of performance on the other for a typical subject. This question is answered by completing a regression analysis that develops an equation for predicting the expected score (with a margin of error for the prediction) on one variable from knowledge of a subject's score on the other variable.

In the regression problem, one variable (or set of variables) is designated as the predic*tor* and another variable (or set of variables) is designated as the predict*ed* variable. As mentioned previously, some researchers designate the predic*tor* and predict*ed* variables as independent and dependent variables, respectively. The terms predictor and predicted variables may provide a more accurate description of the nature of the variables studied in correlational research than do the terms independent and dependent variables. In correlational research, an independent variable is not manipulated to examine its effect on a dependent variable. Rather, two variables are measured and then one is used to try to predict the other one. Consumers should be aware, however, that they may encounter the terms independent and dependent variables used interchangeably with the terms predictor and predicted variables in correlational studies.

An example of such a prediction problem is found in the task of the college admissions office in predicting how well an applicant should do in college, given the applicant's high school background and performance on standardized tests. Variables such as high school grade-point average, college board aptitude and achievement test scores, and interview ratings are designated as predic*tor* variables, and college grade-point average is designated as the predict*ed* variable. The admissions office has correlated the predictor and predicted variables of college students from previous years and developed a regression equation for predicting college grade-point average from high school grade-point average, college board scores, and interview rating. This equation can then be applied to a new applicant's record to predict the expected college grade-point average to help in deciding whether to admit the applicant.

An example of an investigation of the correlation between two variables can be seen in part of the study by Turner and Weismer (1993) concerning speaking rate in the dysarthria associated with amyotrophic lateral sclerosis (ALS). This study included four research questions, one of which dealt with the relationship between physical and perceptual measures of speech rate in persons with ALS and with normal speech. The authors were concerned with this relationship because of previous suggestions that physical measures of speech rate might not predict perceptual measures of speech rate in some instances of dysarthria. Figure 2.24 shows the scatterplots, correlation coefficients, and regression equations for the two variables of speaking rate (in words per minute) and magnitude estimation of perceived speaking rate for twenty-seven normal speakers and twenty-seven dysarthric speakers. Correlations for both speaker groups were strong and positive, and the slightly different regression equations show that perceived speaking rate increased slightly faster with increases in physical speaking rate for the dysarthrics than for the normal speakers.

Carhart and Porter (1971) provide an example of multiple regression analysis in their study of the predictive relation between pure-tone thresholds and speech reception threshold (SRT) with six groups of patients classified according to audiometric configuration. A separate regression analysis was performed for each subject group: patients with flat, gradual, marked high-tone, rising, trough-shaped, and atypical pure-tone configurations. Predictor variables were pure-tone thresholds at 250, 500, 1,000, 2,000, and 4,000 Hz; the

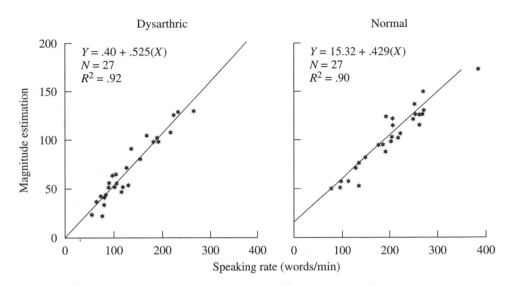

FIGURE 2.24   Results of a Correlational Study of Speaking Rate in Words per Minute and Magnitude Estimation of Perceived Speaking Rate of Normal and Dysarthric Speakers

From "Characteristics of Speaking Rate in the Dysarthria Associated with Amyotrophic Lateral Sclerosis," by G. S. Turner and G. Weismer, 1994, *Journal of Speech and Hearing Research, 36,* p. 1141. Copyright 1994 by the American Speech-Language-Hearing Association. Reprinted with permission.

predicted variable was SRT measured with spondees. Pure-tone threshold at 1,000 Hz emerged as the most important predictor variable for all groups except those subjects with marked high-tone loss; for them, 500 Hz was the best single predictor of SRT. Combinations of frequencies in the multiple prediction equations were also studied, and a noticeable, although not dramatic, improvement in prediction of SRT was achieved by adding a second frequency to the equation; adding a third frequency did not significantly improve the prediction. Also, the second frequency that most improved the prediction differed for various categories of audiometric configuration. The authors summarized the best combinations of predictor variables for each audiometric configuration and suggested an optimal combination for use if separation of patients by audiometric configurations could not be accomplished.

Monsen (1978) provides another excellent example of a multiple correlation study with his research on the relationship between physical characteristics of deaf children's speech (predictor variables) and their speech intelligibility (predicted variable). His multiple regression analysis revealed that the voice onset time differences between /t/ and /d/, the second format difference between /i/ and /ɔ/, and a liquid/nasal contrast measure were the three best predictors of the intelligibility of the deaf children's speech. A number of complex extensions of correlational research strategies are discussed in more detail in Monge and Cappella (1980) and Kerlinger and Pedhazur (1973).

One advantage of correlational research has already been pointed out in referring to Young's (1976, 1993, 1994) criticism of comparative research. Correlational research could be used to estimate the amount of variation in a criterion measure that could be accounted for on the basis of knowledge of group classification rather than simply looking at average differences in a criterion measure between two groups of subjects. Correlational research can be a powerful tool for learning what aspects of human behavior share common properties. If a strong relationship exists between two variables, then a researcher can predict one variable from knowledge of the value of the other. But there are also disadvantages. Correlation does not imply causation, and many people have seemed to miss this fact in applying cause-and-effect statements to correlational data. In addition, correlational studies suffer from problems in the interpretation of the meaning of correlation coefficients. Two variables may be significantly correlated, but this may occur because both variables are correlated with a third variable that may be unknown to the researcher. Knowledge of the third variable may be crucial to understanding the true nature of the correlation between the original two variables. For these and other more technical reasons, it may be difficult to assess the theoretical or practical implications of a correlation. Sometimes correlational studies use a "shotgun" approach in an attempt to intercorrelate many variables, and a large number of significant but fairly small correlation coefficients are found that make it difficult to assess the meaning of the complex interrelation of the variables.

Survey Research

A survey research strategy is used to provide a detailed inspection of the prevalence of conditions, practices, or attitudes in a given environment by asking people about them rather than observing them directly. The instruments used in survey research include questionnaires, interviews, and, sometimes, a combination of the two. From a practical point of view, questionnaires are generally more appropriate for collecting relatively restricted information from a wide range of persons, whereas interviews are generally more appropriate for gathering more detailed information from a more restricted sample. When a balance of depth of information and breadth of respondents is desired, a combination of the two methods may be appropriate. For example, a relatively restricted or superficial questionnaire may be administered to a large number of people and a follow-up interview of a sample of these persons may be conducted.

Surveys do not usually encompass the entire population of interest for a number of practical reasons. For example, the population may be enormous and widely distributed geographically so that the time and expense necessary to study the entire population would be prohibitive. Therefore, a sample is usually drawn from the population for study, and inferences are made concerning the entire population by studying the sample. Such surveys are often called sample surveys, and problems may arise in determining how well the data of the sample survey can be applied to make a generalization about the entire population.

A particular problem with the use of questionnaires should be mentioned. Regardless of whether a questionnaire is sent to the whole population or to a sample of the population, not all the questionnaires are returned, so the ones that are returned may not be an unbiased representation of the population. Interviews and questionnaires both may suffer from problems in determining the accuracy and the veracity of respondents' answers to various questions.

The American Speech-Language-Hearing Association regularly publishes the results of surveys concerning such things as salaries or professional characteristics of its members in its professional journal *Asha.* For example, Lass, Ruscello, Pannbacker, Middleton, Schmitt, and Scheuerle (1995) presented questionnaire results regarding career selection and satisfaction among professionals in the field. In addition to surveys of professional issues, the survey research strategy is often applied to clinical issues. Tye-Murray, Purdy, and Woodworth (1992) provided an example of a questionnaire study in their analysis of survey results concerning the use of various communication strategies by 212 Self Help for the Hard of Hearing (SHHH) members and the relationships among strategies used and attitudinal variables and social interaction indices. Felsenfeld, Broen, and McGue (1994) reported interview data from a twenty-eight-year follow-up survey of educational and occupational accomplishments of adults who had been identified as either phonologically normal or phonologically disordered as children in the 1960s. Blood (1993) provides an example of the use of both interview and questionnaire instruments in survey research for the development of a scale for assessing the communication needs of laryngectomees.

Case Study and Retrospective Research

Two variations of descriptive research encountered in the literature merit discussion. Therefore, some special considerations in the design of case studies and retrospective research are discussed here, with comments on the limitations of these approaches.

Retrospective research is designed to examine data already on file before the formulation of the research problem. A clinic may have kept routine records of patients with a particular disorder and a researcher may review these records to study important independent and dependent variables. Or a researcher may look back at data collected in a previous research study to reexamine old data or to examine some aspect of the data that had not been previously examined.

Some authors (e.g., Plutchik, 1974; Young, 1976) have used the term *retrospective* to describe what we have called comparative research in this chapter, but we believe that a distinction should be made between the two plans of observation. In comparative research, the investigator has control over the selection of subjects and the administration of criterion-variable measures. In retrospective research, however, the investigator depends on subject classifications and criterion-variable measurements that were performed at a different time and possibly by a different person. Thus, there arises the danger in retrospective research that the investigator may not know the reliability and validity of these file data. For example, audiograms in patients' files may have been obtained by a new and unpracticed graduate student who committed procedural errors; the equipment may have been out of calibration on the day of testing; or shortcuts in measurement method may have been taken to save time on a busy day.

Such shortcomings may be overcome to ensure reliable and valid measures in the files if the researcher was responsible for all of the measurements in the first place or is absolutely certain of the conditions under which the data were collected. This could be documented by keeping careful records of calibration and measurement methods. Otherwise, the records used in retrospective research may provide the researcher with incorrect or inaccurate information that, in turn, will be passed on to the profession. Retrospective research, then, should be conducted when the researcher has had administrative control over the collection of the data and when it would be very difficult to collect new data because of financial or other administrative considerations. In the Carhart and Porter (1971) study cited previously (and discussed in greater detail in Chapter 8), retrospective analysis of file data was used and the authors carefully detailed the conditions under which the data were gathered to justify the use of retrospection.

The Carhart and Porter (1971) study illustrates the use of clinical files as the source of previously gathered data in a retrospective study. An alternate source of data for retrospective analysis can be the data of previous research studies. Using old research data may, in fact, be a better approach than using clinical file data because it is probable that old research data would have been collected under more rigorous and standardized conditions than old clinical file data. An example of the use of previously collected research data in retrospective research can be seen in the study of Colburn and Mysak (1982) of developmental disfluency and emerging grammar in young children. Audiotapes of their subjects were available from a previous study of normal language development (Bloom, 1970), and Colburn and Mysak did a retrospective analysis of the development of disfluencies in these longitudinal data. An extra advantage of the retrospective approach in this study is that the subjects proved to have followed a normal course in development of language and fluency over the subsequent ten years between the original data collection and the retrospective analysis, thus allowing the researchers to specify long-term subject characteristics.

The study of speaking fundamental frequency of women's voices by Russell, Penny, and Pemberton (1995) illustrates the combining of retrospective research with currently collected data for a longitudinal study of voice change with aging. Archival recordings made of the women's voices in 1945 and 1981 were available for comparison with recordings made in 1993. Russell et al. presented a method for verification of the accuracy of the recordings in their method section as a rationale for use of the older recordings for comparison of speaking fundamental frequencies at different ages. However, they described why certain measures such as shimmer and jitter could not be used because of lack of information about mouth-to-microphone distance, microphone quality, and microphone angle in the 1945 and 1981 recordings, since these factors had been previously shown to affect perturbation measures. This article is an example of the judicious use and rejection of different retrospective data based on the analysis of the quality and appropriateness of the data for fulfilling specific research purposes.

Case study research is designed to examine in depth specific individuals to illustrate important principles that might be overlooked in examining group data. Several specific reasons for performing case studies are apparent. First, case studies may be used to evaluate phenomena that may occur rarely but that can provide important information. For example, Schiff-Myers (1983) studied the development of personal pronouns from reversal to correct usage in a highly imitative child with otherwise normally developing language and none of the other behavioral characteristics of autism. Kent, Osberger, Netsell, and Hustedde (1987) studied the vocal development of a pair of identical twins, one who had normal hearing and one who had a profound bilateral hearing loss. The authors stated that "these boys offered a rare opportunity to study the effects of hearing loss on vocal development with reasonable control over environmental and genetic factors," and they presented data on phonetic development with implications for early identification and intervention.

Second, the case study approach may aid in the development of insights into the use of certain clinical or research techniques. Shuster, Ruscello, and Toth (1995), for instance, used visual feedback of spectrographic information in an attempt to improve /r/ production in two children who had been unable to attain correct /r/ production during years of traditional treatment. Calculator and Hatch (1995) developed a comprehensive battery of tests to validate facilitators' claims that an individual was able to converse via facilitated communication, applied the protocol to a single case and found that they were unable to validate the claims of facilitators. They stated clearly that their specific results cannot be generalized beyond the single case but proposed guidelines for future validation of claims for successful facilitated communication using the rationale and protocol they developed.

Third, case studies have proven valuable in examining exceptions to generally accepted rules. Chaiklin and Stassen (1968) presented a case in which the fitting of a hearing aid to the indicated ear was not a correct decision and the patient actually preferred to wear the aid in the other ear. Fourth, important case studies have also appeared in the literature to alert the profession to phenomena that have been previously overlooked in clinical practice. Ventry, Chaiklin, and Boyle (1961), for example, first described the condition of collapse of the ear canal during audiometry, and this case report led to numerous research studies on ear canal collapse.

Case studies have their weaknesses in addition to their benefits. Because they are limited in the number of subjects or situations studied, they may allow little generalization. Thus, case studies may need to be combined with follow-up studies of larger numbers of cases that exhibit the same phenomenon. Also, case studies may be contaminated by subjective bias on the part of the investigator. The excitement often generated by dramatic or atypical cases may cause the investigator or the subject to react in a manner that may not be characteristic of typical cases.

Nevertheless, retrospective and case study research are sometimes the only methods available for studying some phenomena. This may happen when few cases are available for study or when financial or administrative considerations preclude the use of other types of research. As long as caution is exerted in the interpretation of retrospective and case study data, they may provide the profession with important information.

Combined Experimental and Descriptive Research

As mentioned in the beginning of this chapter, it is difficult to classify research articles into mutually exclusive categories of research strategies. In reality, many articles that are published in the communicative disorders journals report research that is based on some combination of experimental and descriptive strategy. Because of the prevalence and importance of such investigations in the literature, several examples will be discussed in the following paragraphs.

These articles generally summarize the investigation of the effects of manipulation of one or more independent variables on the performance of subjects who have been selected from groups that differ on the basis of classification variables such as age, gender, or pathology. The effect of the experimental manipulation on the dependent variable for one group is compared with the effect of the experimental manipulation for the other group. The research is partly descriptive because the experimenter cannot directly manipulate the classification of subjects—that is, the experimenter cannot cause a disorder or accelerate maturation or change the gender of a subject. Therefore, the experimenter has to select subjects who fall into preexisting classifications of age, gender, or pathology.

An example of a combined experimental–descriptive investigation is the study by Lahey (1974) on the effects of prosody and syntactic markers on children's comprehension of sentences. She systematically manipulated prosody and syntactic markers in recording three different types of sentences and presented these recordings to four- and five-year-old children. The effects of these manipulations on the comprehension of the sentences of both groups of subjects were examined. The experimental aspect of the study was the researcher's ability to manipulate prosody and syntactic markers in the recordings to study the effects of these manipulations on sentence comprehension. The study was also partly descriptive because Lahey selected subjects from different age groups to examine the development of comprehension in four- and five-year-olds with a cross-sectional plan of observation. In other words, the effects of the experimental manipulations on the four-year-olds were compared with the effects on the five-year-olds.

In another example, Hochberg and Waltzman (1972) studied the effects of presenting pulsed vs. continuous pure tones on the auditory thresholds of persons with and without tinnitus. The study was partly experimental because the researchers could manipulate the manner in which the stimuli were presented to subjects and examine the effect of this manipulation on thresholds. The study was also partly descriptive because they compared the effect that the presentation mode had on listeners with tinnitus with the effect it had on persons without tinnitus. Because they could not manipulate the status of the subjects with regard to tinnitus, they selected subjects who were classified as either having or not having tinnitus.

Examination of some illustrative data from combined experimental–descriptive studies may aid consumers in understanding the importance of combining active and attribute independent variables in this common research strategy. A good example of the combination of attribute and active independent variables in combined experimental–descriptive research is seen in the study by Tomblin, Abbas, Records, and Brenneman (1995) of evoked responses to frequency-modulated (FM) tones in children with specific language impairment vs. children with no language impairment. Averaged cortically evoked potentials were elicited under two conditions: presentation of an unmodulated steady tone of 1,000 Hz and presentation of a modulated tone that varied in frequency between 900 and 1,100 Hz. Frequency modulation was an active independent variable that was manipulated in a bivalent experiment with two levels: modulated vs. unmodulated. Children who were normal language learners were compared to children with specific language impairment in the comparative part of the study. The results showed greater amplitude of auditory evoked response to the modulated than to the unmodulated stimuli for both groups of subjects with no apparent differences found between the two groups. Figure 2.25 shows their results

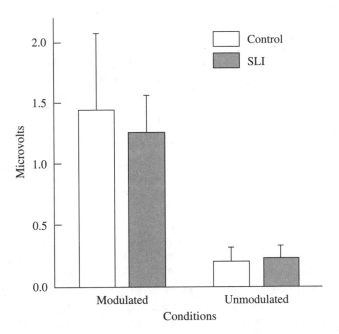

**FIGURE 2.25   Results of a Combined Experimental–
Descriptive Study of the Effects of
Frequency Modulation on Evoked
Responses of Children with Specific
Language Impairment versus Children
with Normal Language**

From "Auditory Evoked Responses to Frequency-Modulated Tones in
Children with Specific Language Impairment," by B. Tomblin, P. Abbas,
N. L. Records, and L. M. Brenneman, 1995, *Journal of Speech and
Hearing Research, 38,* p. 391. Copyright 1995 by the American Speech-
Language-Hearing Association. Reprinted with permission.

plotting evoked response amplitude in microvolts for the control (normal language learners) and SLI (specific language impairment) subjects for the modulated and unmodulated
conditions.

Pashek and Brookshire (1982) studied auditory comprehension of high-level and low-
level adult aphasics. In one of their experiments, they examined the effect of paragraph
presentation rate (normal speech rate vs. slow speech rate) on the auditory comprehension
of the two groups of subjects. Figure 2.26 shows the effect of rate of paragraph presentation on the responses of the two subject groups. Inspection of Figure 2.26 reveals that both
groups of aphasics made more correct responses when the rate of the speech that they listened to was slower than normal. In other words, there was a main effect of rate. There was
also a main effect for subject groups because the high-level subjects always did better than
the low-level subjects. Because both groups of aphasics showed the same main effect of
rate, there was no interaction between rate and subject group.

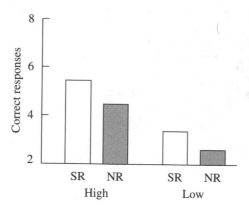

FIGURE 2.26
Results of a Combined Experimental–Descriptive Study of the Effects of Speech Rate on Auditory Comprehension of High-Level and Low-Level Aphasics

From "Effects of Rate of Speech and Linguistic Stress on Auditory Paragraph Comprehension of Aphasive Individuals, by G. V. Pashek and R. H. Brookshire, 1982, *Journal of Speech and Hearing Research, 25,* p. 380. Copyright 1982 by the American Speech-Language-Hearing Association. Reprinted with permission.

In another example, Montgomery (1995) reported two experiments with children exhibiting normal language (NL) vs. children with specific language impairment (SLI). In the first experiment, he studied the effect of syllable length on the children's ability to repeat nonsense words; in the second, he studied the effect of redundancy on a sentence comprehension task. Figure 2.27 shows his results for the first experiment. The figure reveals that the NL children outperformed the SLI subjects, longer stimuli were more difficult, and there was an interaction between stimulus length and subject classification in which the SLI children fell further behind the NL children as stimulus length increased. That is, the graph showing performance on the task as a function of stimulus length fell more sharply for the SLI children than for the NL children. Figure 2.28 shows Montgomery's results for his second experiment with these children. The figure shows (a) NL children outperformed SLI children; (b) NL children performed about the same for both redundant and nonredundant material; (c) SLI children had more difficulty with the redundant than the nonredundant material. Thus, another interaction effect occurred in which the active redundancy variable differentially affected the subjects who differed on the attribute language classification variable.

In another example of a combined experimental–descriptive study, Cohen and Keith (1976) studied the effects of noise on the word-recognition performance of normal-hearing subjects, subjects with flat cochlear hearing loss, and subjects with high-frequency cochlear hearing loss. Word recognition was tested while subjects selected from the three classifications were in a quiet background and while exposed to two different background noise levels. Figure 2.29 presents some of their results and shows how word recognition changed as noise was increased from the quiet condition to signal-to-noise ratios of –4 dB and –12 dB. Figure 2.29 reveals that increased noise levels reduced word-recognition scores but that the amount of reduction was different for each of the three groups of subjects. The high-frequency-loss group showed the greatest reduction, the normal group showed the least reduction, and the flat-loss group was in between these two groups. Also, there was an interaction between subject classification and the independent variable in determining the dependent variable. The manipulation of the independent variable had a different effect on the dependent variable for subjects in the different classifications.

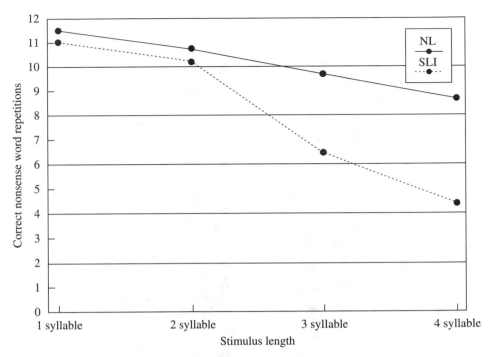

FIGURE 2.27 **Results of a Combined Experimental–Descriptive Study of the Effect of Stimulus Length on Word Repetition of Children with Normal Language (NL) versus Children with Specific Language Impairment (SLI)**

From "Sentence Comprehension in Children with Specific Language Impairment: The Role of Phonological Working Memory," by J. W. Montgomery, 1995, *Journal of Speech and Hearing Research, 38,* p. 191. Copyright 1995 by the American Speech-Language-Hearing Association. Reprinted with permission.

The final example in this section shows the application of a parametric experiment with the manipulation of two active independent variables to four groups of subjects varying in age as part of a series of experiments examining developmental changes in audition in old age. The results of the experiment by Takahashi and Bacon (1992) are shown in Figure 2.30. Four age groups of listeners (young persons in their twenties, and persons in their fifties, sixties, and seventies) listened to speech in modulated and in unmodulated broadband noise at four different signal-to-noise ratios (SNR). The active, manipulated independent variables, then, were noise modulation and SNR, and the attribute variable was age of the subjects. The dependent variable was the percentage of correct speech understanding. The left panel of the figure shows the results of the four groups of subjects at each SNR for the modulated noise condition, and the right panel shows the results for the unmodulated condition. Inspection of the figure reveals main effects of SNR, noise modulation, and age and interactions between SNR and modulation, as well as between modulation and age. As SNR increased, so did speech understanding, as indicated by the slope of the lines upward to the right. Speech

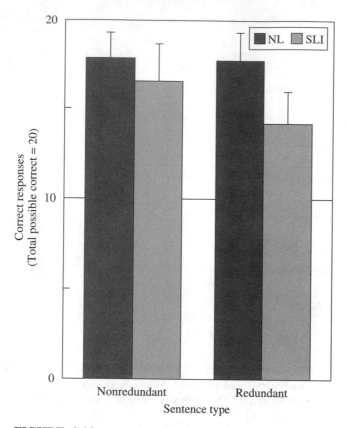

FIGURE 2.28   **Results of a Combined Experimental–
Descriptive Study of the Effect of
Redundancy on Sentence
Comprehension of Children with
Normal Language (NL) versus
Children with Specific Language
Impairment (SLI)**

From "Sentence Comprehension in Children with Specific Language
Impairment: The Role of Phonological Working Memory," by J. W.
Montgomery, 1995, *Journal of Speech and Hearing Research, 38,* p. 192.
Copyright 1995 by the American Speech-Language-Hearing Association.
Reprinted with permission.

understanding was generally better with modulated than with unmodulated noise as indicated
by the higher scores in the left panel. The interaction of SNR and modulation is seen in the
steeper slope of the functions in the right panel than in the left panel, indicating that the modulated and unmodulated functions converged as SNR increased. Finally, the interaction of
modulation and age group is seen in the separation of the young listeners from the older listeners in the modulated condition but not in the unmodulated condition—that is, modulated
noise facilitated young listeners' performance relative to older listeners more than did

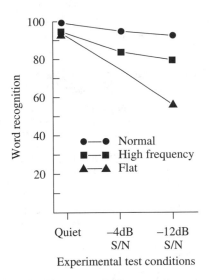

FIGURE 2.29
Results of a Combined Experimental–Descriptive Study of the Effects of Noise on Word Recognition of Subjects with Normal Hearing, Flat Hearing Loss, and High-Frequency Hearing Loss

From "Use of Low Pass Noise in Word Recognition Testing," by R. L. Cohen and R. W. Keith, 1976, *Journal of Speech and Hearing Research, 19,* p. 51. Copyright 1976 by the American Speech-Language-Hearing Association. Reprinted with permission.

unmodulated noise. Such combined experimental–descriptive studies can become quite complex and revealing as more independent variables are introduced and their importance in communicative disorders cannot be stressed enough. Because combined experimental–descriptive research is both a common and important strategy in communicative disorders research, considerable attention will be devoted to it in subsequent chapters of this book.

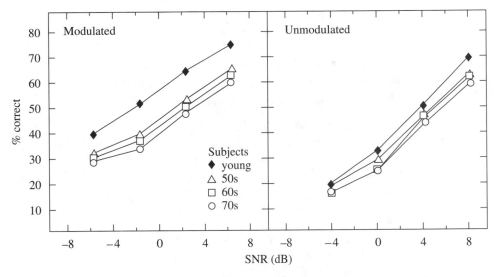

FIGURE 2.30 **Results of a Combined Experimental–Descriptive Study of the Effects of Signal-to-Noise Ratio (SNR) and Noise Modulation on Speech Understanding of Subjects in Four Different Age Groups**

From "Modulation Detection, Modulation Masking, and Speech Understanding in the Elderly," by G. A. Takahashi and S. P. Bacon, 1992, *Journal of Speech and Hearing Research, 35,* p. 1418. Copyright 1992 by the American Speech-Language-Hearing Association. Reprinted with permission.

Study Questions

1. Read the following articles:

   Siren, K. A. (1995). Effects of lexical meaning and practiced productions on coarticulation in children's and adults' speech. *Journal of Speech and Hearing Research, 38,* 351–359.

   Shanks, J. E., Stelmachowicz, P. G., Beauchaine, K. L., & Schulte, L. (1992). Equivalent ear canal volumes in children pre- and post-tympanostomy tube insertion. *Journal of Speech and Hearing Research, 35,* 936–941.

   Bloom, R. L., Borod, J. C., Obler, L. K., & Gerstman, L. J. (1993). Suppression and facilitation of pragmatic performance: Effects of emotional content on discourse following right and left brain damage. *Journal of Speech and Hearing Research, 36,* 1227–1235.

   Write a brief abstract of each article. Outline the four common steps in empirical research described in Chapter 1 that are found in each article and identify the research strategies described in Chapter 2 that are used in each article.

2. Read the following article:

   Abbs, J. H., Folkins, J. W., & Sivarajan, M. (1976). Motor impairment following blockade of the infraorbital nerve: Implications for the use of anesthetization techniques in speech research. *Journal of Speech and Hearing Research, 19,* 19–35.

   a. What research strategy did the authors employ?

   b. Identify the dependent variables that were measured before and after anesthesia.

   c. What differences were observed as a result of anesthesia?

3. Read the following article:

   Walton, J. H., & Orlikoff, R. F. (1994). Speaker race identification from acoustic cues in the vocal signal. *Journal of Speech and Hearing Research, 37,* 738–745.

   a. What research strategy did the authors employ?

   b. Identify the dependent variables that were measured in the two groups.

   c. What differences were observed between the groups?

4. Read the following article:

   Hillenbrand, J., Cleveland, R. A., & Erickson, R. L. (1994). Acoustic correlates of breathy voice quality. *Journal of Speech and Hearing Research, 37,* 769–778.

   a. What research strategy did the authors employ?

   b. Identify the variables that were most highly correlated with breathy voice quality.

5. Read the following article:

   Robbins, J., Fisher, H. B., Blom, E. C., & Singer, M. I. (1984). A comparative acoustic study of normal, esophageal, and tracheoesophageal speech production. *Journal of Speech and Hearing Disorders, 49,* 202–210.

   a. What three groups of subjects were compared (i.e., what was the classification variable)?

   b. Identify the dependent variables that were used to compare the subjects.

   c. What differences were found among the three groups?

6. Read the following article:

   Guitar, B. (1976). Pretreatment factors associated with the outcome of stuttering therapy. *Journal of Speech and Hearing Research, 19,* 590–600.

    a. What were the predictor and predicted variables in this correlational study?

    b. Which variables were identified as the best predictors of each predicted variable?

7. Read the following article:

Gordon-Salant, S., & Fitzgibbons, P. J. (1993). Temporal factors and speech recognition performance in young and elderly listeners. *Journal of Speech and Hearing Research, 36,* 1276–1285.

    a. What research strategies were combined in this study?

    b. Identify the active and attribute independent variables used.

    c. What differences were found among the subject groups as a function of the manipulated independent variables?

8. Read the following article:

Nippold, M. A., & Rudzinski, M. (1993). Familiarity and transparency in idiom explanation: A developmental study of children and adolescents. *Journal of Speech and Hearing Research, 36,* 728–737.

    a. What research strategies were combined in this study?

    b. Identify the dependent variables used.

    c. Explain the effects of idiom familiarity and maturation that are shown in Figure 1.

9. Read the following article:

Quigley, S. P., Wilbur, R. B., & Montanelli, D. S. (1974). Question formation in the language of deaf students. *Journal of Speech and Hearing Research, 17,* 699–713.

    a. What descriptive research strategies were combined in this study?

    b. Identify the dependent variables that were used.

    c. What were the attribute independent variables used?

References

Adams, M. R., & Hutchinson, J. (1974). The effects of three levels of auditory masking on selected vocal characteristics and the frequency of disfluency of adult stutterers. *Journal of Speech and Hearing Research, 17,* 682–688.

Adams, M. R., & Moore, W. H. (1972). The effects of auditory masking on the anxiety level, frequency of disfluency, and selected vocal characteristics of stutterers. *Journal of Speech and Hearing Research, 15,* 572–578.

Ayukawa, H., & Rudmin, F. (1983). Does early middle ear pathology affect auditory perception skills and learning? Comment on Brandes and Ehinger (1981). *Journal of Speech and Hearing Disorders, 48,* 222–223.

Bergman, M. (1971). Hearing and aging. *Audiology, 10,* 164–171.

Blood, G. (1993). Development and assessment of a scale addressing communicative needs of patients with laryngectomies. *American Journal of Speech-Language Pathology, 2(3),* 82–90.

Bloom, L. (1970). *Language development: Form and function in emerging grammars.* Cambridge, MA: MIT Press.

Bordens, K. S., & Abbott, B. B. (1988). *Research design and method: A process approach.* Mountain View, CA: Mayfield.

Brannon, J. B. (1968). Linguistic word classes in the spoken language of normal, hard-of-hearing, and deaf children. *Journal of Speech and Hearing Research, 11,* 279–287.

Calculator, S. N., & Hatch, E. R. (1995). Validation of facilitated communication: A case study and beyond. *American Journal of Speech-Language Pathology, 4*(1), 49–58.

Camarata, S. M., Nelson, K. E., & Camarata, M. N. (1994). Comparison of conversational-recasting and imitative procedures for training grammatical structures in children with specific language impairment. *Journal of Speech and Hearing Research, 37*, 1414–1423.

Carhart, R., & Porter, L. S. (1971). Audiometric configuration and prediction of threshold for spondees. *Journal of Speech and Hearing Research, 14*, 486–495.

Chaiklin, J. B., & Stassen, R. A. (1968). Distorted perception of speech in hearing aid consultation. *Journal of Speech and Hearing Disorders, 33*, 270–274.

Cohen, R. L., & Keith, R. W. (1976). Use of low pass noise in word recognition testing. *Journal of Speech and Hearing Research, 19*, 48–54.

Colburn, N., & Mysak, E. D. (1982). Developmental disfluency and emerging grammar: I. Disfluency characteristics in early syntactic utterances. *Journal of Speech and Hearing Research, 25*, 414–420.

De Filippo, C. L., Sims, D. G., & Gottermeier, L. (1995). Linking visual and kinesthetic imagery in lipreading instruction. *Journal of Speech and Hearing Research, 38*, 244–256.

Elfenbein, J. L., Hardin-Jones, M. A., & Davis, J. M. (1994). Oral communication skills of children who are hard of hearing. *Journal of Speech and Hearing Research, 37*, 216–226.

Ellis Weismer, S., Murray-Branch, J., & Miller, J. F. (1994). A prospective longitudinal study of language development in late talkers. *Journal of Speech and Hearing Research, 37*, 852–867.

Erber, N. P. (1971). Effects of distance on the visual perception of speech. *Journal of Speech and Hearing Research, 14*, 848–857.

Felsenfeld, S., Broen, P. A., & McGue, M. (1994). A 28-year follow-up of adults with a history of moderate phonological disorder: Educational and occupational results. *Journal of Speech and Hearing Research, 37*, 1341–1353.

Geers, A. E., & Moog, J. S. (1992). Speech perception and production skills of hearing-impaired children from oral and total communication education settings. *Journal of Speech and Hearing Research, 35*, 1384–1393.

Helfer, K. S. (1994). Binaural cues and consonant perception in reverberation and noise. *Journal of Speech and Hearing Research, 37*, 429–438.

Hirsh, I. J., Davis, H., Silverman, S. R., Reynolds, E. G., Eldert, E., & Benson, R. W. (1952). Development of materials for speech audiometry. *Journal of Speech and Hearing Disorders, 17*, 321–337.

Hochberg, I., & Waltzman, R. (1972). Comparison of pulsed and continuous tone thresholds in patients with tinnitus. *Audiology, 11*, 337–342.

Jaeger, C. G., & Bacon, H. M. (1962). *Introductory college mathematics.* New York: Harper & Row.

Karsh, D. E., & Brandes, P. (1983). Response to Ayukawa and Rudmin. *Journal of Speech and Hearing Disorders, 48*, 223–224.

Kent, R. D., Osberger, M. J., Netsell, R., & Hustedde, C. G. (1987). Phonetic development in identical twins differing in auditory function. *Journal of Speech and Hearing Research, 38*, 304–314.

Kerlinger, F. (1973). *Foundations of behavioral research.* New York: Holt, Rinehart & Winston.

Kerlinger, F., & Pedhazur, E. J. (1973). *Multiple regression in behavioral research.* New York: Holt, Rinehart & Winston.

Kling, J. W., & Riggs, L. A. (Eds.). (1971). *Woodworth and Schlossberg's experimental psychology.* New York: Holt, Rinehart & Winston.

Lahey, M. (1974). Use of prosody and syntactic markers in children's comprehension of spoken sentences. *Journal of Speech and Hearing Research, 17*, 656–668.

Lass, N., Ruscello, D. M., Pannbacker, M. D., Middleton, G. F., Schmitt, J. F., & Scheuerle, J. F. (1995). Career selection and satisfaction in the professions. *Asha, 37*(4), 48–51.

Lodge, D. N., & Leach, E. A. (1975). Children's acquisition of idioms in the English language. *Journal of Speech and Hearing Research, 18*, 521–529.

Loven, F. C., & Collins, M. J. (1988). Reverberation, masking, filtering, and level effects on speech recognition performance. *Journal of Speech and Hearing Research, 31*, 681–695.

McClellan, M. E. (1967). Aided speech discrimination in noise with vented and unvented earmolds. *Journal of Auditory Research, 7*, 93–99.

Monge, P. R., & Cappella, J. N. (1980). *Multivariate techniques in human communication research.* New York: Academic Press.

Monsen, R. (1978). Toward measuring how well hearing-impaired children speak. *Journal of Speech and Hearing Research, 21,* 197–219.

Montgomery, J. W. (1995). Sentence comprehension in children with specific language impairment: The role of phonological working memory. *Journal of Speech and Hearing Research, 38,* 187–199.

Pashek, G. V., & Brookshire, R. H. (1982). Effects of rate of speech and linguistic stress on auditory paragraph comprehension of aphasic individuals. *Journal of Speech and Hearing Research, 25,* 377–383.

Plutchik, R. (1974). *Foundations of experimental research.* New York: Harper & Row.

Riddel, J., McCauley, R. J., Mulligan, M., & Tandan, R. (1995). Intelligibility and phonetic contrast errors in highly intelligible speakers with amyotrophic lateral sclerosis. *Journal of Speech and Hearing Research, 38,* 304–314.

Russell, A., Penny, L., & Pemberton, C. (1995). Speaking fundamental frequency changes over time in women: A longitudinal study. *Journal of Speech and Hearing Research, 38,* 101–109.

Sapienza, C. M., & Stathopoulos, E. (1994). Respiratory and laryngeal measures of children and women with bilateral vocal fold nodules. *Journal of Speech and Hearing Research, 37,* 1229–1243.

Schiff-Myers, N. B. (1983). From pronoun reversals to correct pronoun usage: A case study of a normally developing child. *Journal of Speech and Hearing Disorders, 48,* 394–402.

Sherman, D. (1954). The merits of backward playing of connected speech in the scaling of voice quality disorders. *Journal of Speech and Hearing Disorders, 19,* 312–321.

Shriberg, L. D., Gruber, F. A., & Kwiatkowski, J. (1994). Developmental phonological disorders III: Long-term speech sound normalization. *Journal of Speech and Hearing Research, 37,* 1151–1177.

Shriner, T. H., Holloway, M. S., & Daniloff, R. G. (1969). The relationship between articulatory deficits and syntax in speech defective children. *Journal of Speech and Hearing Research, 12,* 319–325.

Shuster, L. I., Ruscello, D. M., & Toth, A. R. (1995). The use of visual feedback to elicit correct /r/.

American Journal of Speech-Language Pathology, 4(2), 37–44.

Studebaker, G. A., Taylor, R., & Sherbecoe, R. L. (1994). The effect of noise spectrum on speech recognition performance–intensity functions. *Journal of Speech and Hearing Research, 37,* 439–448.

Takahashi, G. A., & Bacon, S. P. (1992). Modulation detection, modulation masking, and speech understanding in the elderly. *Journal of Speech and Hearing Research, 35,* 1410–1421.

Tomblin, B., Abbas, P., Records, N. L., & Brenneman, L. M. (1995). Auditory evoked responses to frequency-modulated tones in children with specific language impairment. *Journal of Speech and Hearing Research, 38,* 387–392.

Turner, G. S. & Weismer, G. (1994). Characteristics of speaking rate in the dysarthria associated with amyotrophic lateral sclerosis. *Journal of Speech and Hearing Research, 36,* 1134–1144.

Tye-Murray, N., Purdy, S. C., & Woodworth, G. G. (1992). Reported use of communication strategies by SHHH members: Client, talker, and situational variables. *Journal of Speech and Hearing Research, 35,* 708–717.

Underwood, B. J., & Shaughnessy, J. J. (1975). *Experimentation in psychology.* New York: John Wiley & Sons.

Ventry, I. M. (1980). Effects of conductive hearing loss: Fact or fiction? *Journal of Speech and Hearing Disorders, 45,* 143–156.

Ventry, I. M., Chaiklin, J. B., & Boyle, W. F. (1961). Collapse of the ear canal during audiometry. *Archives of Otolaryngology, 73,* 727–731.

Wilder, C. N., & Baken, R. J. (1974). Respiratory patterns in infant cry. *Human Communication, 3,* 18–34.

Young, M. A. (1976). Application of regression analysis concepts to retrospective research in speech pathology. *Journal of Speech and Hearing Research, 19,* 5–18.

Young, M. A. (1993). Supplementing tests of statistical significance: Variation accounted for. *Journal of Speech and Hearing Research, 36,* 644–656.

Young, M. A. (1994). Evaluating differences between stuttering and nonstuttering speakers: The group difference design. *Journal of Speech and Hearing Research, 37,* 522–534.

Chapter 3

Research Design in Communicative Disorders

This chapter considers research designs that are commonly used in communicative disorders. The topics to be discussed are: (1) the meaning of research design, (2) the purposes of research design, (3) general research design principles in experimental and descriptive research, (4) some specific principles of group research design, (5) some specific principles of single-subject research design, and (6) some issues regarding generalization.

Meaning of Research Design

As mentioned in Chapter 2, Bordens and Abbott (1988) distinguished between research design and research strategy by stating that strategy is the general plan of attack and design is the specific set of tactics used to carry out the strategy. Kerlinger (1979, p. 83) has more specifically defined research design as follows:

> The plan and structure of research are often called the design of research. The word "design," as used here, focuses on the manner in which a research problem is conceptualized and put into a structure that is a guide for experimentation and for data collection and analysis. We define research design, then, as the plan and structure of investigation conceived so as to obtain answers to research questions. Modern conceptions of the design of research are founded in experimental research.

Research design, then, is the development of a plan for selecting and measuring the independent and dependent variables in order to answer research questions about their relationships. As Kerlinger stated previously, modern research designs are rooted in the concept of the experiment in which an independent variable is manipulated to determine its effect on a dependent variable. As pointed out in Chapter 2, the *structure* of nonmanipulable independent variables in descriptive research is similar to the *structure* of manipulable independent variables in experiments. Thus, the structure of descriptive research design will be similar in many ways to the structure of experimental design, with the main difference being the manipulability of the independent variables.

Purposes of Research Design

Kerlinger (1973, p. 300) stated that

> *Research design has two basic purposes: (1) to provide answers to research questions and (2) to control variance. . . . Design helps the investigator obtain answers to the questions of research and also helps him to control the experimental, extraneous, and error variances of the particular research problem under study.*

In order to accomplish the first purpose, the investigator must develop an experimental or descriptive research design for obtaining empirical data about the relationship of the independent and dependent variables of interest. In order to accomplish the second purpose, the investigator must structure the research plan in such a way that contamination of the answer to the research question by extraneous variables and measurement error is minimized. Because the relationship between the independent and dependent variable is quantified by describing the degree to which variation or change in one variable is linked to variation or change in the other variable, control of variance is necessary to produce answers to research questions that are as free as possible of contamination by extraneous variables and measurement error. Kerlinger (1973, pp. 306–313) described in detail the concept of research design as variance control by outlining the manner in which efficient research design is used (a) to maximize the systematic variance associated with the independent and dependent variables of interest to the investigator, (b) to minimize error or random variance (including errors of measurement), and (c) to control variance attributable to the influence of extraneous variables on the dependent variable.

The two basic purposes of research design are common to both experimental and descriptive research, but some specific objectives are different for these two types of research. In experimental research, the first design objective is to manipulate the independent variable in order to answer the question "What effect does this have on the dependent variable?" The second design objective is to arrange the experiment so that extraneous variables are controlled and, therefore, cannot have a confounding effect on the dependent variable. In descriptive research, the first objective is to select the variables for observation in order to answer questions such as "What are the dimensions or differences or relationships found in the natural phenomena?" The second objective is to make these observations in a systematic and unobtrusive fashion so that the dimensions, differences, or relationships of the criterion variables are not confounded by extraneous variables.

We have merely rephrased the general purposes of research design into specific objectives to fit the descriptive and experimental models. The main point is that both types of research should be designed to: (1) answer the research question empirically and (2) reduce or eliminate contamination of the answer by extraneous variables.

Kerlinger (1973, pp. 300–301) has indicated that it may be tempting to omit the first purpose (because it is so obvious) and concentrate on the second. He points out, however, that this is a dangerous delimitation because research design could then degenerate into a "sterile technical exercise" in which one may lose sight of the importance of uniting the research questions, the empirical evidence, and the conclusions of the study. The research question should be a common unifying element in the design of research.

General Research Design Principles

As Kerlinger (1973) has pointed out, theoretically at least, there are as many research designs as there are hypotheses to be tested. Therefore, rather than attempt to present an exhaustive taxonomy of descriptive and experimental research designs, we have limited our discussion to some basic principles of research design that have broad applicability in communicative disorders research. Two major classes of research designs are considered here: group designs and single-subject designs. In group designs, one or more groups of subjects are exposed to one or more levels of the independent variable, and the average performance of the group of subjects on the dependent variable is examined to determine the relationship between the independent and dependent variable. Single-subject designs focus on the individual behavior of subjects rather than considering the average performance of a group of subjects. Single-subject designs may, in fact, examine the behavior of more than one person, but the data of each person will be evaluated individually rather than as part of a group average.

In evaluating any research design, there are two important criteria suggested by Campbell and Stanley (1966): *internal validity* and *external validity.* The internal validity of any research design concerns the degree to which the design meets Kerlinger's two purposes within the confines of the study. That is, did the study answer the research question and control variance appropriately to provide an uncontaminated picture of the relationship between independent and dependent variables? The external validity of any research design concerns the degree to which generalizations can be made outside of the confines of the study. Some general comments on the internal and external validity of research designs will be made in this chapter, and a more detailed analysis of the application of these two criteria in treatment efficacy research will be included in Chapter 5.

Group Research Designs

This section will consider group designs for both experimental and descriptive research and briefly address the primary issues affecting internal validity of the major group designs.

Experimental design is concerned with the manipulation of the independent variable and the measurement of its effect on the dependent variable. Descriptive research design is concerned with the classification of subjects and with the application of measurement procedures to subjects in order to assess group differences, developmental trends, or relationships among variables. Experimental and descriptive research designs are often classified as *between-subjects, within-subjects,* or *mixed* (both between-subjects and within-subjects) designs.

In between-subjects designs, different groups of subjects are compared to each other. Within-subjects designs involve the comparison of the same group of subjects in different situations. Mixed designs include both types of comparison in the same study. Some problems are well suited to between-subjects designs, whereas other problems are more logically attacked through within-subjects designs. In some cases, a combination of the two in a mixed design is necessary in order to study the problem appropriately. The selection of an appropriate design is dependent, to a large extent, on a clear understanding of the research problem and a logical analysis of the alternate means for studying the problem.

Between-Subjects Designs

In between-subjects research designs, the performances of separate groups of subjects are measured and comparisons are made between the groups. In experimental between-subjects designs, different groups of subjects are exposed to different treatments or levels of the independent variable. In descriptive between-subjects designs, different groups of subjects are compared with each other with regard to their performance on some criterion variable. We will first discuss some issues in between-subjects experimental designs and then consider points concerning between-subjects descriptive research designs.

In between-subjects experimental designs, the independent variable or experimental treatment is applied to one group of subjects (experimental group) but not applied to another group of subjects (control group). The difference between the performance of the two groups is taken as an index of the effect of the independent variable on the dependent variable. This would be the case, for example, in a treatment experiment in which the experimental group is given treatment and the control group is not given treatment. The two groups are then compared on some dependent variable that is usually some measure of performance improvement.

Ferguson and Takane (1989, p. 238) have summarized the process of designing a between-subjects experiment:

> *In developing the design for an experiment, the investigator (1) selects the values of the independent variable, or variables, to be compared; (2) selects the subjects for the experiments; (3) applies rules or procedures whereby subjects are assigned to the particular values of the independent variable; (4) specifies the observations or measurements to be made on each subject.*

Between-subjects experimental designs may be bivalent, in which case one experimental group is compared to one control group to study the effect of the presence vs. the absence of the experimental treatment (independent variable). These designs may also be multivalent, in which case each of several experimental groups is exposed to a different value of the independent variable and the control group receives no treatment. Finally, between-subjects designs may be parametric, in which case several groups could receive different values of the different independent variables in different combinations and could also be compared with a control group that receives no treatment.

A major consideration in the evaluation of the design of between-subjects experiments is the equivalence of the experimental and control groups. If the two groups of subjects that are exposed to two levels of the independent variable are different from each other in characteristics such as age, intelligence, gender, and prior experience, they may perform differently on the dependent variable because of these subject characteristic differences rather than because they have been exposed to two different levels of the independent variable. The subject characteristic difference, then, is an extraneous, or nuisance, variable that can compete with the independent variable as an explanation for any difference in the dependent variable between the two groups of subjects. In other words, differences in the relative performances of experimental and control groups might be attributable to differences in subject characteristics of the two groups in addition to, or instead of, the effects of the independent variable.

Researchers, then, must attempt to ensure that subjects in the experimental and control groups are equivalent in all respects except for the varied distribution of the independent variable to these groups. There are basically two techniques for attempting to equate experimental and control groups for between-subjects experimental designs: *randomization* and *matching*.

Randomization is usually considered the better of these two techniques and will be discussed first. Christensen (1988, p. 174), in commenting on the importance of randomization as a technique for equating groups, stated:

Randomization, the most important and basic of all the control methods, is a statistical control technique that has the purpose of providing assurance that extraneous variables, known or unknown, will not systematically bias the results of the study. It is the only technique for controlling unknown sources of variation.

Randomization is the assignment of subjects to experimental and control groups on a random basis. Random, in this sense, does not mean that subjects are assigned in a haphazard fashion. Rather, randomization is a technique for group assignment that ensures each subject has an equal probability of being assigned either to the experimental group or to the control group. Christensen (1988, p. 180) summarized the objective of randomization in dealing with extraneous variables in experimental and control groups:

Random assignment produces control by virtue of the fact that the variables to be controlled are distributed in approximately the same manner in all groups (ideally the distribution would be exactly the same). When the distribution is approximately equal, the influence of the extraneous variables is held constant, because they cannot exert any differential influence on the dependent variable.

With a random assignment of subjects to experimental and control groups, extraneous variables (e.g., age, gender, intelligence, or socioeconomic status), which could affect the subjects' performance on the dependent variable, should be balanced among the groups so that there would be no systematic bias favoring one group over another. In such a case, then, the two groups may be considered equivalent at the start of the experiment.

Christensen (1988) points out, however, that randomization may not always result in the selection of experimental and control groups that are equivalent in all respects, especially when a small number of subjects is used. Because random chance determines the assignment of subjects to experimental and control groups (and, therefore, the distribution of extraneous subject-selection variables to experimental and control groups), it is possible occasionally for the two groups to differ on some variables. Researchers often check this possibility by examining the groups after randomization to ascertain the equivalence of the groups on known extraneous variables. Christensen (1988) has indicated, however, that the probability of experimental and control groups being equivalent on extraneous variables is greater with randomization than with other methods of group selection and, therefore, randomization is a powerful technique for reducing systematic bias in subject assignment to experimental and control groups. In addition, randomization is an important prerequisite to unbiased data analysis, and many of the statistical techniques to be described in Chapter 6 are based on the assumption of random assignment to experimental and control groups.

A second technique for attempting to equate experimental and control groups in between-subjects experimental designs is matching. The experimenter could attempt to match the members of the two groups on all extraneous variables that were considered relevant to the experiment. Two groups could be assembled that would be equivalent at the start of the experiment on extraneous variables known to be correlated with the dependent variable. Because the rationale for matching groups is to reduce the possibility of subject-selection differences mimicking the effect of the independent variable on the dependent variable, it makes sense to match the groups on extraneous variables that could influence subjects' performance on the dependent variable. Thus, differences between the experimental and control groups on the dependent variable at the end of the experiment would not be attributable to differences between the groups on these extraneous variables.

A number of techniques are available for matching experimental and control groups on extraneous variables. Two common techniques that are used are *matching the overall distribution* of the extraneous variables in the groups and *matching pairs of subjects* for assignment to experimental and control groups. Christensen (1988) calls the first matching technique the "frequency distribution control technique" because the two groups are matched in their overall frequency distribution (i.e., the frequency of cases occurring at each value of the extraneous variable) rather than comparing subjects on a case-by-case basis on a number of characteristics. Christensen (1988) calls the second matching technique the "precision control technique" because matching subjects on a case-by-case basis not only reduces subject differences as an extraneous variable, but also increases the sensitivity of the experiment to small effects of the independent variable on the dependent variable when subjects are equated on extraneous variables that are highly correlated with the dependent variable.

Overall matching is accomplished by assembling experimental and control groups that have similar distributions of the extraneous variables—that is both groups have about the same average and spread of each of the extraneous variables. For example, factors such as age, intelligence, level of education, and gender would be distributed about equally in the experimental and control groups. Each group could be assembled so that it would contain equal numbers of males and females; the age range and average age would be the same in each group; the average IQ and the range from the lowest to the highest IQ in each group would be about the same, and so on.

Although overall matching on the surface may appear to be an adequate technique for ensuring group equivalence, consumers of research should be aware that there are disadvantages to this technique. For example, one distinct disadvantage is that the combinations of extraneous variables in individual subjects may not be well matched for two groups. Although age and IQ may be the same on the average in the two groups, the older subjects may be more intelligent than the younger subjects in one group, whereas the younger subjects may be more intelligent than the older subjects in the other group. Although individual nuisance variables may seem to be equivalent in the two groups, the interaction of the nuisance variables in each subject in the two groups may not necessarily be the same.

Matching pairs of subjects for subsequent assignment to experimental and control groups is a more effective technique than overall matching. Matching pairs is accomplished by first selecting a subject for assignment to one group and then searching for another subject whose constellation of extraneous variables is essentially the same as for the first subject. Because no two people are exactly alike in all respects, matching is usually accomplished within certain limits on the extraneous variables. For example, the first subject may be a twenty-one-year-old female college senior with an IQ of 115. To find her matched pair member for assignment to the other group, the experimenter would then look for a female college senior with an IQ between 112 and 118 in the age range from twenty to twenty-two years. The rest of the subjects would be paired in a similar fashion, with each pair having a unique pattern of the extraneous variables.

Once matched pairs have been assembled, the next step is to assign the pair members to the experimental and control groups. Although pair matching would equate experimental and control groups on the known extraneous variables selected for matching, it would not equate them with respect to any other extraneous variables overlooked by the experimenter. Therefore, assigning pair members to experimental and control groups only on the basis of some convenience may result in nonequivalent groups with respect to unknown extraneous variables. Suppose, for example, that the pairs were assembled by selecting subjects from two different clinical settings and matching one member from each setting to one member of the other setting. Then, for the sake of convenience, all pair members from one setting are assigned to the experimental treatment, and all pair members from the other setting are assigned to the control group. The problem is that if there were any differences between the groups of subjects in the two settings on unknown extraneous variables, then these differences would result in a differential subject-selection threat to internal validity, despite the matching of the groups on the known extraneous variables.

Campbell and Stanley (1966) and Van Dalen (1966) have suggested, however, that matching pairs can be a powerful technique for ensuring group equivalence if that technique is *combined with randomization.* Members of matched pairs could be subsequently assigned *at random,* one pair member being assigned randomly to the experimental group and the other pair member to the control group. This combination of matching pairs and randomization would be used (1) to match pairs on extraneous variables that are known to be correlated with the dependent variable and (2) to reduce the probability of group differences on unknown extraneous variables through the random assignment of pair members to the two groups.

Consumers of research should be aware of some of the advantages and disadvantages both of randomization and of matching. Randomization is often preferred, for example, if a large number of subjects is available because it is difficult to match numerous pairs, especially if they must be matched on several extraneous variables. Therefore, it would be more efficient to randomize group assignment at the outset, because randomization alone decreases the probability of group differences with respect to both known and unknown extraneous variables.

Randomization is also generally preferred when more than one experimental group is to be compared with the control group. If, for example, three experimental groups were to be compared with one control group, then matched quadruplets rather than matched pairs would be needed. Matching quadruplets of subjects would present considerable difficulty to any experimenter, especially if the quadruplets were to be matched on several extraneous variables. It would be much more efficient to assign subjects randomly to each of the four groups at the outset than to try to match groups of four subjects for subsequent randomization.

The combination of matching pairs with subsequent randomization of pair members to experimental and control groups may be preferred by some investigators when only a small number of subjects is available for inclusion in the experiment. As indicated by Christensen (1988), the risk for failure to equate groups as a result of randomization is greater with a small number of subjects than it is with a larger number of subjects. Therefore, experimenters may often feel more confident about group equivalence on known extraneous variables if pair matching is combined with subsequent randomization. Despite the disadvantages of overall matching and pair matching, many experimenters apparently believe that matching alone is better than nothing at all, as evidenced by the prevalence of articles in the research literature that use matching alone for assembling experimental and control groups.

Between-subjects designs have been discussed so far only with regard to experimental research. Between-subjects designs are also common in descriptive research, and some of the foregoing considerations are applicable to descriptive research designs. In addition, there are other specific considerations unique to descriptive research that need to be addressed.

Between-subjects designs are found in comparative research, cross-sectional developmental research, and surveys that compare the responses of different groups. Comparative research involves the description of dependent variable differences between groups of subjects who differ with respect to some classification variable (e.g., children with palatal clefts vs. children without palatal clefts). Cross-sectional developmental research uses a between-subjects design because separate groups of subjects who differ with respect to age are compared. Some surveys are conducted for the purpose of comparing the interview or questionnaire responses of subjects who fall into different classifications (e.g., hearing-aid users vs. nonusers).

Between-subjects descriptive research designs may be bivalent, in which case the classification variable is broken into two mutually exclusive categories (e.g., laryngectomees vs. speakers with normal larynges). Between-subjects descriptive designs may also be multivalent, in which case the classification variable is divided into categories that are ordered along some continuum (e.g., mild vs. moderate vs. severe hearing loss). Finally, between-subjects descriptive designs may include comparisons of subjects who are simultaneously categorized with respect to more than one classification variable (e.g., male vs. female; mild vs. moderate vs. severe mental retardation).

As is the case with between-subjects experimental designs, subject selection is the major consideration in between-subjects descriptive research designs. Consumers should recognize, however, that researchers cannot randomly assign subjects to different classifications in a descriptive study. Instead, the researcher has to select subjects who already fall within the various classifications (e.g., normal hearing vs. hearing-impaired subjects). The main strategy in between-subjects descriptive research design, then, is selection of subjects who fall into distinctly different categories of the classification variable but who are otherwise equivalent with regard to known extraneous variables. This is, indeed, a formidable task. A comparison of some problems encountered and some strategies used in designing between-subjects research studies with manipulable independent variables vs. classification variables may be found in Ferguson and Takane (1989, pp. 237–247).

The first step in this design is the definition of criteria for selecting subjects from each category of the classification variable. Consumers of research should pay careful attention to the manner in which subject-selection criteria are defined. Classifications must be constructed that are mutually exclusive, that is, subjects should fall into only one category with regard to each classification variable. For example, in a comparison of patients with cochlear hearing loss and patients with conductive hearing loss, all subjects must fit the definition of only one of the two groups. Patients who were found to have both a cochlear and a conductive component to their losses would have to form a third comparison group, that is, patients with mixed hearing losses. Consumers are likely to notice that researchers vary in the strictness with which they define subject-selection criteria. Compromises are often necessary in trying to establish well-defined groups and remain reasonably consistent with the actual characteristics of the subjects that are available for study.

Although some classification variables are relatively easy to categorize, others may require more elaborate criteria for defining mutually exclusive groups of subjects. Sometimes it may be necessary to use several measures in a battery of selection tests in order to classify subjects. In many cases, a range of scores on a particular measure may be used to define arbitrary boundaries for classification. Consumers should examine the reliability and validity of tests used for subject classification in order to evaluate the effectiveness with which the researcher has assembled the groups of subjects.

The second design step in between-subjects descriptive research is the attempt to equate subjects on extraneous variables. Because subjects cannot be assigned randomly to the various classifications, consumers of research should realize that equivalence of groups on all extraneous variables is quite difficult to achieve. The inability to eliminate this subject selection threat to internal validity is one of the reasons that many researchers are reluctant to infer cause–effect relationships from descriptive studies.

Because random assignment to classifications is impossible, the best alternative is to try to minimize group differences on extraneous variables known to correlate with the dependent variable. A common method for reducing extraneous variable differences is to match the various groups on the extraneous variables known to be most highly correlated with the dependent variable. Both overall matching and pair matching have been used for this purpose in between-subjects descriptive research. The advantages and disadvantages of these two techniques were discussed earlier. Neither technique fully eliminates subject characteristic differences between comparison groups, but many researchers consider using these techniques to be better than ignoring the problem of extraneous variables. The greatest problem, of course, is in overlooking relevant extraneous variables that could influence performance on the dependent variable.

In summary, between-subjects designs compare the performance of different groups of subjects in experimental or descriptive research. In experimental work, the comparison is made between groups of subjects who are exposed to different treatments or levels of the independent variable. In descriptive research, the performances of subjects in different classifications are compared. Effective between-subjects designs include efforts to select groups that are equivalent regarding extraneous subject characteristic variables.

Within-Subjects Designs

In within-subjects designs, the performance of the *same* subjects is compared in different conditions. In experimental research, the subjects are exposed to all levels of the independent variable. Longitudinal developmental studies are within-subjects descriptive designs because the same subjects are studied as they mature. Correlational studies also include within-subjects designs because each subject is measured on all of the variables that are correlated. Experimental within-subjects design will be considered first, and additional comments will be made about within-subjects descriptive research designs.

In the preceding discussion of between-subjects experimental design, emphasis was placed on evaluation of attempts to equate groups of subjects on extraneous variables. There is no problem with extraneous variables affecting the performance of one group of subjects and not the other in a within-subjects design because only one group of subjects participates. In other words, assignment of subjects to experimental and control groups is not a problem. The basic concern in evaluation of a within-subjects design is that all conditions should be equivalent except for the application of the various levels of the independent variable. Action should be taken to ensure that observed changes in the dependent variable can be attributed to the effect of the independent variable rather than to the effect of nuisance or extraneous variables that can emulate the effect of the independent variable.

Many of these threats to internal validity may be related to the temporal arrangements or sequence of the conditions of a within-subjects experiment. Therefore, a necessary tactic in within-subjects experimental design is the attempt to control what is sometimes termed *sequencing effect* or *order effect*. Sequencing effect and order effect are not used consistently in the various textbooks on research design, but two distinct effects are usually identified regarding the temporal arrangement of experimental conditions. We will use the terminology employed by Christensen (1988) in describing these effects.

Christensen uses *sequencing effect* to describe the overall problem that occurs when subjects participate in a number of treatment conditions and their participation in an earlier condition may affect their performance in a subsequent condition. He differentiates between two types of sequencing effects. The first effect is called an *order effect,* that is, a general performance improvement or decrement that may occur between the beginning and end of an experiment. For example, subjects' performances might improve toward the end of an experiment because of the practice in the task that they receive or because of familiarity with the experimental environment. On the other hand, subjects may show a decrease in performance in the latter part of an experiment because of fatigue.

Christensen calls the second sequencing effect a *carry-over effect*. A carry-over effect is not a general performance change from the beginning to the end of an experiment but rather the result of the influence of a specific treatment condition on performance in the next condition. In other words, the results of one treatment condition may be carried over into the next condition. For example, in studies of temporary threshold shift (TTS) induced by presentation of intense noise, it is important that subjects be given sufficient time to recover from TTS before experiencing a subsequent noise exposure. Otherwise, performance in the subsequent condition would be affected by the carryover of TTS remaining from the first exposure. This carry-over effect may occur whenever exposure to one treatment condition either permanently or temporarily affects performance in subsequent conditions. Temporary carryover can often be minimized with a rest period between experimental conditions, but permanent carryover is a more serious problem that will be discussed later in this section.

There are two major techniques for reducing sequencing effects: *randomizing* and *counterbalancing* the sequence of experimental treatments. Randomization is the presentation of the experimental treatment conditions to the subjects in a random sequence. Random distribution of the treatments in the time course of the experiment would essentially wash out most sequencing effects in a within-subjects design. Sometimes, however, the experimenter may wish to examine the nature of a sequencing effect, and this cannot be done with randomization. Counterbalancing is a technique that enables the experimenter to control and measure sequencing effects by arranging all possible sequences of treatments and, then, randomly assigning subjects to each sequence. Any differences in performance attributable to the sequencing of treatment conditions could then be measured by examining the performances of subjects who participated in the different sequences. In a sense, the sequence of treatment conditions would become another independent variable that is manipulated by the experimenter.

In some cases, sequencing effects may involve such severe or permanent carryover that within-subjects designs are not appropriate. For example, Underwood and Shaughnessy (1975) list experiments on the effects of instructions as being generally inappropriate for within-subjects designs. Suppose an experimenter wished to study the differential effect of two types of instructions on subjects' performance of a certain task. One set of instructions contains information that may influence performance, but this information is withheld from the other set of instructions. If subjects always received the informative instructions last, a possible order effect might be introduced (i.e., subjects might warm up or become fatigued from the first to the second condition). If the sequence of instructions were randomized or counterbalanced, however, those subjects who received the informative instructions first would not be likely to forget those instructions when tested later with the noninformative instructions. In other words, there would be a permanent carry over effect from the informative to the noninformative instructions.

Whenever carryover is likely to be permanent, a between-subjects design is more appropriate than a within-subjects design. In the example of the effects of instructions on performance, subjects could be randomly assigned to one of two groups: one group would receive the informative instructions, and the other group would receive the noninformative instructions. Whenever a sequencing effect cannot be controlled by randomization or counterbalancing, between-subjects designs are usually considered more appropriate. Whenever sequencing can be well controlled, within-subjects designs are often considered to be more powerful than between-subjects designs because the subjects act as their own control group by participating in all experimental conditions.

Longitudinal developmental research is an example of the application of a within-subjects design to descriptive research. The longitudinal design differs from the between-subjects cross-sectional design because the researcher follows the same subjects as they age or mature rather than measuring the performance of different groups of subjects selected from each age range. This within-subjects developmental design allows the researcher to study the rate of development directly for each subject as time passes and the subjects age or mature.

Correlational studies are also examples of within-subjects designs in descriptive research because they involve the application of a number of different measures to a group of subjects. Sequencing effects can usually be controlled through randomization or counterbalancing the sequence of the tests administered.

Mixed Designs

In many research studies more than one independent variable is considered. The effects of two or more independent variables on a dependent variable may be examined in an experimental study. More than one classification variable may be investigated in a descriptive study. In many of these cases, one independent variable is studied with a between-subjects comparison, and the other independent variable is studied with a within-subjects comparison. Hence, a mixed design that incorporates each of the two tactics is used.

In an experiment in which two independent variables are manipulated, it may sometimes be better to measure the effects of one independent variable with a between-subjects design and measure the effects of the other independent variable with a within-subjects design. A descriptive study may incorporate a comparison of the correlation between two variables in one type of subject with the correlation between these two variables in another type of subject. A descriptive study may also incorporate a comparison of the longitudinal development of two different types of subjects. Combined descriptive–experimental studies often involve a within-subjects experimental study of the effect of an independent variable on a dependent variable with two different types of subjects. The experimental effect for one group would be compared to the experimental effect for the other group. All of these research studies would involve mixed designs because they incorporate both within-subjects and between-subjects comparisons.

Because mixed designs incorporate the tactics of both between-subjects and within-subjects designs, the foregoing discussion of both types of designs applies to the mixed designs. The cautions required to ensure group equivalence for between-subjects designs apply to groups compared in mixed designs. Similarly, the comments on randomizing or counterbalancing techniques apply to the within-subjects component of a mixed design.

It is important for consumers of research to be aware of the nature of mixed designs because of their prevalence in the communicative disorders literature. Consumers should be able to identify which part of a mixed design is a within-subjects comparison and which part is a between-subjects comparison in order to evaluate the attempts made by the researcher minimize the influence of extraneous variables.

Single-Subject Research Designs

In addition to the group research designs discussed previously, there are many single-subject research designs that are prevalent in the research literature in communicative disorders. Single-subject designs may be applied to only one subject or to a small number of subjects who are evaluated as separate individuals rather than as members of a larger group to be averaged together. Group research designs are based on comparison of the average behavior of one group of subjects to the average of another group in between-subjects designs or are based on the comparison of the average behavior of one group of subjects in two different conditions in a within-subjects design. Usually there is only one measurement of the dependent variable made per subject in each group or condition. Statistical comparisons of the averages of these measurements in different groups or different conditions form the basis for conclusions about the relationships of the independent and dependent variables. In single-subject designs, however, the focus is on a detailed analysis of the behavior of each individual subject under highly controlled and specified conditions. Rather than measuring each subject's behavior just once in each condition, multiple measurements of the dependent variable are made under different experimental conditions. Single-subject designs are often called *time-series* designs because a series of measurements of the dependent variable are made over a period of time.

Single-subject designs are similar in some respects to within-subjects designs in the sense that each subject participates in all conditions of the experiment that represent all levels of the independent variable. However, single-subject designs differ from within-subjects designs in that the focus is on the analysis of the performance of the individual subject in each condition rather than on how the group performed on the average in each condition. Single-subject designs include at least two time segments: a *baseline* segment of behavioral observation and a *treatment* segment in which the independent variable is manipulated. A simple time-series design with one baseline and one treatment segment is often referred to as an *A-B* design, with the letter *A* referring to the first, or baseline, segment and the letter *B* referring to the second, or treatment, segment. Figure 3.1 diagrams a hypothetical AB single-subject design and illustrates the kind of small fluctuation in the dependent variable often seen in baseline and a dramatic increase in the dependent variable during the treatment segment. Single-subject designs often include other segments that incorporate design elements to improve control over extraneous variables; some of these design elements will be discussed later in this section and in Chapter 5.

In a baseline segment, the subject's behavior is measured over time with no intervention, changing of conditions, or manipulation of the independent variable. Some variability over time is expected in behavior, but the baseline segment is continued until

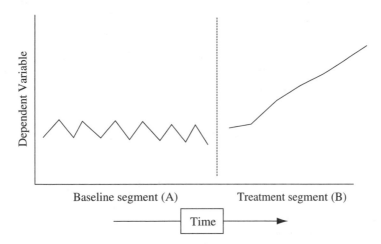

**FIGURE 3.1   Results of a Hypothetical Single-Subject
                Experiment**

reasonable stability is observed in the subject's behavior. Setting criteria for baseline stability is a controversial issue, but several characteristics of the single-subject's behavior in
the baseline segment have been considered including *level, trend, slope,* and *variability*
(Christensen, 1988; Kratchowill & Levin, 1992; McReynolds & Kearns, 1983; Hersen &
Barlow, 1976). Level refers to the overall value of the dependent variable. Trend refers to
whether the graph of the behavior in the baseline segment is flat, increasing, or decreasing
over time. Slope is the rate of change over time, if any trend is evident. Variability is the
range over which behavior fluctuates during the baseline segment. In general, a stable
baseline implies no extensive changes in level and a reasonably small range of variability.
Sidman (1960) has suggested a range of 5 percent as acceptable baseline variability, but
this criterion may be too stringent for research in clinical, as opposed to laboratory, settings (Christensen, 1988). Baseline stability also implies either no systematic trend upward
or downward in the behavior or, if a trend is evident, a constant slope against which
changes in behavioral trend during a treatment segment can be compared. Figure 3.2 illustrates hypothetical baseline data showing upward trends with different slopes (lines 1 and
2), a change in level (line 3), and large variability (line 4) and small variability (line 5)
without a systematic level change or directional trend. More detailed analyses of possible
outcomes of baseline measurements and their effects on the validity of single-subject
designs can be found in Campbell and Stanley (1966; see especially Figure 3 on page 38),
Hersen & Barlow (1976; see especially pages 74–82), and Kratchowill & Levin (1992; see
especially Chapters 2 and 3).

   Once the baseline segment has been completed, the treatment segment is introduced
and the subject is exposed to the independent variable. Measurement of the dependent variable at specific intervals is continued during treatment in the same manner as during the
baseline segment. Changes in the subject's behavior over time during the treatment are
compared to the measurements taken during the baseline segment as an indication of the

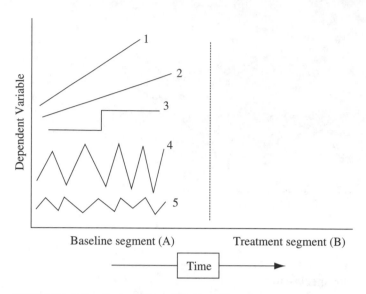

FIGURE 3.2   Several Possible Baseline Outcomes in a Hypothetical Single-Subject Experiment

effect of the independent variable on the dependent variable. In group within-subjects designs, each subject's behavior is measured once under each level of the independent variable, and the average behavior of the group of subjects is compared among conditions to see the effect of the independent variable on the dependent variable. In the single-subject design, the subject's behavior is measured several times under each level of the independent variable but no averaging takes place: the pattern of behavior over time is compared between the baseline and treatment conditions.

As stated previously, the simple time-series design with one baseline and one treatment segment is often referred to as an *A-B* design. A common extension of this simple design is the *ABA* (or *reversal*) design in which a reversal to a second baseline condition is made after behavior change has been observed in the treatment condition. The ABA design is commonly used to determine whether behavior that has been temporarily changed will revert to baseline level if the treatment is removed. Another common extension is the *ABAB* design in which the reversal includes a second treatment segment following the second baseline segment. In an ABAB design, behavior changed during the first treatment segment should revert to baseline level in the second *A* segment and should show change again in the second *B* segment if the independent variable introduced during the treatment segment affected the dependent variable. Figure 3.3 diagrams a hypothetical ABAB single-subject design and illustrates a first baseline with moderate variability and no systematic level changes or trends, increase in the dependent variable during the first treatment segment, return to the original baseline level during the second baseline segment, and another increase in the dependent variable during the second treatment segment.

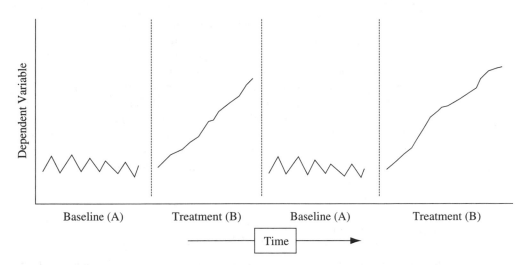

Dependent Variable

Baseline (A)   Treatment (B)   Baseline (A)   Treatment (B)

Time

FIGURE 3.3   Results of a Hypothetical ABAB Single-Subject Experiment

In addition to these reversal designs, a number of other design elements are available for incorporation into single-subject designs to examine changes in one dependent variable as a result of application of different independent variables or to examine changes across different dependent variables, subjects, or settings caused by introduction of an independent variable. A variety of alternating treatment designs, changing-criterion designs, and multiple baseline designs for accomplishing these objectives are discussed in more detail in a number of texts on single-subject design (e.g., Christensen, 1988; Kratchowill & Levin, 1992; McReynolds & Kearns, 1983; Hersen & Barlow, 1976). Christensen (1988) has outlined methodological considerations in the design of single-subject experiments and compared them to considerations in the group designs. Whereas the group designs achieve control over extraneous variables by random assignment of subjects to groups or randomization and counterbalancing of conditions to subjects, single-subject designs use multiple time-series measures in both baseline and treatment segments to compare treatment effects to temporal fluctuations in behavior without treatment. In addition, reversal designs are implemented to compare withdrawal of the independent variable to its application.

Christensen (1988) outlined the specifics of several other variations commonly employed in single-subject designs. Briefly, alternating treatment designs examine the effects of more than one independent variable (and their interactions) by applying different treatments to a single subject in alternating sequences that are counterbalanced after baseline measurement. Multiple baseline designs involve collection of baseline data on different behaviors of the same subject or on the same behavior of different subjects. After baseline measurement, treatment is introduced at staggered times to different subjects or different behaviors. The effects of treatments on different behaviors or subjects are then examined in the various treatment segments. In changing criterion designs, treatment is introduced in successive segments with a higher criterion for improvement of behavior introduced in each segment as treatment continues. The effectiveness of the independent variable is demonstrated by successive replications of changes in the dependent variable as the standard for acceptance of a change in behavior increases (i.e., more is expected of the subject as a result of treatment in each successive segment).

Single-subject designs have become more and more prevalent in the communicative disorders literature over the past three decades in both basic and applied research, and the popularity of this approach is likely to continue. Several research method books (e.g., Christensen, 1988; Kratchowill & Levin, 1992; McReynolds & Kearns, 1983; Hersen & Barlow, 1976) are available that cover single-subject design in more detail than can be presented here. Interested readers are referred to these sources for further detail concerning the single-subject approach to research design.

External Validity Issues in Research Design   packet p. 11 & 12

The preceding discussion has focused on issues of internal validity in research design. Some comments are now in order regarding external validity or generalizability of results. Campbell and Stanley (1966, p. 5) stated that

 external validity *asks the question of generalizability: To what populations, settings, treatment variables, and measurement variables can this effect be generalized?*

Much of the effort to strengthen the internal validity of a research design is aimed at specifying the independent and dependent variables, reducing the influence of extraneous variables, controlling random variability and measurement error, narrowing subject characteristics, limiting the setting involved, and following a strict measurement protocol. These efforts constrain the ability to generalize results to other subjects, settings, measurements, or treatment variables. Efforts to extend the generalizability of results can weaken the internal validity of a single study through relaxation of control over relevant extraneous variables. Yet both types of validity are important in any area of research, particularly in communicative disorders and other fields in which generalization to a variety of populations in different settings is critical. As Campbell and Stanley (1966, p. 5) stated:

> *While* internal validity *is the* sine qua non, *and while the question of* external validity, *like the question of inductive inference, is never completely answerable, the selection of designs strong in both types of validity is obviously our ideal. This is particularly the case for research on teaching, in which generalization to applied settings of known character is the desideratum.*

Internal validity, as the *sine qua non,* must be dealt with in any study before external validity can be considered. Trying to generalize results that are not internally valid would waste both time and effort. As Pedhazur and Schmelkin (1991, p. 229) have said:

> *Clearly, when internal validity of a study is in doubt, it makes little sense to inquire to what or across what, are its findings generalizable.*

External validity is more difficult to deal with than internal validity in a single research study and often better addressed in a series of studies as part of a systematic research program. Although researchers try to limit their generalizations, their results *may be* generalizable. However, external validity cannot be assumed until some evidence for generalization is presented. In the interim, consumers of research need to *limit* the degree to which they try to generalize the results of an individual research article.

The main concern for consumers of research is the manner in which researchers try to find solutions to the problem of generalizing results beyond the confines of an individual study. There are basically two ways of conceptualizing generalization. Pedhazur and Schmelkin (1991, p. 229) have characterized them as follows:

> *External validity refers to generalizability of findings* to *or* across *target populations, settings, times, and the like.*

Pedhazur and Schmelkin (1991, p. 229) further specified the process of "generalizing to":

> *The term* generalizing to *concerns validity of generalizations from samples to populations of which the samples are presumably "representative." Consequently, whatever the target population (e.g., people, times, settings), the validity of this type of generalization is predicated on the sample-selection procedures.*

There are basically two procedures for improving the external validity of results for generalizing to other populations such as people, settings, and times. The first is selecting random samples of people, settings, and times to be included in the study. Random sampling helps to improve generalization to the specific target because all of the subjects (or stimuli) in the population have an equal probability of being selected for inclusion in the study. A random sample comprises a group of subjects that is likely to be more representative of the characteristics of the target population than a nonrandom sample. Random sampling is often discussed only with respect to subjects in a study but can also be considered for settings, values of the independent variable, times of measurement, stimulus materials, measurement procedures, and so on.

Unfortunately, most investigators are unable to select random samples from the population of interest because of practical constraints. Pedhazur and Schmelkin (1991, p. 329) have summarized this problem as follows:

> *In spite of its appeal and seeming simplicity, simple random sampling is not used often in research. From a practical point of view, the task of selecting a random sample from a list can be extremely tedious and time consuming. More often than not, lists (let alone numbered lists) of elements of relatively large populations are difficult, if not impossible, to come by. Additional constraints arise when the population of interest resides in geographically wide areas. For example, a simple random sample of the population of the United States would probably yield a sample so dispersed as to make it an economic and physical nightmare.*

Despite the practical constraints that limit the ability of most researchers to select simple random samples, there are alternate tactics for improving generalizability. First, there are several techniques for targeting a specific subpopulation by examining clusters or stratified groups of subjects and then taking random samples within local subgroups (see, for example, Kerlinger, 1973, pp. 117–132 or Pedhazur and Schmelkin, 1991, pp. 318–341 for discussion of these methods). Second, generalization can also be improved by increasing sample size; in general, a larger sample more closely approximates the characteristics of a population. The specific concern of how large a sample should be selected may be approached with a technique called *power analysis* that can determine a sample size based on the notion of what the probability is of detecting a hypothesized degree of effect of an independent variable on a dependent variable, or *effect size.* In general, increasing to a larger sample size leads to a higher probability of detecting an effect of a given size in the population. Power analysis is discussed in more detail in Pedhazur and Schmelkin (1991) and Cohen (1988).

Third, generalization can be improved with replication. A finding that can be replicated in a subsequent study is stronger in external validity than a finding that has not yet been replicated. Sidman (1960) has discussed two major types of replication and calls the replication that would extend generalization to the same population, setting, or variables a *direct replication.* In a direct replication, the investigator repeats the research with the same subjects or a new group of subjects to confirm the reliability of the original results and test their generality within the limits of type of subjects, settings, and measurements. Direct replication is an important and practical technique for improving generalization when it is impractical for an investigator to select a large or random sample.

In summary, generalization *to* the population, setting, or other variables is a difficult task, but this type of external validity can be improved with larger and more representative samples of the population of interest. Now we turn to the problem of generalization *across* populations, settings, or other variables of interest.

Pedhazur and Schmelkin (1991, p. 229) further specified the process of "generalizing across":

> Generalizing across *concerns the validity of generalizations* across *populations. For example, results obtained with a sample from a given population (e.g., males, blacks, blue-collar workers), are generalized to other populations (e.g., females, whites, white-collar workers), or results obtained in one setting (e.g., classroom, laboratory) are generalized to another setting (e.g., playground).*

Generalizing across populations, settings, or other variables should be limited until evidence is presented that indicates the validity of a result beyond the confines of an individual study. Evidence for generalization across these variables of interest may be derived from *systematic replication* studies (Sidman, 1960).

In systematic replication, the research may be repeated under different conditions or with different types of subjects in order to extend generalization to other subjects, settings, measurements, or treatments. Some aspect of the subjects, setting, measurement, or treatment would be varied to include some new subject, setting, measurement, or treatment to which the investigator would like to generalize results. Systematic replication is, therefore, a powerful tool for extending external validity beyond the limits of a single research study. Consumers of research should consider the generalizability of research results as limited to the particular kinds of subjects, settings, measurements, and treatments used until such time as systematic replications demonstrate that the results are, in fact, more general. In some cases, of course, the limited generality of results may not pose a problem to consumers of research. The results of a study that used a particular measurement with a particular type of subject in a specific setting may be easily applied by professionals who normally use that particular measure with that kind of subject in that setting. Many research consumers, however, are interested in broadening the generality of research findings and will, therefore, be more interested in the implications of replication for the extension of external validity.

Unfortunately, replication has not always been as common a practice in behavioral research as it has been in biological, medical, or physical sciences. But in recent years, more and more replication studies have appeared in the literature, perhaps indicating more sensitivity to the need for replications to extend the external validity of behavioral research findings. Smith (1970) identified several reasons why researchers do not often replicate studies, including such factors as lack of time, funds, or available subjects; reluctance of some journals to publish replications of previous work; and development of new research interests by the investigator. In commenting on many of these reasons, Smith (1970, p. 971) stated that

> *if the goal of scientific research is to render established truths, then the neglect of replication must be reviewed as scientific irresponsibility.*

Smith further suggested that many of these barriers to replication can be overcome by obtaining replication data when the original study is conducted. A section on replication could then be added to the original article. Muma (1993) has issued a call for more replication research in communicative disorders. He surveyed research journals in the field over a ten-year period and found relatively few replications published, raising the possibility that there may be some unreplicable findings in the research literature.

Many combined experimental-descriptive studies involve a form of systematic replication because they compare experimental effects for different kinds of subjects. The examples cited in Chapter 2 in the section entitled Combined Experimental-Descriptive Research show how the experimental effect on one type of subject may be compared with the experimental effect on another type of subject.

There are some excellent examples of replications that extend external validity in the communicative disorders literature. Guitar (1976) included a direct replication in his correlational study of pretreatment factors associated with improvement in stuttering treatment and Monsen (1978) included a direct replication in his regression analysis of acoustic variables used to predict the intelligibility of deaf speakers. In both cases the direct replications showed results that were quite consistent with the results of the original studies, thus strengthening the generality of the original results within the limits of the same type of subjects, settings, and measures.

Systematic replications have also appeared as follow-up articles or have been included in an article reporting the replication along with the original results. Silverman (1976) provides an excellent example of a systematic replication in which an experiment on listener reactions to lisping was replicated with a different kind of subject used as listeners in order to extend generality regarding other subjects. Costello and Bosler (1976) evaluated generality to four other settings in their study of the efficacy of articulation treatment. Cottrell, Montague, Farb, and Throne (1980) examined generality to other measurements in their study of operant conditioning for improvement of vocabulary definition of developmentally delayed children by testing the degree to which their original results generalized to untrained vocabulary words within the same semantic classes. Courtright and Courtright (1979) examined external validity in regard to other treatments. They extended their earlier findings regarding imitative modeling as a language-intervention strategy by replicating an earlier study of modeling vs. mimicry and examining two other treatment variables associated with modeling—reinforcement and origin of the model—to determine their influence on the effectiveness of modeling.

In summary, external validity, or generality of results, is usually limited in any single research article. Random sampling and direct replication can help to improve generalization within the limits of type of subject, setting, measurement, and treatment. Systematic replication can help extend generalization to other kinds of subjects, settings, measurements, or treatments. As Hunter, Schmidt, and Jackson (1982, p. 10) have stated:

> *Scientists have known for centuries that a single study will not resolve a major issue. Indeed, a small sample study will not even resolve a minor issue. Thus, the foundation of science is the cumulation of knowledge from the results of many studies. There are two steps to the cumulation of knowledge: (1) the cumulation of results across studies to establish facts and (2) the formation of theories to place the facts into a coherent and useful form.*

Hunter et al. (1982), then, have emphasized not only the empirical importance of external validity but also its theoretical importance, which is in consonance with Stevens's (1968) reminder of the schemapiric view of science. In other words, external validity is not only important in research design but also in the integration of rational and empirical evidence in the explanation of the laws of behavior.

Study Questions

1. Read the following article:

    Swanson, L. A., Leonard, L. B., & Gandour, J. (1992). Vowel duration in mothers' speech to young children. *Journal of Speech and Hearing Research, 35,* 617–625.

    a. Did this study use a between-subjects or within-subjects design to study changes in mothers' speech?

    b. What steps did the authors take to strengthen internal validity in this design?

2. Read the following article:

    Stevens, L. J., & Bliss, L. S. (1995). Conflict resolution abilities of children with specific language impairment and children with normal language. *Journal of Speech and Hearing Research, 38,* 599–611.

a. Did this study use a between-subjects or within-subjects design to study conflict resolution abilities in these children?

b. What steps did the authors take to strengthen internal validity in this design?

3. Read the following article:

Mirolles, J. L., & Cervera, T. (1995). Voice intelligibility in patients who have undergone laryngectomies. *Journal of Speech and Hearing Research, 38,* 564–571.

a. Did this study use a between-subjects or within-subjects design to study intelligibility in these patients?

b. What steps did the authors take to strengthen internal validity in this design?

4. Read the following article:

Edwards, J., & Lahey, M. (1993). Auditory lexical decisions in children and adults: An examination of response factors. *Journal of Speech and Hearing Research, 36,* 996–1003.

a. Describe the between-subjects and within-subjects components of this study.

b. Identify which independent variables were manipulable and which were not.

5. Read the following article:

Gordon-Salant, S., & Fitzgibbons, P. J. (1995). Comparing recognition of distorted speech using an equivalent signal-to-noise ratio index. *Journal of Speech and Hearing Research, 36,* 706–713.

a. How were between-subjects and within-subjects research designs mixed in this study?

b. Identify the active and attribute independent variables that were used.

c. Which of these variables was examined between-subjects and which within-subjects?

6. Read the following article:

Blood, G. W. (1994). Efficacy of a computer-assisted voice treatment protocol. *American Journal of Speech-Language Pathology, 3,* 57–66.

a. What kind of research design did the author employ?

b. Identify the steps taken to improve internal validity.

7. Read the following article:

Guitar, B. (1976). Pretreatment factors associated with the outcome of stuttering therapy. *Journal of Speech and Hearing Research, 19,* 590–600.

a. What steps did the author take to improve external validity?

b. Did this improve generalization *to* or *across* populations?

8. Read the following article:

Muma, J. (1993). The need for replication. *Journal of Speech and Hearing Research, 36,* 927–930.

a. What were the results of Muma's survey of replications in a decade of published studies?

b. According to Muma, how would replication improve research in communicative disorders?

References

Bordens, K. S., & Abbott, B. B. (1988). *Research design and methods: A process approach.* Mountain View, CA: Mayfield Publishing Company.

Campbell, D. T., & Stanley, J. C. (1966). *Experimental and quasi-experimental designs for research.* Chicago: Rand-McNally.

Christensen, L. B. (1988). *Experimental methodology* (4th ed.). Boston: Allyn & Bacon.

Cohen, J. (1988). *Statistical power analysis for the behavioral sciences* (2nd ed.). Hillsdale, NJ: Lawrence Erlbaum Associates.

Costello, J., & Bosler, S. (1976). Generalization and articulation instruction. *Journal of Speech and Hearing Disorders, 41,* 359–373.

Cottrell, A. W., Montague, J., Farb, J., & Throne, J. M. (1980). An operant procedure for improving vocabulary definition performances in developmentally delayed children. *Journal of Speech and Hearing Disorders, 45,* 90–102.

Courtright, J. A., & Courtright, I. C. (1979). Imitative modeling as a language intervention strategy: The effects of two mediating variables. *Journal of Speech and Hearing Research, 22,* 389–402.

Ferguson, G. A., & Takane, Y. (1989). *Statistical analysis in psychology and education* (6th ed.). New York: McGraw-Hill.

Guitar, B. (1976). Pretreatment factors associated with the outcome of stuttering therapy. *Journal of Speech and Hearing Research, 19,* 590–600.

Hersen, M., & Barlow, D. H. (1976). *Single case experimental designs: Strategies for studying behavior change.* New York: Pergamon.

Hunter, J. E., Schmidt, F. L., & Jackson, G. B. (1982). *Meta-analysis: Cumulating research findings across studies.* Beverly Hills, CA: Sage Publications.

Kerlinger, F. (1973). *Foundations of behavioral research* (2nd ed.). New York: Holt, Rinehart & Winston.

Kerlinger, F. (1979). *Behavioral research: A conceptual approach.* New York: Holt, Rinehart & Winston.

Kratchowill, T. R., & Levin, J. R. (Eds.). (1992). *Single-case research design and analysis: New directions for psychology and education.* Hillsdale, NJ: Lawrence Erlbaum Associates.

McReynolds, L. V., & Kearns, K. P. (1983). *Single-subject experimental designs in communicative disorders.* Baltimore: University Park Press.

Monsen, R. B. (1978). Toward measuring how well hearing-impaired children speak. *Journal of Speech and Hearing Research, 21,* 197–219.

Muma, J. (1993). The need for replication. *Journal of Speech and Hearing Research, 36,* 927–930.

Pedhazur, E. J., & Schmelkin, L. P. (1991). *Measurement, design, and analysis.* Hillsdale, NJ: Lawrence Erlbaum Associates.

Sidman, M. (1960). *Tactics of scientific research.* New York: Basic Books.

Silverman, E. M. (1976). Listeners' impressions of speakers with lateral lisps. *Journal of Speech and Hearing Disorders, 41,* 547–552.

Smith, N. C. (1970). Replication studies: A neglected aspect of psychological research. *American Psychologist, 25,* 970–975.

Stevens, S. S. (1968). Measurement, statistics, and the schemapiric view. *Science, 161,* 849–856.

Underwood, B. J., & Shaughnessy, J. J. (1975). *Experimentation in psychology.* New York: John Wiley & Sons.

Van Dalen, D. B. (1966). *Understanding educational research.* New York: McGraw-Hill.

Chapter **4**

Measurement Issues in Communicative Disorders Research

This chapter considers some general issues regarding behavioral and instrumental measures of speech, language, and hearing used in communicative disorders research. The topics to be discussed are: (1) definition of measurement, (2) levels of measurement, (3) quality of measurement, (4) reliability of measurement, and (5) validity of measurement.

Measurement in communicative disorders research takes many forms. We may classify these measures generally as (a) instrumental measures of physical variables and (b) observer measures of behavioral variables. For example, electronic instrumentation is used for measurement of physiological variables such as airflow or acoustical variables such as formant frequency, and behavioral observation is used for measurement of language variables such as mean length of utterance or speech variables such as frequency of nonfluency. In many cases there are clear correlations between physical and behavioral variables, such as between vocal fundamental frequency and perceived vocal pitch. In many other instances, there are no clear correlations between physical and behavioral variables.

Measurement of many speech, language, and hearing behaviors depends on human observation of behavior in the form of self-reports (e.g., questionnaires or interviews), perceptual judgments of speech samples, transcription and analysis of language samples, auditory tests (e.g., SRT and speech discrimination), and formal language and speech tests. Young (1969, p. 135) has stated that "a measurement of a speech disorder is primarily a perceptual event, and the observer's response necessarily represents the 'final' validation for any measurements." Gerratt, Kreiman, Antonanzas-Barroso, and Berke (1993, p. 14) have further expanded on Young's statement in their discussion of voice quality measurement:

> *Voices can be objectively measured in many ways (see, e.g., Baken, 1987; Hirano, 1981). However, voice quality is fundamentally perceptual in nature. Patients*

seek treatment for voice disorders because they do not sound normal, and they often decide on whether treatment has been successful based on whether they sound better or not. For this and other reasons, speech clinicians use and value perceptual measures of voice and speech far more than instrumental measures (Gerratt, Till, Rosenbek, Wertz, and Boysen, 1991). Further, listeners' judgments are usually the standard against which other measures of voice (acoustic, aerodynamic and so on) are evaluated.

On the other hand, the importance of instrumental analysis in communicative disorders cannot be denied. As Decker (1990, p. xviii) has pointed out:

While it is true that some will always have more use than others for electronics, no one in speech pathology and audiology can say that electronics has no place in what they do. Electronics has become a fact of life in modern society and its application to an enormous variety of human endeavors has helped to expand our knowledge exponentially. In the fields of speech pathology and audiology, electronic applications have not only broadened the reach of the basic and applied scientist but have created a whole new clinical armamentarium for the practitioner. So it is important to understand how these electronic tools work and, more importantly, how they can be made to work for us.

In the conclusion of their survey of electronic instrumentation systems for speech analysis, Read, Buder, and Kent (1990, pp. 371–372) stated:

We have entered into a new era in speech analysis, with sophisticated systems accessible even to small clinics, laboratories, and college departments. Even some secondary schools now include speech analysis in their physics or computing curricula. We must anticipate some basic changes in our field as a result of this access. A wider range of observers will be able to make and test claims about the physical structure of speech. Speech analysis will be applied to problems in communication and languages for which physical evidence has never before been readily available.

It should be obvious from the foregoing that *both* instrumental and behavioral measurements play an important role in clinical and research activity in communicative disorders. The main issue here for consumers of research is the importance of evaluating the quality of any measurements used in communicative disorders research. Regardless of whether measurements are instrumental or behavioral, accurate quantification of communication variables can only be achieved through careful measurement procedures that are designed to yield valid and reliable results.

Definition of Measurement

We must first define *measurement* and identify some important properties of measurement that are required for valid quantification of communication variables. Stevens (1946, p. 677) presented a succinct definition of measurement when he stated that:

measurement, in the broadest sense, is defined as the assignment of numerals to objects or events according to rules. The fact that numerals can be assigned under different rules leads to different kinds of scales and different kinds of measurement. The problem then becomes that of making explicit (a) the various rules for the assignment of numerals, (b) the mathematical properties (or group structure) of the resulting scales, and (c) the statistical operations applicable to measurements made with each type of scale.

Nunnally (1978, p. 3) has reinforced Stevens' definition with a similar statement:

Although tomes have been written on the nature of measurement, in the end it boils down to something rather simple: measurement consists of rules for assigning numbers to objects in such a way as to represent quantities of attributes. *The term* rules *indicates that the procedures for assigning numbers must be explicitly stated. In some instances the rules are so obvious that detailed formulations are not required. . . . Such examples are, however, the exception rather than the usual in science. . . . Certainly the rules for measuring most psychological attributes are not intuitively obvious.*

Nunnally further stated that measurement is a process of abstraction about an object or event because we measure their various *attributes* or *features*. In behavioral science, the objects that we measure are people who have many different attributes, and the events that we measure are their behaviors that have many attributes. Nunnally has emphasized the importance of careful consideration of the nature of each attribute before trying to measure it and careful attention to the rules of measurement to be sure that they are clear, practical to apply, and do not require different kinds and amounts of skills by persons who use the measurement procedure. When different people employ the measuring instrument, or supposedly alternate measures of the same attribute, they should obtain similar results.

Thus, an important goal in communicative disorders research is the measurement of speech, language, and hearing variables with a clear and practical set of rules. Nunnally (1978, p. 5) summarized the process of development of measurement rules succinctly:

In establishing rules for the employment of a particular measure, the crucial consideration is that the set of rules must be unambiguous. The rules may be developed from an elaborate deductive model, they may be based on much previous experience, they may flow from common sense, or they may spring from only hunches; but the proof of the pudding is in how well the measurement serves to explain important phenomena. Consequently, any *set of rules that unambiguously quantifies properties of objects constitutes a* legitimate *measurement method and has a right to compete with other measures for scientific usefulness.*

Levels of Measurement

In addressing the issue of explicit measurement rules, Stevens (1946, 1951) specified four scales or levels of measurement on the basis of the operations performed in assigning numerals to objects or events. Although there is some debate among statisticians (Haber, Runyon, and Badia, 1970) regarding the number, characteristics, and appropriateness of Stevens' scales, his original measurement scheme has remained influential in modern statistical treatment of data (Siegel, 1956) and will be used in this discussion. Knowing what level of measurement has been used to assign numerals to objects or events is an important step in ascertaining the appropriateness of procedures used to organize and analyze the results of a study.

The four levels of measurement outlined by Stevens are: *nominal, ordinal, interval,* and *ratio* levels arranged from simplest to most complex. Table 4.1 shows defining characteristics and examples of each of the four levels of measurement. As Stevens (1951) has pointed out, these scales reflect various degrees of correspondence between the properties of the number scale and the empirical operations performed to assign numbers to attributes of objects and events. Graziano and Raulin (1989) have discussed four characteristics of the abstract number system that match empirical operations used in measurement of an attribute: identity, magnitude, equality of interval, and a true zero (or absence of the attribute measured). The four characteristics may be used to define the four levels of measurement and are cumulative in their application from nominal to ordinal to interval to ratio.

Nominal Level of Measurement

The nominal level is the simplest level of measurement. The word *nominal* is derived from the Latin word for *name,* and the process of nominal measurement is essentially the naming of attributes of objects or events. At the nominal level of measurement, attributes of objects or events are classified into mutually exclusive categories by determination of the equality of the attribute measured for the members of each category. The only mathematical property applied to nominal measurements is identity: each member of a named class is identical in the attribute measured. Examples would include gender (male vs. female), screening test result (pass vs. fail), or diagnostic category (stutterer vs. nonstutterer). In the three examples, each member of each category is considered identical for purposes of nominal measurement. Thus all males are identical as a group and all females are identical as a group with respect to measurement of gender. All passes are identical as a group and all failures are identical as a group with respect to performance on the screening test. All stutterers are identical as a group and all nonstutterers are identical as a group with respect to diagnostic category.

The only mathematical operation accomplished with nominal level measurements is counting the frequency of occurrence of members of each category. Sometimes the categories are assigned numbers (e.g., fail = O and pass = 1; female = 1 and male = 2), but these numbers are just labels used for identification purposes and do not specify magnitude. Telephone numbers, social security numbers, or numbers on football players' jerseys are good examples of the use of numbers for identification at the nominal level. You cannot perform meaningful mathematical manipulations of these identification numbers other than counting frequency of occurrence of items in each category. For example, you cannot add two telephone numbers together, dial the result, and reach both parties. You cannot state that a football player numbered nineteen is better than a player numbered twelve

TABLE 4.1   Levels of Measurement

Scale	Defining Characteristics	Examples
Nominal	Mutually exclusive categories or named groupings	Pass/fail criterion on screening test Type of nonfluency (prolongation vs. repetition) Type of hearing loss (conductive, sensorineural, or mixed) Stimulus categories (meaningful vs. meaningless syllables) Subject characteristics (stutterer vs. nonstutterer) Phoneme production (correct vs. incorrect)
Ordinal	1. Mutually exclusive categories or named groupings 2. Ranks or ordered levels	Ranked severity groups (mild, moderate, severe) Stimulus complexity (easy, moderate, difficult) Socioeconomic status (low-, middle-, upper class) Rank in class (e.g., first, second, third, etc.) Ranking of members of a group by rated degree of any subject attribute (e.g., perceived degree of vocal hoarseness)
Interval	1. Mutually exclusive categories or named groupings 2. Ranks or ordered levels 3. Equivalence of units throughout scale or constant distance between adjacent intervals	Standard scores on behavioral tests (e.g., PPVT-R, TOLD Standard scores, ITPA PLQ) Ratings obtained with many equal-appearing interval scales Fahrenheit and Celsius temperatures
Ratio	1. Mutually exclusive categories or named groupings 2. Ranks or ordered levels 3. Equivalence of units throughout scale or constant distance between adjacent intervals 4. Equivalence of ratios among scale values can be determined 5. A true zero point exists on the scale	Vowel duration Voice onset time Sound frequency Sound intensity Air pressure Air flow Stuttering frequency Number of misarticulations Diadochokinetic rate Speech intelligibility score

because his number is higher. A person with a higher social security number does not pay a higher premium or receive a higher benefit because of the higher social security number.

Ordinal Level of Measurement

The ordinal level of measurement considers not only the identity of members of a category but also the magnitude of the attributes of objects or events by allowing us to rank these magnitudes from least to most. At the ordinal level of measurement, objects or events are put into a relative ranking by determination of a greater or lesser value of the attribute to be measured. An ordinal scale of height, for example, could be constructed by visually arranging a group of children from shortest to tallest without actually using a ruler to determine the height of each child. Attributes such as vocal hoarseness or stuttering severity could be ordered from least to most severe using a listener judgment procedure. With an ordinal scale, we know how the objects or events line up with respect to the attribute, but we do not know the size of the differences between each object measured. Class rank is a good example: the difference between the first and second student is not necessarily the same as the difference between the second and third student in their actual grade-point averages, which might be 95, 94, and 90. They rank 1, 2, and 3, but the difference between 1 and 2 is one point whereas the difference between 2 and 3 is four points.

Interval Level of Measurement

The interval level of measurement includes identity and magnitude and allows us to specify the equality of the intervals between adjacent examples of the attribute measured. The interval level of measurement involves the determination of the equality of the distance between the objects or events on the attribute to be measured but does not include a true zero point that indicates the absence of the attribute. The most common example of an interval scale is temperature measurement with the Celsius or Fahrenheit scales: the temperature markings on the thermometer are equal interval distances painted on the glass surface to represent changes in the volume of mercury as temperature rises and falls. However, the zero point is arbitrary and does not represent the absence of temperature. We can say that the difference between sixty and seventy degrees is the same as the difference between seventy and eighty degrees, but we cannot specify equality of ratios between temperatures. Some variables in communicative disorders (e.g., speech naturalness; see Martin, Haroldson, and Triden, 1984) can be measured with equal-appearing interval scales (say, for example, a one- to nine-point scale). Many standardized behavioral test scores are measured at the interval level, including psychological tests of intelligence, personality, and achievement that have scores based on deviation away from the average but that do not have a true zero. Many language tests have standard scores that are constructed in this way and result in interval level measurements (e.g., ITPA PLQ, standard scores on PPVT-R, TOLD).

Ratio Level of Measurement

Ratio level measurements include identity, magnitude, and equality of intervals and allow for specification of ratios between numbers. The ratio level of measurement requires the establishment of a true zero and the determination of the equality of ratios between the objects or events in the attribute to be measured. Most physical measures are ratio level measurements (e.g., length, height, weight, pressure, velocity). Many behavioral attributes can also be measured at the ratio level, especially those that are based on summing the number of occurrences of a specific behavior. Stuttering frequency, for example, can be counted in a speech sample. It is possible to have zero nonfluencies (absence of stuttering behavior), and twenty nonfluencies in a sample represent twice the stuttering frequency as ten nonfluencies. In another example, speech intelligibility can be measured with a word-recognition test by counting the number of words spoken by a speaker that are heard correctly by a listener. A speaker can have an intelligibility score of zero, indicating that none of his or her words can be recognized correctly; and a listener can recognize twice as many words spoken by a speaker who is 80 percent intelligible as by a speaker who is 40 percent intelligible.

When a choice of levels is available, the preferred order is ratio, interval, ordinal, and nominal. Stevens (1951) has argued for this order of preference because more statistical operations are permissible with the ratio than with the interval, with the interval than with the ordinal, and with the ordinal than with the nominal level (Stevens, 1951; see especially Table 6, page 25). As Stevens (1958, p. 384) has said:

> *Each of these scales has its uses, but it is the more powerful ratio scale that serves us best in the search for nature's regularities. . . . Why, it may be asked, do we bother with the other types of scales? Mostly we use the weaker forms of measurement only* faute de mieux. *When stronger forms are discovered we are quick to seize them.*

Although researchers try to reach the highest level of measurement available (i.e., ratio), practical limitations or the lack of a suitable higher level measurement may force the use of a lower level of measurement. The statistical operations permissible with each level of measurement will be discussed in Chapter 6.

Factors That Affect Quality of Measurement

A number of factors can affect the quality of measurements made in communicative disorders research. As Campbell and Stanley (1966) pointed out, instrumentation is one of the most important factors that can jeopardize the internal validity of treatment efficacy research. An exhaustive discussion of factors that can affect the quality of measurements in communicative disorders research is beyond the scope of this book, but mention of a few key factors can provide an important guide for consumers of research to follow in evaluating the quality of measurements made in research studies they read. Several sources are available that review specific factors to be considered in speech, language, and hearing measurements (see Baken, 1987; Cudahy, 1988; Decker, 1990; Haynes, Pindzola, and Emerick, 1992; Peterson, and Marquardt, 1994; Rintelmann, 1991). We will first consider some specific factors that need to be controlled in making measurements in communicative disorders research and then discuss the two general qualities of reliability and validity that are fundamental requirements in any behavioral or instrumental measurements.

Test Environment

A poor test environment can easily jeopardize any behavioral or instrumental measurement of speech, language, or hearing. For example, research data may be contaminated by distractions, noise, interruptions, poor lighting, or inappropriate stimuli in a test environment.

The degree to which the test environment affects a measure will vary depending on the measure, but several obvious examples come to mind immediately. Measures of auditory threshold may be affected by background noise, a problem in educational settings or industry, but one that is capable of much better control in research conducted in laboratories or clinics. Research measurements for children may be more prone to problems of distraction in an environment that is new, colorful, or filled with stimuli that can attract their attention. Any measurements that require adequate visual perception for correct responses must be made in an environment that has adequate lighting. Thermal comfort is necessary for subjects to pay attention to tasks that require vigilant responses. In addition, it is important to keep such factors as those mentioned constant across subjects so as to not differentially affect the performances of different subjects. In short, the test environment must be appropriate to the task and kept constant across subjects to avoid contamination of measurements.

Instrument Calibration

Electronic and mechanical instruments must be kept in good working order and meet current calibration standards. For example, audiometers should be calibrated according to the current standard (ANSI, 1989). Calibration should not be faulty because of malfunction nor should it drift during the course of an experiment. Therefore, it is important for a researcher to check the calibration of instrumentation periodically during the course of a study. Instrumentation should not be changed during a study because measurements taken with one instrument may not necessarily match those from another (Read, Buder, and Kent, 1990; 1992). The method section of a research article should contain sufficient information for the consumer of research to ascertain the adequacy of the instrumentation and its calibration.

Instructions to Subjects

Instructions to subjects for the completion of their tasks must be clear and appropriate for the population being measured. Cronbach (1984, pp. 56–57), for example, outlined several effective techniques for giving directions to formal test takers, stressing the need to be firm, audible, and polite in standardizing the instructions given to all subjects. He stressed that directions should be "complete and free from ambiguity" and that testers should attempt to "standardize the state of examinees." Much like the test environment, instructions should remain constant across subjects. Of great concern in recent years have been the issues of measurement with multicultural populations and individuals with disabilities (see Thorndike et al., 1991, pages 16–17 and Chapters 14 and 15). The implication of linguistic differences and differential abilities for clarity of instructions is obvious in both issues. For example, measurements with deaf children whose first language is ASL should include instructions in ASL, not in signed English.

Observer Bias

When human beings are judges, there is ample opportunity for their judgments to be confounded by bias in observing or rating samples of behavior of different subjects or of subjects participating in different experimental conditions. For example, judges' standards may change from one experimental session to another, raters may be influenced by knowledge of the purpose of the investigation, or observers may make judgments based partially on their expectations about the behavior of subjects in different groups (e.g., children with and without cleft palate).

Rosenthal (1966) has written extensively about the effects on research results of the human experimenter as part of the measurement instrumentation system, and many writers now call the problem of biased human observations the "Rosenthal Effect." Rosenthal and Rosnow (1984) categorized these experimenter effects as "interactional" vs. "noninteractional" observer bias based on whether the experimenter actually affects the subject's behavior or simply errs in observing it. A *noninteractional* effect occurs when the observer does not influence the subject's performance but does affect the *recording* of the subject's behavior. This class of experimenter effect includes error or bias in the experimenter's observation of behavior, unintentional error in mathematical calculation or interpretation of responses, and intentional fabrication of data. As an example of noninteractional observer bias, consider what might happen if judges were asked to rate hypernasality in speech samples recorded by children with cleft palates before and after pharyngeal flap surgery. Observers might expect less hypernasality after surgery and thereby unconsciously rate the postsurgery tape recordings with lower hypernasality ratings. An *interactional* effect occurs when the observer's interaction with the subject actually changes the subject's behavior during the experiment. This class of experimenter effect includes a number of factors associated with human observers that may affect the behavior of subjects in experiments. For example, Rosenthal and Rosnow (1984) have summarized *biosocial* attributes of experimenters (e.g., gender, age, race, bodily activity), *psychosocial* attributes of experimenters (e.g., personality characteristics such as anxiety, hostility, authoritarianism), and *situational* variables (e.g., experimenter's experience in prior experiments or on earlier trials of the same experiment, familiarity with subjects) that may influence the way subjects behave in an experiment.

It is obvious from the foregoing that a number of specific factors can affect the quality of measurements made in communicative disorders research. The specific constellation of factors that need careful attention will depend on the nature of the specific measurement to be made. Consumers of research will need to depend somewhat on their measurement experience in evaluating the quality of measurements made in the research articles they read. We now turn to two particularly important and general topics concerning what Thorndike et al. (1991) have termed "qualities desired in any measurement procedure"—reliability and validity.

Reliability of Measurements

 Reliability is an integral part of any research undertaking; it generally refers to the degree to which we can depend on a measurement. Two definitions of reliability are currently used in behavioral research. First, reliability means measurement *precision* (Kerlinger, 1979; Thorndike et al. 1991; Pedhazur and Schmelkin, 1991). A precise measure can be expected to remain reasonably stable if the measurement procedure is repeated with the same subject. An imprecise measure will show more fluctuation with remeasurement over time. Cordes (1994, p. 265) has stated that the most common use of the term *reliability* in communicative disorders research is related to the "general trustworthiness of obtained data," that common synonyms for reliability include "dependability, consistency, predictability, and stability," and that this view of reliability concerns the question of whether the observed "data could be reproduced if the same subjects were tested again under similar circumstances."

A second definition of reliability refers to measurement *accuracy* and stems from the mathematical *true score* model (also called *classical test theory*). Cordes (1994, p. 265) suggested that this second definition is a "subtype of the more general reliability, when that term is defined as consistency, dependability, reproducibility, or stability." In classical test theory, reliability of measurement is defined as the ratio of true-score variance to observed-score variance. As Pedhazur and Schmelkin (1994, p. 83) state:

According to the true-score model, an observed score is conceived of as consisting of two components—a true component and an error component. In symbols:

$$X = T + E$$

where X is the fallible, observed score; T is the true score; and E is random error.

They further explain that:

Conceptually, the true score can be thought of as the score that would be obtained under ideal or perfect conditions of measurement. Because such conditions never exist, the observed score always contains a certain amount of error (Pedhazur and Schmelkin, 1994, p. 84).

The concept of true scores and random (measurement) errors is illustrated schematically in the two hypothetical measurements shown in Figure 4.1. This illustration shows the partitioning of an observed score into a true score and measurement error and indicates the relative contribution of each to the observed score. One can see that the first measurement procedure has less error than the second. Observed scores obtained from the first measurement procedure will clearly be closer to the individual's true score than those obtained from the second measurement procedure. In classical test theory, then, the measurement with less error is more reliable because its observed score provides a more accurate (i.e., less error-prone) approximation of the true score.

Pedhazur and Schmelkin (1991) discussed two types of errors that may influence the reliability of the measurement process. The first type of measurement error is systematic. Systematic errors recur consistently with every repeated measurement. An example of systematic measurement error is an improperly calibrated audiometer that consistently produces an output of 20 dB HTL when the intensity dial is set at 10 dB HTL. The second type of measurement error is unsystematic error that occurs in unpredictable ways during repeated measurements. We can use the audiometer once again as an example of unsystematic measurement error. Suppose that this audiometer has an intermittent malfunction

Measurement 1

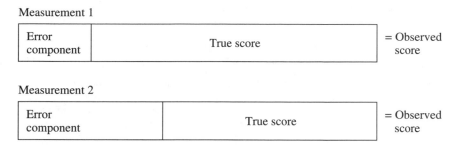

FIGURE 4.1   **Schematic Illustration of the Relationship of True Score and Error Component to Observed Score for Two Different Measurements**

in the circuitry that controls the frequency of the sound being produced. When the frequency dial is set at 1,000 Hz the malfunction intermittently results in frequency outputs that vary anywhere between 900 Hz and 1,100 Hz unbeknownst to the examiner. In this situation the examiner would not know exactly what the actual output frequency is without monitoring each presentation with a frequency meter.

Measurement error emanates from many different sources and various authors have described potential reliability influencing factors from different perspectives. Lyman (1978) listed five general sources of measurement error that may affect reliability: (1) characteristics of the examinee, (2) behavior of the examiner-scorer, (3) aspects of the test content, (4) time factors, and (5) situation factors. Thorndike and Hagen (1977) identified three important classes of reasons for poor measurement reliability: (1) the person who is being measured may actually change from day to day; (2) the task may be different in two forms of the same measure or in different parts of one measure; and (3) the measure may provide a limited sample of behavior that may not yield dependable characterizations of the behavior over the long run. Isaac and Michael (1971, p. 88) presented a table that categorized sources of measurement error as general vs. specific and temporary vs. lasting characteristics of the persons who are measured. Ebel (1965) discussed six ways of improving test characteristics in order to reduce measurement error associated with the instrument itself. Kerlinger (1973) listed a number of factors reflecting the influence of temporal changes in the subject such as mood, memory, and fatigue; the influence of changes in the measurement situation; and the influence of a very important source of measurement error: *unknown causes.*

Several different methods have been used to estimate the reliability of measurements in behavioral research, and these methods can be considered within three broad categories of reliability estimation: (a) *stability* (b) *equivalence,* and (c) *internal consistency.* The specific method chosen will depend largely on the specific sources of error being considered (Pedhazur and Schmelkin, 1994). Each of these approaches has certain advantages and disadvantages, and Cordes (1994) provides an excellent discussion of the limitations of each approach to reliability estimation in communicative disorders research. The different methods for estimating measurement reliability within each of the three broad categories are summarized in Table 4.2.

TABLE 4.2   Categories of Reliability and Methods of Assessment

Categories of Reliability		
Stability	*Equivalence*	*Internal Consistency*
Test-retest	Alternate or parallel forms	Split-half
		Cronbach's alpha
		Kuder-Richardson 20

Stability

The primary method for estimating the stability of measurement is known as the test-retest method. Pedhazur and Schmelkin (1991, p. 88) state that the test-retest method most closely relates to the "view of reliability as consistency or repeatability of measurement." This approach involves performing a complete repetition of the exact measurement and correlating the results of the two measurements. The resultant correlation coefficient, sometimes called the *coefficient of stability,* is taken as an estimate of measurement reliability. Cordes (1994) and Pedhazur and Schmelkin (1991) contend that the test-retest method of reliability estimation is particularly vulnerable to carry-over effects that may lead to overestimation of reliability.

Equivalence

The primary method for estimating the equivalence of measurement is called the *alternate* or *parallel forms* method. This method of reliability estimation is sometimes used to avoid the potential carry-over effects associated with the test-retest method. Reliability estimation using equivalent forms is accomplished by correlating the scores of two different forms of a measure of the same attribute. The resultant correlation coefficient, sometimes called the *coefficient of equivalence* or *alternate form reliability,* is taken as an estimate of reliability. The principle limitation of using equivalent forms for the estimation of reliability is the difficulty associated with construction of equivalent forms and in the determination of the actual equivalence of measurements (Pedhazur and Schmelkin, 1991; Thorndike et al., 1991).

Internal Consistency

One common method for estimating the internal consistency of measurement is known as the *split-half* method. This approach to measurement reliability was developed out of the confluence of theoretical limitations of the test-retest and equivalent forms methods and of certain practical limitations that dictate a single administration of measurements. Split-half reliability is, in a sense, a variation on alternate form reliability in which the two halves of a measure may be seen as constituting two alternate forms. The split-half approach requires that the items that constitute a given measure be split in half (e.g., even- vs. odd-numbered questions of a test); each half is then correlated with the other for the measurement of the reliability coefficient (Pedhazur and Schmelkin, 1991).

A correlation coefficient used frequently with split-half data to express internal consistency reliability is derived from the Spearman-Brown formula (Thorndike et al., 1991). Using the split-half method to estimate the reliability of a one hundred-item test will result in a correlation coefficient that is based on only fifty item pairs; the effective length of the test is cut in half. The Spearman-Brown formula is based on the assumption that increasing the length of a test will, in turn, increase its reliability because larger samples of behavior permit more adequate and consistent measurements (Anastasi, 1988). In essence, the Spearman-Brown formula mathematically corrects for the split-half reduction in test items and yields an estimate of the correlation coefficient that would be expected for the correlation of two versions of the whole one hundred-item test. For this reason, the Spearman-Brown formula is sometimes referred to as the Spearman-Brown *prophecy formula.*

Two other methods for internal consistency estimation of reliability are Cronbach's alpha and the related Kuder-Richardson #20 Formula (KR-20), which provide reliability coefficients that estimate the average of all possible split-half correlations among the items of a measure. Cronbach's alpha procedure is used for test items that are scored with multiple answers (e.g., multiple-choice items, answer ensembles such as "always, sometimes, never" or "strongly agree, agree, neutral, disagree, strongly disagree," or five-point rating scales), and the KR-20 is conceptually and computationally similar to Cronbach's alpha but is used for dichotomously scored items (e.g., "correct-incorrect" such as the word-recognition scores of speech audiometry). Both methods provide indications of the homogeneity of test items relative to overall performance on a measure as an index of reliability.

The three categories of reliability estimation methods discussed previously are concerned with measurement error associated with temporal fluctuations (i.e., stability), differences between parallel forms (i.e., equivalence), and interitem consistency (i.e., internal consistency). These three methods, however, do not account for measurement errors that may emanate from the observer or observers who are making the measurements. A method that has become quite common in behavioral research for the estimation of measurement error associated with the observer is called "*inter*observer" or "interrater" agreement. Kearns (1990, p. 79) described the interobserver method of estimating measurement error as follows:

> *Interobserver agreement coefficients are used to evaluate the level of variability or inconsistency among observers who score the same behaviors. An acceptable level of agreement between observers is generally taken as an indication that changes in the observed behavior are true changes and not a result of variability in the way that target behaviors were scored.*

Interobserver agreement coefficients are typically derived from measurements made by two or more observers measuring the same event. In some instances, however, it is important to know how stable one observer is in measuring the same event on two different occasions. In that case, the measures made by one observer at two different times are compared and an "*intra*observer" agreement coefficient is calculated.

It is tempting to consider observer agreement coefficients in light of the categories of measurement listed in Table 4.1. In this regard, interobserver agreement would be placed under the general category of equivalence and intraobserver agreement under the category of stability. Despite the intuitive appeal for such categorization, it is conceptually unwise to do such. As Kearns (1990, p. 79) suggests, "Although the terms reliability and interobserver agreement have been used interchangeably in the applied literature, these terms actually differ in their conceptual and statistical properties."

Similarly, Cordes (1994, p. 270) pointed out that interobserver agreement methods of reliability estimation do not use the conceptual underpinnings of the true score model and that they do not address reliability in terms of "dependability or reproducibility." Rather, interjudge agreement reliability estimates address only measurement consistency, or lack thereof, that can be attributed to "differences among observers." Cordes (1994, p. 276) issued a caveat regarding observer agreements that should be heeded by the prudent consumer of research:

> *The reliability of observational data is more complex than reporting that some vaguely described observer agreement statistic fell at some certain numeric level.*

Intraobserver and interobserver agreement measures, then, are important only because they tell us that the observer(s) measured the same thing. They do not, however, tell us if the measure itself is accurate in a "true score" sense. Two observers could be in perfect agreement in providing an inaccurate measure. Intraobserver and interobserver agreement can, therefore, be considered an important first step in establishing reliability because they show that observers are consistent with each other, but more information about the accuracy and precision of the measure itself must accompany any observer agreement index.

A question frequently asked is "How high should the reliability coefficient be? Is 0.6 a sufficient reliability coefficient or should it be higher before I put my faith in the measurement?" Pedhazur and Schmelkin (1991) suggested that various researchers have used guidelines regarding minimally acceptable levels of reliability that tolerate low coefficients in the early stages of research but require high reliabilities when measurements are used for making important selection and placement decisions about individuals. Questioning the wisdom of such formulations, Pedhazur and Schmelkin (1991, p. 110) pointed out that an acceptable reliability coefficient cannot be achieved by decree, but, rather, "it is for the user to determine what amount of error he or she is willing to tolerate, given the specific circumstances of the study (e.g., what the scores are to be used for, cost of the study)."

The interpretation of reliability data is sometimes facilitated by the computation of the *standard error of measurement.* Thorndike et al. (1991, p. 102) defined the standard error of measurement as "the standard deviation that would be obtained for a series of measurements of the same individual." In practice, the standard error of measurement is an estimate of the standard deviation of observed scores (Pedhazur and Schmelkin, 1991) that is used to assess the precision of a given measurement. Estimates of the standard error of measurement give an indication of the variability that might be expected in the score of any individual if the measurement were to be repeated a number of times. In general, small standard errors of measurement are associated with higher measurement reliability. Thorndike et al. (1991) have provided an excellent discussion regarding the computation and the interpretation of the standard error of measurement.

In evaluating the reliability of a measure, then, the consumer of research should look for both reliability coefficients and standard errors of measurement. A measure with good reliability will have a high reliability coefficient and a low standard error of measurement. A measure with poor reliability will have a lower reliability coefficient and a higher standard error of measurement.

As discussed previously, measurement errors may arise from a variety of sources. Cordes (1994, p. 273) pointed out that traditional reliability estimation methods that appear frequently in communicative disorders research are not comprehensive and may fail to capture and differentiate among these sources of error. Cronbach, Gleser, Nanda, and Rajaratnam (1972) advanced the notion of generalizability theory that has been described as the most comprehensive method available for estimating measurement reliability (Cordes, 1994). Generalizability theory extends classical test theory by enabling one to simultaneously "identify and distinguish among several sources of error (e.g., subjects, occasions, raters, items, time)" in a measurement (Pedhazur and Schmelkin 1991, p. 115). Cordes (1994) and Pedhazur and Schmelkin (1991) pointed out that generalizability theory has been used fairly infrequently, probably because of its computational complexities. A readable discussion of generalizability theory and its applications is provided by Shavelson, Webb, and Rowley (1989). One notable recent use of generalizability theory in communicative disorders research was a study by Demorest and Bernstein (1992) regarding speechreading skills assessment. The introduction of more generalizability theory studies in our literature will advance our understanding of the reliability of measurements commonly used in communicative disorders research and will ultimately lead to improvement in the form of more reliable measures.

Validity of Measurements

The validity of a measurement generally refers to the "truthfulness" of the measurement (Shaughnessy and Zechmeister, 1985). The validity of a measurement, then, can be defined as the degree to which it measures what it purports to measure (Kerlinger, 1973; Thorndike et al., 1991). As Shaughnessy and Zechmeister (1985, p. 15) stated, "A valid measure is one that measures what it claims to measure." Whereas reliability is the consistency or precision or accuracy of measurement, validity is truthfulness or correctness or reality of measurement. A reliable measure may be quite repeatable or precise but may not be true or correct. For example, a scale in a butcher shop may consistently and precisely weigh the meat put on it at a half-pound over the true or correct weight. Such a scale would be reliable but not valid, and customers of this shop would consistently and repeatedly pay the price of an extra half-pound for all of the meat they purchased. Reliability, then, does not ensure validity, but it is a necessary prerequisite for validity. That is to say, to be valid, a measure must first be reliable. Once reliability has been established, then the validity of a measure can be assessed.

As Kerlinger (1973, pp. 456–457) has pointed out, if the measure in question is a physical one (e.g., measuring the sound pressure level of a pure tone), there is usually little difficulty in determining its validity. Physical measures generally present a more or less direct analogue of the property that the researcher wishes to measure. The validity of behavioral or cognitive measures, however, is often more difficult to determine. In some cases, it may be so difficult to measure directly certain human behaviors or characteristics that researchers may have to resort to indirect measures to make inferences about them. This has often occurred, for instance, in language research when data concerning linguistic performance have been used to make inferences about linguistic competence or language-processing strategies. The validity of such indirect measures may be difficult or even impossible to establish.

There are basically three ways in which to examine the validity of a measurement: (a) content validity; (b) criterion validity; and (c) construct validity (Anastasi, 1988; Kerlinger, 1973; Thorndike, et al., 1991).

Content Validity

The content validity of a measurement may be established by logical examination of the content of test items to see how well they sample the behavior or characteristic to be measured. The various parts of the measure should be representative of the behaviors or characteristics that it is supposed to measure. This is usually determined by first describing all of the behaviors or characteristics to be measured and then checking the measure to see how well it samples these behaviors or characteristics. Suppose, for example, that researchers wanted to measure the language performance of a group of children. First, the researchers would have to outline all of the behaviors that would constitute those aspects of language performance they wished to sample (e.g., use of past and future tense of certain verbs or comprehension of grammatical relation between subject and object). Then they would have to determine how well their measure sampled this universe of possible behaviors.

Content validation, then, is basically a subjective procedure for logically or rationally evaluating the measurements to see how well they reflect what the researcher wishes to measure. This analysis is usually done by the researcher or by a panel of judges assembled by the researcher for this task. As such, the analysis is not a strictly empirical measure of validity, but more a rational one, and it may be subject to error arising from the particular bias of the judges. There are many situations, however, in which content validity is the only type of validity that can be established.

Occasionally, the term *face validity* is confused or used interchangeably with *content validity.* Anastasi (1988, p. 144) has made the distinction between the two very clear by stating that face validity

> *is not validity in the technical sense; it refers, not to what the test actually measures, but to what it appears superficially to measure. Face validity pertains to whether the test "looks valid" to the examinees who take it, the administrative personnel who decide on its use. . . . Fundamentally, the question of face validity concerns rapport and public relations.*

The fact that the face validity of a measurement is not considered validity in a technical sense in no way implies that it is a trivial concern. Anastasi (1988, p. 144) pointed out that face validity is a desirable feature of a particular measurement in that "if test content appears irrelevant, inappropriate, silly, or childish, the result will be poor cooperation, regardless of the actual validity of the test."

Criterion Validity

The criterion validity of a measurement may be established by empirical examination of how well the measure correlates with some outside validating criterion. The degree to which the measure correlates with a known indicator of the behavior or characteristic it is supposed to measure gives an indication of its criterion validity. There are two types of criterion validity that differ from one another only with respect to the time of administration of the outside criterion.

The first is *concurrent validity*. Concurrent validity is assessed when a measure and an outside validating criterion are administered at the same time. It might be important, for example, to develop a measure that is less time-consuming, cumbersome, and expensive than an existing one. The concurrent validity of the shorter version would be established by examining how well it correlates with the longer version. Concurrent validity may also be important in determining how well a measure is related to some concomitant occurrence in the real world outside the testing situation. For example, the concurrent validity of selected acoustic measurements of voice production could be established by examining them in relationship to listener judgments of voice quality.

The second type of criterion validity is *predictive validity*. Predictive validity is assessed when a measure is used to predict some future behavior. In such a case, the measure is administered first, time elapses, and then the criterion measure is administered. For example, college admissions officers may use college board scores to predict how well high school students might be expected to do in college. A treatment study may involve the use of certain pretreatment measures to predict how much patients might be expected to improve during the course of treatment.

The greatest difficulty in determining criterion validity lies in the selection of an appropriate outside validating criterion. There may be none in existence or it may be very difficult to measure one. The outside criterion itself needs to be valid and reliable and available for measurement. Many measures have never been subjected to examination of their criterion validity simply because no suitable outside criteria are available for measurement.

Construct Validity

The construct validity of a measurement may be established by means of both empirical and rational examination of the degree to which the measure reflects some theoretical construct or explanation of the behavior or characteristic being measured. Kerlinger (1973, p. 461) calls construct validity "one of the most significant advances of modern measurement theory and practice" because it brings both empirical and theoretical considerations together in examining *why* a measure is valid. As we emphasized in Chapter 1, a theory is an explanation of empirical knowledge of some phenomenon. If such an explanation exists, then the results of a measure should confirm the theory if the measure is valid *and* the theory is correct.

Construct validity could be established in several ways. For instance, a theory might predict that a particular behavior should increase with age. The measure could be administered to persons of different ages, and if the measured behaviors were found to increase with age, the construct validity of the measure with respect to the age aspect of the theory would be established. The theory might also predict that different kinds of subjects (e.g., pathological vs. normal) should score in certain ways. If empirical testing with the measure confirmed this, then the measure would have construct validity with respect to that aspect of the theory. The theory might also state that certain experimental manipulations should affect the measure; for example, drug administrations should reduce scores, whereas reinforcement should increase scores on the measure. If experiments were carried out that confirmed these effects, the measure would have construct validity with respect to this aspect of the theory. Factor analysis, a statistical technique for reducing a large number of variables to a smaller number of clusters of common variables that identify common traits, might also be used to establish construct validity. This would involve the determination of how much the measure has in common with other measures known to fit certain theoretical constructs. Also, the internal consistency of the measure might be assessed by item analysis, a statistical technique for correlating each item in the measure with the overall score to see if each item measures the construct as well as the overall measure does.

The greatest problem in establishing construct validity lies in the validity or the correctness of the theoretical constructs used to predict performance. This is analogous to the problem finding a suitable outside validating criterion in predictive and concurrent validity. As Thorndike et al. (1991) have pointed out, the construct validity of a test or measure is borne out if measurements agree with the theoretical prediction, but if the prediction is not verified, it may be the result of an invalid measure *or* an incorrect theory *or* both. A variety of sources are available to those interested in test validity and reliability, test development and standardization, and similar topics (Anastasi, 1988; Cronbach, 1984, and Thorndike et al. 1991). The reader is urged to consult these sources.

An excellent review of the reliability and validity of language and articulation tests was published by McCauley and Swisher (1984). They applied ten psychometric criteria to thirty articulation and language tests for preschool children and found many of the tests lacking in specificity regarding the ten criteria. The criteria included aspects of test construction such as description of the normative sample, sample size, evidence of test-retest reliability, information about criterion validity, and so on. Their results were not particularly encouraging and they concluded that:

> *the reviewed tests failed to provide compelling evidence that they can reliably and validly be used to provide information concerning the existence of language or articulation impairment. These findings suggest important limitations on the use of such tests that must be considered by investigators and by speech-language clinicians (McCauley and Swisher, 1984, pp. 40–41).*

McCauley and Swisher suggested that test authors and publishers should be encouraged to gather empirical evidence of test reliability and validity as an integral part of test development and that test users can wield considerable influence as consumers by evaluating the adequacy of tests before purchasing them. More recently Sturner, Layton, Evans, Heller, Funk, and Machon (1994) conducted a psychometric examination of speech and language screening tests and drew conclusions similar to those of McCauley and Swisher regarding diagnostic tests.

Study Questions

1. Read pages 21–30 in Chapter 3 of Siegel, S. (1956). *Nonparametric statistics for the behavioral sciences.* New York: McGraw-Hill.

    a. Write a brief summary of Siegel's discussion of each level of measurement.

    b. Siegel's examples of each level of measurement come from psychology and sociology. Find examples of each level of measurement in communicative disorders.

2. Read the following article:

    McCauley, R. J., & Swisher, L. (1984). Psychometric review of language and articulation tests for preschool children. *Journal of Speech and Hearing Disorders, 49,* 34–42.

    a. What were the ten criteria suggested for reviewing language and articulation tests?

    b. Identify the consequences of each unmet criterion.

3. Read the following article:

    Sturner, R. A., Layton, T. L., Evans, A. W., Heller, J. H., Funk, S. G., & Machon, M. W. (1994). Preschool speech and language screening: A review of currently available tests. *American Journal of Speech-Language Pathology 3,* 25–36.

    a. What psychometric characteristics of screening tests did the authors review?

    b. Which of the tests reviewed met the criteria for first level screening outlined by the authors?

4. Read the following article:

    Punch, J., & Rakerd, B. (1993). Loudness matching of signals spectrally shaped by a simulated hearing aid. *Journal of Speech and Hearing Research 36,* 357–364.

    a. How did the authors simulate a monaural hearing aid with multiple frequency response?

    b. What steps did the authors take to ensure proper calibration of this listening system?

5. Read the following article:

    Kreiman, J., Gerratt, B. R., Kempster, G. B., Erman, A., & Berke, G. S. (1993). Perceptual evaluation of voice quality: Review, tutorial, and a framework for future research. *Journal of Speech and Hearing Research, 36,* 21–40.

    a. What problems with voice quality ratings are raised by the authors?

    b. What suggestions for improving the reliability of perceptual measures of voice quality are outlined by the authors?

6. Read the following articles:

    Preminger, J. E., & Van Tasell, D. J. (1995). Quantifying the relation between speech quality and speech intelligibility. *Journal of Speech and Hearing Research, 38,* 714–725.

    Preminger, J. E., & Van Tasell, D. J. (1995). Measurement of speech quality as a tool to optimize the fitting of a hearing aid. *Journal of Speech and Hearing Research, 38,* 726–736.

    a. What procedures did the authors use to measure intrasubject and intersubject reliability?

    b. What practical implications of their reliability results did they discuss?

7. Read the following article:

    Nicholas, L. A., & Brookshire, R. H. (1995). Presence, completeness, and accuracy of main concepts in the connected speech of non-brain-damaged adults and adults with aphasia. *Journal of Speech and Hearing Research, 38,* 145–156.

a. How did the authors validate the main concepts?

b. What different measures of reliability and agreement were used by the authors?

8. Read the following article:

Hixon, T. J., & Weismer, G. (1995). Perspectives on the Edinburgh study of speech breathing. *Journal of Speech and Hearing Research, 38,* 42–60.

a. What questions did the authors raise about the validity of the measurements reported in the Edinburgh speech breathing research?

b. What alternate measurement procedures were suggested by the authors?

References

American National Standards Institute. (1989). *American National Standard specifications for audiometers (ANSI s3.6-1989).* New York: American National Standards Institute.

Anastasi, A. (1988). *Psychological testing* (6th ed.). New York: Macmillan.

Baken, R. J. (1987). *Clinical measurement of speech and voice.* Boston: Allyn & Bacon.

Cordes, A. K. (1994). The reliability of observational data: I. Theories and methods for speech-language pathology. *Journal of Speech and Hearing Research, 37,* 264–278.

Cronbach, L. J. (1984). *Essentials of psychological testing* (4th ed.). New York: Harper & Row.

Cronbach, L. J., Gleser, G., Nanada, H., & Rajaratnam, N. (1972). *The dependability of behavioral measurements: Theory of generalizability of scores and profiles.* New York: John Wiley & Sons.

Cudahy, E. (1988). *Introduction to instrumentation in speech and hearing.* Baltimore: Williams & Wilkins.

Decker, T. N. (1990). *Instrumentation: An introduction for students in the speech and hearing sciences.* New York: Longman.

Demorest, M. E., & Bernstein, L. E. (1992). Sources of variability in speechreading sentences: A generalizability analysis. *Journal of Speech and Hearing Research, 35,* 876–891.

Ebel, R. L. (1965). *Measuring educational achievement.* Englewood Cliffs, NJ: Prentice Hall.

Gerratt, B. R., Kreiman, J., Antonanzas-Barroso, N., & Berke, G. S. (1993). Comparing internal and external standards in voice quality judgments. *Journal of Speech and Hearing Research, 36,* 14–20.

Graziano, A. M., & Raulin, M. L. (1989). *Research methods: A process approach.* New York: Harper & Row.

Haber, A., Runyon, R. P., & Badia, P. (Eds.). (1970). *Readings in statistics.* Reading, MA: Addison-Wesley.

Haynes, W. O., Pindzola, R. H., & Emerick, L. L. (1992). *Diagnosis and evaluation in speech pathology.* Englewood Cliffs, NJ: Prentice Hall.

Isaac, S., & Michael, W. B. (1971). *Handbook in research and evaluation.* San Diego: Edits.

Kearns, K. (1990). Reliability of procedures and measures. In L. B. Olswang, C. K. Thompson, S. F. Warren, & N. J. Minghetti (Eds.), *Treatment efficacy research in communicative disorders.* Rockville, MD: American Speech-Language-Hearing Foundation.

Kerlinger, F. (1973). *Foundations of behavioral research* (2nd ed.). New York: Holt, Rinehart & Winston.

Kerlinger, F. (1979). *Behavioral research: A conceptual approach.* New York: Holt, Rinehart & Winston.

Lyman, H. B. (1978). *Test scores and what they mean* (3rd ed.). Englewood Cliffs, NJ: Prentice Hall.

Martin, R. R., Haroldson, S. K., & Triden, K. A. (1984). Stuttering and speech naturalness. *Journal of Speech and Hearing Disorders, 49,* 53–58.

McCauley, R. J., & Swisher, L. (1984). Psychometric review of language and articulation tests for preschool children. *Journal of Speech and Hearing Disorders, 49,* 34–42.

Nunnally, J. C. (1978). *Psychometric theory.* New York: McGraw-Hill.

Pedhazur, E. J., & Schmelkin, L. P. (1991). *Measurement, design, and analysis.* Hillsdale, NJ: Lawrence Erlbaum Associates.

Peterson, H. A., & Marquardt, T. P. (1994). *Appraisal and diagnosis of speech and language disorders.* Englewood Cliffs, NJ: Prentice Hall.

Read, C., Buder, E. H., & Kent, R. D. (1990). Speech analysis systems: A survey. *Journal of Speech and Hearing Research, 33,* 363–374.

Read, C., Buder, E. H., & Kent, R. D. (1992). Speech analysis systems: An evaluation. *Journal of Speech and Hearing Research, 35,* 314–332.

Rintelmann, W. F. (Ed.). (1991). *Hearing assessment.* Austin, TX: Pro-ed.

Rosenthal, R. (1966). *Experimenter effects in behavioral research.* New York: Appleton-Century-Crofts.

Rosenthal, R., & Rosnow, R. L. (1984). *Essentials of behavioral research.* New York: McGraw-Hill.

Shavelson, R. J., Webb, N. M., & Rowley, G. L. (1989). Generalizability theory. *American Psychologist, 44,* 922–932.

Shaughnessy, J. J., & Zechmeister, E. B. (1985). *Research methods in psychology.* New York: Alfred A. Knopf.

Siegel, S. (1956). *Nonparametric statistics for the behavioral sciences.* New York: McGraw-Hill.

Stevens, S. S. (1946). On the theory of scales of measurement. *Science, 103,* 677–680.

Stevens, S. S. (1951). Mathematics, measurement, and psychophysics. In S. S. Stevens (Ed.), *Handbook of experimental psychology* (pp. 1–49). New York: John Wiley & Sons.

Stevens, S. S. (1958). Measurement and man. *Science, 127,* 383–389.

Sturner, R. A., Layton, T. L., Evans, A. W., Heller, J. H., Funk, S. G., & Machon, M. W. (1994). Preschool speech and language screening: A review of currently available tests. *American Journal of Speech-Language Pathology, 3,* 25–36.

Thorndike, R. L., & Hagen, E. P. (1977). *Measurement and evaluation in psychology and education* (3rd ed.). New York: John Wiley & Sons.

Thorndike, R. M., Cunningham, G. K., Thorndike, R. L., & Hagen, E. P. (1991). *Measurement and evaluation in psychology and education* (5th ed.). New York: Macmillan.

Young, M. A., (1969). Observer agreement: Cumulative effects of rating many samples. *Journal of Speech and Hearing Research, 12,* 135–143.

Chapter 5

Evaluating Treatment Efficacy Research

Treatment efficacy research in communicative disorders is gaining widespread attention as witnessed by two recent publications on the topic, one sponsored by the American Speech Language-Hearing Foundation (Olswang, Thompson, Warren, & Minghetti, 1990) and the other sponsored by the National Institute on Deafness and Other Communication Disorders that was published in its entirety in volume 18, numbers 2 and 3, of the *Journal of Fluency Disorders* (1993). In addition, The Academy of Rehabilitative Audiology included in its recent monograph "Research in Audiological Rehabilitation: Current Trends and Future Directions," a chapter on treatment efficacy by Montgomery (1994) that reviews the federal government perspective on the topic and discusses the nature of outcome measures in efficacy research. As such, the purpose of this chapter is to review the internal and external validity of treatment research designs and some factors that jeopardize internal and external validity.

Much of the material in this chapter is based on the survey of research designs in educational psychology research by Campbell and Stanley (1966) entitled *Experimental and Quasi-Experimental Designs for Research.* Their classification of research designs and of the factors that threaten the internal and external validity of these designs has had a strong impact on behavioral research. The popularity of their classification is evident in the many textbooks on behavioral research that have adopted it (e.g., Bordens & Abbott, 1988, Isaac & Michael, 1971; Levine & Elzey, l976, Pedhazur & Schmelkin, 1991).

The Campbell and Stanley classification comprises experimental and quasi-experimental designs commonly used in educational psychology, especially in research on teaching. Because we are dealing with research in communicative disorders that includes some other designs and that excludes some of the designs they used, some modification of their classification is necessary. Our discussion, however, is mainly based on their system, and we wish to express our debt to them for the influence that their work has had in shaping our thinking about the evaluation of research designs.

The next two sections of this chapter will be concerned with the two major criteria of internal and external validity formulated by Campbell and Stanley (1966) for evaluation of research designs on the effects of teaching methods and with the factors that jeopardize internal and external validity. These criteria were intended to be used for the evaluation of both experimental designs in which the independent variable could be manipulated easily and extraneous variables well controlled and quasi-experimental designs in which the independent variable could not be manipulated easily and extraneous variables could not be well controlled. The latter designs were compromise attempts to approximate experiments in situations that would not allow for the easy manipulation of the independent variable and control of extraneous variables. These criteria are easily applied to treatment efficacy research in communicative disorders.

Campbell and Stanley (1966, p. 5) stated that internal validity concerns the question: "Did in fact the experimental treatments make a difference in this specific experimental instance?" If an experiment has internal validity, the experimenter can conclude that manipulation of the independent variable (experimental treatment) caused the change in the dependent variable and competing explanations from lack of control of extraneous variables are minimized within the confines of the specific experiment. If, indeed, a study has internal validity, the next concern is the degree to which the results of the experiment can be generalized. External validity according to Campbell and Stanley (1966, p. 5) "asks the question of generalizability: To what populations, settings, treatment variables, and measurement variables can this effect be generalized?"

Campbell and Stanley have formulated a list of twelve factors, of which eight jeopardize internal validity and four jeopardize external validity. An examination of the degree to which an experimental design minimizes these twelve factors indicates the degree to which the experiment has internal and external validity. In summarizing these important criteria, Campbell and Stanley (1966, p. 5) have stated:

> *Both types of criteria are obviously important, even though they are frequently at odds in that features increasing one may jeopardize the other. While* internal validity *is the sine qua non, and while the question of* external validity, *like the question of inductive inference, is never completely answerable, the selection of designs strong in both types of validity is obviously our ideal.*

Internal Validity and Factors That Affect It

A major consideration in the evaluation of research designs is whether the researcher has controlled or accounted for the variety of factors that could have a significant effect on the validity of the data collected. The experimenter (and the consumer) needs to be certain that the change in the dependent variable was, in fact, caused by the experimental treatment and *not* by factors that can mimic the effect of the treatment. That is, the experimenter needs to eliminate alternate explanations that might account for the treatment effect. The fewer the alternate explanations, the greater the internal validity of the experiment. It is to the factors that can affect internal validity in both experimental and descriptive studies that we now turn.

History

The first factor that can have an effect on internal validity is *history*. History, in an experimental context, is defined as events occurring between the first and second (or more) measurements in *addition* to the experimental variable. In other words: Has some event occurred to a subject or group of subjects between measurements to confound the effect of the experimental variable or treatment? In such an instance, the experimenter cannot determine whether the result was a function of the extraneous events alone, the extraneous events interacting with the experimental treatment, or the experimental treatment alone.

An example should help clarify the impact that history can have on validity. Assume that an experimenter is evaluating a particular treatment approach for a group of young children who stutter. Unbeknownst to the experimenter, several of the subjects are receiving treatment in their local schools. The experimenter evaluates fluency before and after treatment and concludes that the particular treatment produced increased fluency. The conclusion is suspect because an equally plausible explanation for the improved fluency is that the treatment received in school, rather than the experimental treatment, accounted for the decreased stuttering or, even more likely, the two treatment approaches (one in school, the other given by the experimenter) interacted to produce the observed result.

Some types of experimental designs are more prone to the contaminating effects of history than others. Long-term studies are more likely to be contaminated by history effects than are studies in which data are collected over a short time. In such cases, the longer the interval between the pretest and the posttest, the greater the likelihood that history will serve to contaminate the results.

Maturation

The effect of maturation is similar to the effect associated with history. History refers to events that occur outside the experimental setting and, thus, outside the control of the experimenter. Maturation, on the other hand, refers to changes in subjects themselves that cannot be controlled by the experimenter, changes that may cause effects that are attributed, incorrectly, to the experimental treatment. Examples of maturational factors are age changes, changes in biological or psychological processes that take place over time, and the like.

Obviously, maturation effects can play an important role in long-term treatment research. Take, for example, a language-stimulation program designed to improve expressive language in young children. The program might be introduced to two-year-old children whose language performance is evaluated before the initiation of the program. Then, the effects of the treatment program might be evaluated when the group of children reaches three years of age. Because of changes that occur in language performance (pretest at two years vs. posttest at three years), the experimenter concludes that the language stimulation program was successful in enhancing language development for young children. It is hardly likely, although not impossible, that such a study would appear in print because it is obvious that maturational processes—neurological, physiological, psychological—could have a role in changes in language performance. Furthermore, the interaction between maturational factors and the experimental treatment could have produced the improved performance rather than either maturational processes or the treatment operating singly.

Maturation has served to confuse certain types of research in communicative disorders or, at the very least, has made these kinds of research difficult to perform. A good illustration deals with the efficacy of early treatment for stroke patients. There is still controversy over whether early intervention for aphasic patients produces benefits over and above what might be expected merely as the result of spontaneous recovery. The major difficulty confronting the researcher is to isolate or eliminate the effects of maturation (spontaneous recovery) so that changes in language performance can be attributed to the treatment program.

Testing or Test-Practice Effects

A third factor that can affect internal validity is the effect that merely taking a test may have on scores achieved on subsequent administrations of the same test. This effect may be due to the practice afforded by the first test, familiarity with the test items or format, reduction of test anxiety, and so on. By their very nature, pretest–posttest designs are especially vulnerable to test-sensitizing effects or test-practice effects. As a simple illustration, take the measurement of speech discrimination in the audiology clinic. Let us assume that the investigator wishes to determine if auditory training will improve speech discrimination. The subject is tested for the first time with a standard discrimination test and then retested after treatment. The subject's score improves significantly and the investigator concludes that the treatment is beneficial. An equally plausible alternate hypothesis, however, is that the improvement in discrimination is simply a function of testing or practice with the discrimination test and that some improvement might have been observed if the subject had been merely retested without the treatment. It may also be, of course, that a portion of the change was due to the treatment. Obviously, in these circumstances, it would be extremely difficult to know which was which. Any time pretreatment tests are used, the reader must ask whether posttreatment changes are due to treatment effects, testing effects, or a combination of the two.

Brief mention should be given here to reactive vs. nonreactive measures. Huck, Cormier, and Bounds (1974), among others, have noted that tests, inventories, and rating scales are referred to as *reactive* measures. They are reactive because they may change the phenomenon that the researcher is investigating. Huck et al. (1974, p. 235) emphasize that

> *any measure is reactive if it has the potential for modifying the variables under study, it may focus attention on the experiment, if it is not part of the normal environment, or if it exercises the process under study.*

As Campbell and Stanley (1966, p. 9) point out, "the more novel and motivating the test device, the more reactive one can expect it to be." Videotapes and tape recordings may also be reactive measures. As a result, special care must be taken by the investigator to reduce the reactive effects of these recording devices.

A *nonreactive* measure, on the other hand, does not change what is being measured. Isaac and Michael (1971) put nonreactive measures into three categories: (1) *physical traces*—for instance, examining the condition of library books to determine their actual use rather than giving students a questionnaire on book usage; (2) *archives and records*—

such as clinic folders, attendance records, and school grades; and (3) *unobtrusive obser-vation*—in which the subject may not know that a particular behavior is being observed.[1] Although Isaac and Michael emphasize that nonreactive measures are not impervious to sampling bias and other kinds of distortion, Campbell and Stanley (1966) urge the use of such measures whenever possible.

Instrumentation

Campbell and Stanley (1966, p. 5) define the instrumentation threat to internal validity as one "in which changes in the calibration of a measuring instrument or changes in the observers or scorers used may produce changes in the obtained measurements." It should be clear from the following discussion that this threat to validity transcends types of research in communicative disorders. Instrumentation effects can be a threat to the internal validity of any research study.

The most obvious instrumentation threat to the validity of studies in communicative disorders is faulty, inadequate, or changing calibration of the equipment used in the research. Because all students in communicative disorders are taught about the importance of calibration in their clinical work, there is no need to belabor the point here. Appropriate calibration and ongoing monitoring of calibration are absolutely essential ingredients in the collection of valid data, whether the data are for research purposes *or* for clinical purposes.

How does the reader of a research article determine whether the equipment was calibrated or maintained in calibration throughout the duration of the study? In many instances, the researcher provides a detailed description of the equipment employed and the calibration techniques used. Provided that the reader has some knowledge of instrumentation and calibration procedures, the adequacy of the instrumental array can be assessed by a careful reading of the method section. Often, however, only sketchy information is available on the instrumentation used and the calibration procedures employed. Because journal space is at a premium, editors have a tendency to prune procedures to a bare minimum. As a result, we may run across such statements as, "the equipment was calibrated and remained in calibration throughout the study" or "calibration checks were conducted periodically during the course of the investigation."

Although it is readily apparent that mechanical and electrical instruments can be sources of error that pose threats to validity, it may be less obvious that such devices as rating scales, questionnaires, attitude inventories, and standardized language tests are also instruments and that their use or misuse can have a profound influence on the adequacy of the data collected in either experimental or descriptive research. A poor pencil-and-paper test, one that has not been standardized, one that has inadequate reliability, or one that was standardized on a sample different from that under investigation can have serious consequences for internal validity. For communicative disorders and other behavioral disciplines as well, considerable attention and research effort have been given to the development and evaluation of rating scales. These efforts have been made in recognition of the need to develop valid and reliable rating scale instruments to reduce the chances that the rating scale itself would pose an instrumentation threat to validity.

---

[1]For the interested reader, unobtrusive measures are discussed at length by Webb, Campbell, Schwartz, and Sechrest (1966), and Bordens and Abbott (1988).

Statistical Regression

Statistical regression is a phenomenon in which subjects who are selected on the basis of atypically low or high scores change on a subsequent test so that their scores are now somewhat better (in the case of the low scorer) or somewhat poorer (in the case of the high scorer) than they were originally. The investigator may conclude that the treatment produced the change when, in reality, the scores have simply moved or regressed toward a more typical, mean score—that is, the scores have become less atypical. This occurs primarily because of measurement errors associated with the test instrument used in selecting and evaluating the subjects. The more deviant or atypical the score, the larger the error of measurement it probably contains (Campbell & Stanley, 1966).

To illustrate, let us say that an experimenter is interested in assessing the value of an articulation treatment program in a school setting. After screening all the children with an articulation screening test, the experimenter selects for study those ten children who performed the poorest on the test, that is, had the lowest scores. The treatment program is initiated for the children and a month later, the children are retested. An improvement is noted and the experimenter concludes that the treatment program is a success. The conclusion may be unwarranted if changes could have been caused by the extreme, atypical performance becoming less atypical (regressing toward the mean). If no intervention had been provided, the retest scores might still have shown some improvement without treatment.

To give another example, a group of hearing-impaired people might be evaluated and chosen to participate in a counseling study on the basis of their high scores on the Hearing Handicap Scale (HHS). In this case, a high score represents considerable handicap and a low score represents little handicap. A counseling program is initiated and after four counseling sessions, the subjects are retested with the HHS. The investigator finds that after counseling the scores are lower than they were before counseling and concludes, again erroneously, that the counseling program was successful in reducing self-assessed hearing handicap. An equally plausible explanation is that the improved scores simply represent statistical regression and that the atypical scores would have become more typical scores even without counseling. It should be emphasized that statistical regression is not always a concomitant of extreme scores. As Campbell and Stanley (1966) pointed out, if a group selected for independent reasons turns out to have extreme scores, there is less likelihood that the data will be contaminated by regression effects.

Differential Selection of Subjects

The selection of subjects to form experimental and control groups in experimental research can affect internal validity if subject selection is not done properly. Internal validity may be threatened because differences between subjects in the experimental and control groups may account for the treatment effects rather than the treatment itself. In most experimental research, one important requirement is that the subjects should be equal, on important dimensions, before experimental treatment or manipulation. The experimenter attempts to ensure equality by random assignment of subjects to experimental and control groups. The absence of equality prior to treatment poses a subject-selection threat to the internal validity of experimental research.

To further explain, let us use an example dealing with an experimental study of phonological processing treatment. Assume that a researcher wishes to conduct an experiment to evaluate the efficacy of a new method of phonological processing treatment with young children. The researcher selects a sample of children with phonological processing deficits and assigns subjects *randomly* to one of three groups: (1) a nontreatment group, (2) a standard-treatment group, and (3) a new-treatment group. Through random assignment, the researcher attempts to reduce the effects of any pretreatment differences among subjects by distributing these differences randomly among the three groups. In this way, the effects of differences between experimental and control subjects on treatment outcomes are minimized and differential selection of subjects poses little threat to internal validity.

Mortality

Mortality simply refers to the differential loss of subjects between experimental and control groups or between other comparison groups. Mortality can threaten the internal validity of both experimental and descriptive studies. This occurs because the subjects who fail to complete the research procedure may be quite different in important respects from those subjects who continue to participate in the study. It is difficult for an investigator to know how the dropouts may differ from those subjects who remain.

Mortality in an experimental study may differentially affect experimental and control-group composition by posttest time to such a degree that meaningful and valid comparison of posttest scores is impossible. It might be possible, for example, that subjects who dropped out were the ones who might have benefitted the least (or the most) from the experimental treatment. Because these possibilities remain unknown to the experimenter, the only ways to account for them would be to find all the dropouts or to replicate the entire study with a new sample.

Follow-up studies are especially prone to the problems of mortality in studying the long-term success of treatment programs. Is the stuttering adult still reasonably fluent six months after the termination of treatment? This type of research is among the most difficult to do, and the problem of experimental mortality is at the core of the difficulty. If we cannot locate or follow all, or a significant majority of, the subjects, then there is no way of determining if the subjects who cannot be followed are different on any number of dimensions from the subjects who can be located. The investigator might simply choose to reevaluate those subjects who can be located, but the data will hardly be representative.

Interaction of Factors

The final threat to internal validity deals with the possible interaction effects among two or more of the previously described jeopardizing factors. Although these factors have been treated singly in this discussion, there is little question that they can interact with one another to cause an effect greater than each operating independently and, more important, greater than the experimental effect under investigation. As noted earlier, each of the jeopardizing factors or a combination of factors may also interact with the experimental variable to produce an effect that can be mistaken for the experimental effect alone. Oftentimes, however, it is the interaction between subject selection and some other factor, especially maturation, that confounds the interpretation of the data.

One example may suffice. Let us say that we have an experimental group composed of second graders with specific language impairment on whom we wish to assess the efficacy of an experimental language treatment program. We use third-grade children with specific language impairment as the control group. The treatment program is initiated, significantly greater gains are noted for the experimental group than are noted for the control group; we conclude that our experimental treatment program is a success. Note, however, that maturational influences may be operating differentially for the two groups so that more rapid maturation and change in language development may have occurred for the younger children. Thus, the effect of the treatment program could be in large part due to subject-selection-maturation-interactions rather than to the program itself. The picture is further clouded if a history threat has also occurred so that a significant portion, or perhaps any portion, of the experimental group is receiving treatment outside school. Instrumentation can interact with maturation and history if the language tests used to evaluate performance had low reliability, especially for second-grade children. The major point is that the factors that can jeopardize internal validity can act singly or in concert to produce changes in performance or behavior that can be mistaken for the effect of the experimental treatment.

External Validity and Factors That Affect It

As noted earlier in this chapter, external validity, as defined by Campbell and Stanley (1966), simply refers to the generalizability of the data, that is, the extent to which the results of a research study can be generalized to other subjects, settings, measurements, and treatments. Each of these four ways of generalizing results will be considered in this section. Four threats to external validity that were identified by Campbell and Stanley (1966) are outlined here. Each of these four threats provides an example of a problem in generalizing in one of these four ways: to other subjects, settings, measurements, or treatments.

Bracht and Glass (1968) have extended Campbell and Stanley's (1966) discussion of external validity to include twelve threats to generalization that they classified under the rubrics of population validity and ecological validity. Population validity factors concern the populations of subjects to which results can be generalized. Ecological validity factors concern the environments to which results can be generalized (i.e., settings, measures, treatments). Consideration of all twelve factors is beyond the scope of this chapter, and we have chosen to review the four Campbell and Stanley threats as examples of threats to each of the main areas of generalization: subjects, settings, measures, and treatments. Interested readers are referred to the Bracht and Glass (1968) article for a fuller treatment of external validity.

It should also be pointed out that threats to external validity are qualitatively different from threats to internal validity. Serious threats to internal validity render results meaningless and uninterpretable and preclude the drawing of valid conclusions about the relations among the variables studied. Threats to external validity, however, only *limit* the degree to which internally valid results can be generalized. No single research study is expected to have wide-ranging generalizability to many different kinds of subjects, settings, measures, or treatments. Generalizations grow from cumulative research centered on a given topic. Researchers build a case for generalization from comparison of the results of many studies. Also, efforts to control threats to internal validity often reduce external validity by introducing greater specificity to the population and environment of the research design. Therefore, the accumulation of several internally valid research studies is necessary to overcome limitations to external validity.

Subject Selection

The first threat to external validity presents a problem in generalizing to other subjects. This threat concerns the degree to which the subjects chosen for the study are representative of the population to which the researcher wishes to generalize. If there are important differences between the two (and these differences may not always be apparent to the experimenter), then meaningful generalizations will be limited. We have emphasized earlier the importance of subject selection to internal validity. It should be clear that subject selection procedures can pose an equally important threat to external validity, especially because subject selection may interact with the experimental variable to produce positive results only for certain types of subjects and not for others. Brookshire (1983, p. 342) has discussed the problems of generalization of results of experiments with aphasics and stated:

> In any experiment, the population to which experimental findings can be generalized is determined by the characteristics of the subjects who participate in the experiment. In order for the results of an experiment to be generalizable to a given population, the sample of subjects which participates in the experiment must be representative of the population. That is, the sample must resemble the population with regard to those variables which are likely to affect the relationship between the independent and dependent variable(s).

Brookshire further stated that investigators should report both the relevant variables used to select subjects and the characteristics of the subjects on these variables in order to make legitimate generalizations to a specific population. He discussed eighteen specific subject characteristics (e.g., age, severity of aphasia, handedness, visual acuity, time post onset) that could be relevant in specifying an intended target population of aphasics for generalization.

The important point is that generalization should be limited to subjects who have characteristics in common with the subjects studied. In other words, the subjects must be representative of the population to which the researcher wishes to generalize and the relevant characteristics of the subjects that determine their degree of representativeness should be specified in the article to allow readers to evaluate the generality of results to other subjects.

Reactive or Interactive Effects of Pretesting

The second threat to external validity presents a problem in generalizing to other measures. This threat concerns the degree to which a reactive pretest may interact with an independent variable in determining the subjects' performance on the dependent variable. In other words, subjects who are exposed to a reactive pretest may react to an experimental treatment in a way that is different from people who have not been exposed to the pretest. The effect of the treatment may be demonstrated only for subjects who were tested just before treatment and not for the population at large who might receive the treatment without the specific pretest.

Suppose a researcher is interested in assessing a particular aspect of stuttering treatment designed to reduce a stutterer's fear of speaking situations. The pretest involves an interview in which various measures of speaking fear are taken. The treatment program is initiated and following its completion, the subject is again required to answer questions about fear or to demonstrate his or her mastery of fear. The experimenter notes a significant decrease in fear of speaking situations and concludes that the program is successful. Although it may be true for the subjects in the experiment, it may very well be that the treatment program would not be successful or would be less successful if administered to individuals who have not had the pretest experience. In this example, external validity is in jeopardy because of the interaction of the pretest and the experimental treatment.

Reactive Arrangements

The third threat to external validity presents a problem in generalizing to other settings. This threat concerns the degree to which the setting of the research is reactive or interacts with the independent variable in determining the subjects' performance on the dependent variable. Campbell and Stanley (1966, p. 6) note that the "reactive effects of experimental arrangements" are such that they "would preclude generalization about the effect of the experimental variable upon persons being exposed to it in nonexperimental settings." For example, a child is taken from the classroom to the speech clinician's office to be given an experimental language stimulation program. Is the effect of that language stimulation program specific to the experimental setting of the clinician's office or can the language stimulation program be equally effective in the normal classroom environment? How does the experimental arrangement interact with the treatment to produce the observed effect? If there is an interaction, then the treatment effects cannot be generalized to people who have not experienced the experimental arrangement. In this example, the experimental language stimulation program might be modified so that it could be administered in the classroom and its effect there directly evaluated. If the treatment program is designed specifically to be administered by the speech clinician working in an office and no claims are made about the efficacy of the program in the classroom, then the experimenter would be justified in generalizing the treatment to all similar "experimental arrangements," that is, *limiting* the generalization to similar settings rather than trying to extend it to a large variety of settings without sufficient evidence. Some texts refer to reactive arrangements as the Hawthorne effect. The Hawthorne effect refers to changes in a subject's behavior that occur simply because the subject knows that he or she is participating in a research study. The increased attention that the subject receives, the change in routine, the experimental setting itself may all act to cause a performance change that may mimic or accompany the change attributed to the independent variable alone. This effect was first noticed in studies of worker performance at a Hawthorne Illinois, Western Electric Company telephone-assembly plant in the 1920s, hence, the name, Hawthorne effect.

Parsons (1974) completed an exhaustive reanalysis of the Hawthorne research and concluded that the key elements of the Hawthorne effect are feedback to subjects about their performance and reinforcement of performance. Parsons (1974, p.930) concluded by defining the Hawthorne effect as "the confounding that occurs if experimenters fail to realize how the consequences of subjects' performance affect what subjects do." In other words, the Hawthorne effect is not just the simple problem of subjects' awareness that they are participating in a research study but is related to how they perceive the consequences of their behavior during the course of the research. The control of the Hawthorne effect is best accomplished by ensuring comparability of treatment between groups in their knowledge of the nature of experimental treatments.

Multiple-Treatment Interference

The fourth threat to external validity presents a problem in generalizing to other treatments. This threat concerns the degree to which various parts of a multiple treatment interact with each other in determining subjects' performance on the dependent variable. This effect is likely to occur when more than one experimental treatment is administered to the same subjects or when a treatment consists of a carefully sequenced set of steps. The threat to external validity lies in the fact that the results of a multiple-treatment study can only be generalized to people who would receive the same sequence and number of treatments.

An example might be a study in which fluency is reinforced and nonfluency is punished during a conditioning segment of an experiment on stuttering. It would be difficult to ferret out the individual effects of the punishment and the reinforcement in examining any reduction in nonfluency because of the multiple-treatment effect. Separate studies would be needed of the individual effects of punishment of nonfluency, reinforcement of fluency, and the combined punishment of nonfluency and reinforcement of fluency. In other words, the treatment must be representative of the kind of treatment to which the results can be generalized.

Evaluation of Some Experimental Designs for Studying Treatment Efficacy

In this section, much of the material discussed previously will be applied to the evaluation of experimental designs for studying treatment efficacy. Many individuals express an interest in the analysis of treatment efficacy research because of the direct applicability of such research to clinical work. Also, much has been written about the validity of these designs (e.g., Campbell & Stanley, 1966). These designs incorporate within subjects, between-subjects, or mixed comparisons and, therefore, serve to illustrate many of the concepts advanced in the earlier sections of this book.

In outlining the paradigms of the experimental designs to follow, we will adopt Campbell and Stanley's notation system (1966). The left-to-right orientation will indicate the progression of time from before to after treatment, and the vertical orientation will indicate simultaneous occurrences. X will be the symbol for the administration of the experimental treatment, and O will refer to the observation and measurement of the dependent variable. When subjects are randomly assigned to groups, *R* will precede the appropriate groups. When subjects are matched on known extraneous variables and subsequently assigned to groups at random, *MR* will precede the appropriate groups. When there are no formal means for certifying either of these attempts to equate groups in an experiment, dashed lines (- - - - - - -) will separate the groups.

Weak Designs

Campbell and Stanley (1966) have identified several weak designs in educational research that may be applicable to the investigation of treatment efficacy in communicative disorders. These experimental designs are weak in both internal and external validity. They are presented here to help the consumer of research to identify weak treatment research. They also may serve as a frame of reference for understanding the manner in which the stronger designs represent improvements on the weaker designs.

The One-Shot Case Study

The first weak design is what Campbell and Stanley called the one-shot case study, and it can be diagrammed as follows:

$$X \ O$$

In such a study, a single group is observed only once, after having been exposed to some treatment. For example, children with articulation disorders might be given an articulation test after treatment had been administered and their scores on this measure (dependent variable) used as an indication of the success of the treatment (independent variable). The major problem is that there is no reference point for comparison of the posttreatment scores on the articulation test; no pretest was administered and no control group was used. The *effects* of the articulation treatment cannot be evaluated because no comparison can be made to either pretreatment articulation performance or the performance of some group that did not receive treatment. Even if the articulation test scores were compared to existing norms, there is no basis for the conclusion that treatment affected the scores without pretreatment or control-group comparisons because no evidence is shown to indicate that articulation was better after treatment than it was before treatment. Campbell and Stanley have also pointed out that this design may suffer from the "error of misplaced precision" because careful data collection represents a wasted effort without the opportunity for comparison of the posttest scores with control group or pretest scores. The one-shot case study is fraught with threats to both internal and external validity when used as an experimental design for studying the treatment efficacy. It is extremely difficult, if not impossible, to draw valid conclusions from the results of a one-shot case study.

One-Group Pretest–Posttest Design

A second weak design discussed by Campbell and Stanley is the one-group pretest–posttest design, which may be diagrammed as follows:

$$O_1 \ X \ O_2$$

In such a design, one group is assembled, pretested, exposed to the experimental treatment, and posttested. This is a within-subjects design because all subjects are tested under two conditions: before and after treatment. For example, a group of children might be pretested on a language test and then tested again after treatment on the language test. This design is more commonly found in the research literature and represents some improvement over the one-shot case study. However, there are still numerous drawbacks to this design because of the threats to its internal and external validity.

The first problem concerns the effects of history because many events that could affect the posttest outcome may have occurred during the course of the experiment in addition to the experimental treatment. A child may participate in language activities in school that could influence his or her performance after treatment. Maturation is also a threat because growth and development during the course of a study might affect the posttest, regardless of the application of the experimental treatment. Testing represents still a third threat because the pretest may have increased the subjects' ability to perform well on the posttest.

Instrumentation could be a threat if care is not taken to be sure that the pretest and posttest measures are equivalent. This is especially important when judgments of human observers are used in the pretest and posttest. For instance, the Rosenthal Effect could operate if the human observers were biased in their observations by the belief that a change should have taken place as a result of the experimental treatment.

Statistical regression is a threat to internal validity when groups with extreme scores are retested. This would be important when subjects are selected because they had extremely poor pretest scores and were thereby considered good candidates for treatment. In such a case, regression toward the mean on a second test would be expected and could be a competing explanation for any performance gains after treatment. Threats to external validity would be primarily the interaction of selection or pretesting with the experimental variable, factors that are better controlled in the stronger designs to follow. Therefore, even though this design appears to be an improvement over the one-shot case study, it is still a weak design with many threats to both internal and external validity.

The Static-Group Comparison

Another weak design is called the static group comparison and can be diagrammed as follows:

$$\begin{array}{c} X \quad O_1 \\ \hline O_2 \end{array}$$

In such a study, a group that has been exposed to the experimental treatment is compared to another group that has not, but no attempt is made to pretest the groups or to equate them by randomization or matching. This is a between-subjects design because two different groups are compared to each other. For example, children exposed to language treatment might be compared with children not exposed to such treatment to study the effects of treatment on their language performance.

There are two major problems with such a design. First, there is no pretest against which to compare posttest scores. Second, there is no formal means of certifying the equivalence of the groups on relevant extraneous variables, so any differences between the two groups may not be a result of the treatment program alone. Differential selection of subjects in the two groups would, therefore, be the greatest threat to internal validity because of lack of knowledge about extraneous variables in both groups. Also, any experimental mortality would seriously affect the internal validity of this design because there would be no way of certifying extraneous variables associated with mortality or what effect such variables would have had on the dependent variable in addition to the experimental treatment. Interaction of selection and mortality with the other factors would also threaten internal validity. The interaction of selection with the experimental variable would be the greatest threat to external validity, again because of the lack of knowledge about extraneous variables.

Nonequivalent Control-Group Design

A fourth weak design is the nonequivalent control group design, which can be diagrammed as follows:

$$\begin{array}{ccc} O_1 & X & O_2 \\ \hline O_3 & & O_4 \end{array}$$

In such a study, one group is formed, pretested, exposed to the experimental treatment, and posttested, whereas another group is formed, pretested, not exposed to the experimental treatment, and posttested. This is a mixed design because it has both a within-subjects component (pretest vs. posttest) and a between-subjects component (experimental vs. control group). A difference between the two groups in the *improvement from pretest to posttest* is an index of the effect of the experimental treatment. This type of study might be done with naturally assembled groups because of the convenience of using one group intact as the experimental group and the other group intact as the control group. For instance, groups of subjects in two different clinics or schools might be compared. The subjects in one school would be exposed to the experimental treatment, whereas the subjects at the other school would be the control group receiving no treatment to compare the effect of treatment to no treatment. Sometimes this design is seen with the control group receiving a regularly scheduled treatment to compare the effectiveness of a new treatment against the effect of an old treatment. Some studies have also used two control groups, one without treatment and another with the older treatment in order to make both comparisons.

This design may eliminate contamination of internal validity by the effects of history, maturation, and pretesting because of the introduction of a control group and may appear, therefore, to be a better design than the previous three, especially if the two groups perform similarly on the pretest. But there are problems involving the subject-selection factor and its interaction with the other factors that jeopardize internal validity. Because the groups have been selected on the basis of convenience rather than assembled on the basis of randomization or matching, it is possible that certain biases may arise from group composition that the experimenter cannot account for or measure. For example, if patients from a private clinic constituted one group and patients from a public clinic constituted the other, there might be important differences that related to their decision to attend a private vs. a public clinic. More affluent patients might attend the private clinic so that socioeconomic status would not be controlled as an extraneous variable. Private patients might be more motivated in therapy because they pay more for services rendered by the private clinic than do those patients in the public clinic. On the other hand, less affluent patients in a public clinic might be more motivated because they were striving to achieve better financial conditions and believed that better communication would help them to obtain better jobs. The effects of these possible threats to internal validity as a result of differential selection of subjects are unknown. In addition, interaction of subject selection and other factors such as history, maturation, or mortality could also jeopardize internal validity.

Even though this design represents an obvious improvement over the previous three designs, it is not as strong in either internal or external validity as the designs in the next section. Unfortunately, the nonequivalent control-group design will probably find continued use in the literature because of its convenience, and readers should, therefore, be aware of the limitations inherent in this design.

Stronger Designs

Now that we have examined the pitfalls of some weak designs for studying treatment efficacy, let us turn to the evaluation of stronger designs that illustrate some methods of reducing threats to internal and external validity.

Randomized Pretest–Posttest Control-Group Designs

Campbell and Stanley (1966) have outlined designs that include steps to ensure that (1) experimental and control groups are equivalent at the outset and (2) experimental and control groups are tested at equivalent time intervals to reduce threats to internal validity arising from factors such as maturation or regression.

The basic randomized pretest–posttest control-group design may be diagrammed as follows:

$$R \quad O_1 \quad X \quad O_2$$
$$R \quad O_3 \qquad O_4$$

In this mixed design, two groups are formed by randomly assigning half of the subjects to the experimental group and half to the control group. Both groups are pretested and posttested in the same manner at the same times. The factors that could jeopardize internal validity are well controlled in this design as the following discussion indicates.

History should be controlled because general historical events should theoretically have as much effect on the $O_1 - O_2$ difference as it does on the $O_3 - O_4$ difference because the groups are randomly assembled at the same time. There may be the possibility, however, of specific historical events differentially affecting one group and not the other (e.g., subjects in the experimental group meet for coffee between experimental sessions and influence each other's attitudes toward the experiment). Careful monitoring of such events can often preclude their threats to internal validity. Maturation and pretesting effects should be equivalent in both groups and affect the O_2 and O_4 scores by approximately the same amounts if randomization is used. Regression is not a threat, even if both groups have extreme scores on the pretest because both groups should evidence the same amount of regression as a result of random assignment. Differential subject selection is controlled because the groups have been randomly assembled and, therefore, extraneous variables should be randomly distributed among the subjects.

Attention must be paid to instrumentation and mortality, of course. Instrumentation problems would be minimized if careful calibration of equipment is achieved and if human observers are carefully employed by the researcher to preclude bias in their use of measurements. If mortality exists in any experiment, it poses a threat to internal validity. In this design, mortality should not generally affect one group more than the other because it should be present to the same extent in both groups if it is related to any extraneous variable (e.g., motivation). If, however, the researcher should note that the mortality rate is high or, perhaps, that it is unevenly distributed between groups, he or she should undertake a replication of the experiment and also try to determine if any subject characteristics are related to mortality. Whenever mortality rates are high or unevenly distributed among groups in this or any research design, a serious threat may be posed to internal validity. But differential mortality is much less likely to occur with random assignment to experimental and control groups because the potential for attrition is randomly distributed.

In general, then, this design is strong in internal validity. There are also several variations on the randomized pretest–posttest control group design that may be considered. For example, matching may be used in conjunction with randomization to assemble the groups if there are certain extraneous variables that experimenters know should be controlled. The experimental and control groups would be formed by matching pairs of subjects on the known extraneous variables and, then, randomly assigning one member of each pair to the experimental group and the other member to the control group. Such a design could be diagrammed as follows:

$$\text{MR} \quad O_1 \quad X \quad O_2$$
$$\text{MR} \quad O_3 \quad\quad O_4$$

The matching would equate pair members on extraneous variables known to be correlated with the dependent variable, and the random assignment of pair members to experimental and control groups should ensure that overlooked extraneous variables would be randomly distributed.

The randomized control-group design has been conceptualized by some researchers as a mixed design with a between-subjects independent variable (experimental vs. control groups) and a within-subjects independent variable (pretesting vs. posttesting). In this case, the *score* on whatever behavior is tested in the pretests and posttests would be the dependent variable. It has also been suggested (Campbell & Stanley, 1966) that the *gain in score* from pretest to posttest be considered the dependent variable. In that case, the *gain* of the control group would be compared to the *gain* of the experimental group and the experiment could be considered a simple bivalent experiment with just a between-subjects comparison of the control-group gain to the experimental-group gain as an index of the effectiveness of treatment. The bivalent independent variable is treatment and assumes two values: presence vs. absence of treatment (analogous to the presence vs. absence of noise or earmold-venting samples shown in Chapter 2).

Using the pretest-to-posttest gain as the dependent variable, this design could be extended to a multivalent experiment by assembling groups that receive different values or different amounts of the experimental treatment (independent variable). For example, if the treatment involved training a certain behavior, several groups could each receive different amounts of training. Rather than simply comparing practice drills to no practice drills, the experimenter would be able to demonstrate changes in the dependent variable as a function of amount of practice drill. Such a design could be diagrammed as follows:

$$
\begin{array}{llllll}
\text{Group 1} & R & O_1 & X_1 & O_2 \\
\text{Group 2} & R & O_3 & X_2 & O_4 \\
\text{Group 3} & R & O_5 & X_3 & O_6 \\
\text{Group 4} & R & O_7 & & O_8 \\
\end{array}
$$

In this case, Group 1 might receive a certain amount of practice, Group 2 twice as much practice, Group 3 three times as much practice, and Group 4 would receive no practice and serve as the control group.

The design could be extended to a parametric design by studying the effects of two types of practice drills with varying amounts of each. For example, massed practice vs. distributed practice in three different amounts could be studied in the following paradigm:

$$
\begin{array}{llll}
\text{Group 1} & R & O_1 & X_{\text{Massed 1}} & O_2 \\
\text{Group 2} & R & O_3 & X_{\text{Massed 2}} & O_4 \\
\text{Group 3} & R & O_5 & X_{\text{Massed 3}} & O_6 \\
\text{Group 4} & R & O_7 & X_{\text{Distributed 1}} & O_8 \\
\text{Group 5} & R & O_9 & X_{\text{Distributed 2}} & O_{10} \\
\text{Group 6} & R & O_{11} & X_{\text{Distributed 3}} & O_{12} \\
\text{Group 7} & R & O_{13} & & O_{14} \\
\end{array}
$$

The first three groups would receive massed practice, with Group 1 receiving a certain amount, Group 2 twice as much, and Group 3 three times as much. Groups 4 through 6 would receive distributed practice, with Group 4 receiving the same amount of practice as Group 1 did, Group 5 receiving twice as much, and Group 6 receiving three times as much. Group 7 would receive no practice and would act as the control group. These designs may be expensive and difficult to administer, but they can be worth the effort because of the advantages of multivalent and parametric experiments discussed in Chapter 2.

Although these equivalent pretest–posttest control-group designs are strong in internal validity, there are some restrictions on their external validity, mainly because of the interactions of some jeopardizing factors with the experimental treatment. The first problem with external validity involves the interaction of subject selection with the experimental variable. Although the simple main effect of subject selection as a threat to internal validity is minimized by random assignment of subjects to the experimental and control groups, it is possible that any demonstrated treatment effect may be valid only for the particular type of subjects studied in the investigation. For example, the results of a treatment study done with adult, male, college students who stutter attending a university clinic may be generalizable only to persons who stutter and are males, adults, college students, and attending a university clinic. Attempts to generalize to females, to children, to persons with less than a college education, or to persons attending other types of clinics may be unwarranted. Successful experiments in language treatment with mentally retarded children may not be generalizable to deaf or cerebral-palsied children. There is no guarantee, then, that generalization across subjects who are different from those studied in the original experiment will be valid. This does not mean that generalization never occurs; it simply means that it cannot be assumed until it has been proven. The possibility of the interaction of subject selection and the experimental treatment *limits* the generalizability to subjects who are equivalent to those in the original study until subsequent research demonstrates broader generalizability of the results.

One way to overcome this limitation and thereby extend generalization across subjects is to perform replications with other types of subjects. Replication of the experiment with different types of subjects would help to delineate the extent to which subject selection and the experimental treatment interacted by demonstrating the relative effectiveness of the treatment with various types of subjects.

Readers should recognize that such replication could be considered a combination of descriptive and experimental research because the experimental treatment would be manipulated by the researcher but the subject classification would not. The experiment would be replicated with subjects who differed in some classification variables such as age, gender, socioeconomic status, or type of pathology.

Such a replication of a randomized pretest–posttest control-group design could be diagrammed as follows:

$$
\begin{array}{llll}
\textit{Initial experiment:} & R & O_1 \quad X \quad O_2 \\
\textit{Adults} & R & O_3 \qquad\quad O_4 \\
\textit{Replication:} & R & O_5 \quad X \quad O_6 \\
\textit{Children} & R & O_7 \qquad\quad O_8
\end{array}
$$

In such a replication, the $O_1 - O_2$ difference would be compared with the $O_3 - O_4$ difference in the first experiment to examine the effect of the experimental treatment for the adult subjects. The replication with children would then be run and the $O_5 - O_6$ difference compared to the $O_7 - O_8$ difference to examine the effect of the experimental treatment for the children. The replication would then be compared with the initial experiment to see whether the same effect that was obtained with the adults could be generalized to children. Such systematic replication is the most promising method of reducing the threat to external validity posed by the interaction of subject selection and the experimental treatment. Otherwise, experimental results remain applicable only to subjects with essentially the same characteristics as those who participated in the original investigation.

A second threat to the external validity of the preceding designs is posed by the reactive effect of experimental arrangements. Experiments are usually novel events in the lives of subjects who participate in them, and experimental settings or situations are usually somewhat artificial. Subjects are often aware that they are participating in experiments, and they may differ in their attempts to discern the purpose of the experiment and in their conclusions regarding what the purpose is. The Hawthorne effect has always been thought to operate in experiments on human subjects as a threat to external validity. Government agencies now insist on protection of the rights of experimental subjects, and researchers must obtain informed consent from subjects before the experiment begins. Even if subjects agree to wait until after the experiment to be informed of its true purpose, they may have a preconceived notion of the purpose of the experiment and behave according to what they think the experimenter wants them to do (or does *not* want them to do).

In many cases, it is not possible to control such reactive arrangements entirely, but they may be somewhat attenuated. For example, some studies may compare a placebo group to both the experimental and control groups to examine the effect of the suggestion to subjects that they are participating in an experiment. If the placebo group shows more improvement than the control group, a reactive arrangement may have accentuated improvement in the experimental group. Reactive arrangements are probably present in most experiments to the extent that subjects behave differently than they would if they did not know or believe they were in an experiment and the degree to which the experimental setting can be made more "natural" is important in reducing this threat to external validity. Systematic replication of the experiment in more "natural" settings may also help to extend the generalization of the results.

Still a third threat to external validity of the designs we have discussed so far is the interaction of pretesting with the experimental variable. It is possible that the pretest itself may sensitize the subjects to the possible effects that could be caused by the independent variable and make them more likely to show improvement. If the pretest sensitizes subjects to respond more to the experimental variable than would subjects who were not pretested, then the results cannot be generalized to subjects who have not had the same pretest. If the experimenter wishes to generalize only to subjects who will always have the same pretest, there is little problem with this factor. But suppose that someone in another clinic that does not use the same pretest wishes to use the treatment of an experiment. Can it be assumed that the same results will obtain without using the same pretest? Such generalization from any of the previous designs cannot be made and only the next design is able to deal with the interaction of pretesting with the experimental treatment.

The Solomon Randomized Four-Group Design

Campbell and Stanley (1966, 24–25) have discussed a design first used by Solomon in 1949 that is not only strong in internal validity but also makes a successful attempt to control one factor affecting external validity—the interaction between pretesting and the experimental treatment. The Solomon Randomized Four-Group Design may be diagrammed as follows:

$$
\begin{array}{lllll}
\text{Group 1} & \text{R} & O_1 & \text{X} & O_2 \\
\text{Group 2} & \text{R} & O_3 & & O_4 \\
\text{Group 3} & \text{R} & & \text{X} & O_5 \\
\text{Group 4} & \text{R} & & & O_6 \\
\end{array}
$$

In the Solomon design, the subjects are randomly assigned to one of four groups. Group 1 receives the pretest, the experimental treatment, and the posttest. Group 2 is pretested, is *not* exposed to the experimental treatment, and is posttested (i.e., Group 2 acts as a traditional control group). Group 3 is *not* pretested, *does* receive the experimental treatment, and *is* posttested. Group 4 is *not* pretested, is *not* exposed to the experimental treatment, but is posttested. Because this design is an extension of the randomized pretest–posttest control-group design, comparison of Groups 1 and 2 is used to show the effect of the experimental treatment and has the same internal validity as the randomized pretest–posttest control-group design. In addition, by paralleling Groups 1 and 2 with

Groups 3 and 4 (groups that are not pretested), the interaction of pretesting and the experimental treatment can be evaluated.

The statistical analysis of the results of the pretests and posttests of a Solomon design is complex and controversial because of the asymmetry caused by removing the pretest for Groups 3 and 4. It is assumed that randomization should have resulted in essentially equivalent pretest scores (or *potential* pretest scores for the unpretested groups). Campbell and Stanley (1966, p. 25) suggest examining posttest scores only. Comparing the average scores on O_2 and O_5 to the average scores on O_4 and O_6 gives an index of the effectiveness of treatment. Comparing the average scores on O_2 and O_4 to the average scores on O_5 and O_6 gives an index of the influence of the pretest as a threat to internal validity. Comparing all four scores will indicate whether there is an interaction between the pretest and the experimental treatment that threatens external validity. If the $O_2 - O_4$ difference is greater than the $O_5 - O_6$ difference, this would indicate that pretesting interacted with the experimental treatment, thereby precluding generalization to unpretested groups.

The Solomon design has been used in a number of investigations in educational psychology and it was recently used in an investigation of self-assessed sign language skills among beginning signers (Lodge-Miller and Elfenbein 1994). We hope that the Solomon design will find more application in the communicative disorders literature in the near future because it will pay off handsomely in improving treatment research.

Time-Series Designs

A great deal of interest in the use of time-series designs in treatment efficacy research has developed in recent years. Rather than using a single pretest and a single posttest with a large number of subjects, time-series designs employ repeated measurements of the dependent variable over an extended period of time with a single subject or a small number of subjects. The designs have found wide application in behavior modification research, and a number of examples of these designs can now be found in the communicative disorders literature.

Our interest here is in describing some of the basic principles in the design of time-series experiments for studying treatment efficacy. General discussions of the application of behavioral principles in communication disorders are provided by Brookshire (1967), Sloane and MacAulay (1968), Girardeau and Spradlin (1970), Lloyd (1976), Starkweather (1983), Ingham (1984), McReynolds and Kearns (1983), and Gow and Ingham (1992).

In describing the time-series design as a quasi-experiment, Campbell and Stanley (1966, p. 37) stated:

> *The essence of the time-series design is the presence of a periodic measurement process on some group or individual and the introduction of an experimental change into this time series of measurements, the results of which are indicated by a discontinuity in the measurements recorded in the time series.*

The simplest time-series design is the AB design, which may be diagrammed as follows:

$$\underbrace{O_1 \quad O_2 \quad O_3 \quad O_4}_{\text{A segment}} \quad X \quad \underbrace{O_5 \quad O_6 \quad O_7 \quad O_8}_{\text{B segment}}$$

In this design, repeated measurements of the dependent variable are made in the A segment ("baseline") before the experimental treatment is introduced. In the B segment ("experimental segment"), the experimental treatment is introduced and several more repeated measurements of the dependent variable are made. This is a within-subjects design because all subjects participate in two conditions—baseline and experimental segments. Comparison of a subject's performance in the baseline with his or her performance in the experimental segment indicates the effect of the experimental treatment on the dependent variable.

This design has many strengths. It also has a few weaknesses that may be overcome with simple modifications. The strengths center on the fact that the repeated measurements of the dependent variable in the baseline provide relatively good control over the threats to internal validity posed by maturation, pretesting, regression, and instrumentation. In a sense, the subjects act as their own control group during the A (or baseline) segment of the design because the experimenter can examine their performances on the repeated measurements without an experimental intervention. If these baseline data are stable, maturation, pretesting, regression, and instrumentation should not threaten internal validity. Although this time-series design may appear, on the surface, to be similar to the one-group pretest–posttest design, the repeated measurements in the baseline make it a substantially stronger design by reducing these threats to internal validity.

The AB time-series design, however, does have a few weaknesses that merit attention. Even with a stable baseline, history may pose a threat because a historical event that does not occur during baseline but that does occur during the experimental segment may compete with the experimental treatment in affecting the dependent variable. Maturation could also pose a possible threat because it may not always start to affect performance at the outset of the A segment and progress in a linear fashion throughout the course of the experiment. Delayed maturation could, perhaps, begin toward the initiation of the B segment and mimic the effect of the experimental treatment on the independent variable.

Campbell and Stanley (1966) have suggested that the addition of control subjects to a time-series design is one possible method for improving its internal validity. An AB randomized control-subjects design may be diagrammed as follows:

$$R \quad O_1 \quad O_2 \quad O_3 \quad O_4 \quad X \quad O_5 \quad O_6 \quad O_7 \quad O_8$$
$$R \quad O_9 \quad O_{10} \quad O_{11} \quad O_{12} \qquad O_{13} \quad O_{14} \quad O_{15} \quad O_{16}$$

$$\underbrace{\qquad\qquad} \qquad \underbrace{\qquad\qquad}$$
$$\text{A segments} \qquad\qquad \text{B segments}$$

In this AB randomized control subjects design, subjects would be randomly assigned to participate as experimental and control subjects. This design would now be a mixed design because it has both within-subjects and between-subjects components. The experimental subjects would be observed several times in the baseline (A segment), and the experimental treatment would be applied in conjunction with more repeated measurements of the dependent variable in the B segment. The control subjects would be observed in baseline and also observed during a "pseudo-B segment" with no experimental treatment applied. In essence, they would be observed in two baseline segments. If the experimental subjects showed performance change in the B segment, but the control subjects did not, the possibility of history or delayed maturation affecting the behavior of one group of subjects and not the other would be greatly reduced.

The AB design may also be strengthened by its extension to an ABA design that incorporates another baseline segment after the experimental treatment. As mentioned in Chapter 3, the ABA design is often called a "reversal design" because of the reversal to baseline after completion of the experimental segment. An ABA design may be diagrammed as follows:

$$\underbrace{O_1 \quad O_2 \quad O_3 \quad O_4}_{\text{A segment}} \quad \underbrace{X \quad O_5 \quad O_6 \quad O_7 \quad O_8}_{\text{B segment}} \quad \text{(X Removed)} \quad \underbrace{O_9 \quad O_{10} \quad O_{11} \quad O_{12}}_{\text{A segment}}$$

In this design the A segment is followed by the B segment and then another baseline is introduced for observation of the subject's performance without the presence of the experimental treatment. This is a within-subjects design since all subjects participate in all conditions. A reversal design is often used to study a dependent variable that may be temporarily affected by the experimental treatment. If the treatment causes a temporary change in the dependent variable, removal of the treatment should cause performance to return to baseline level. Some dependent variables, on the other hand, are permanently affected by the experimental treatment and do not return to baseline levels in the second A segment. In treatment studies, it is desirable to produce a performance change that is maintained after the experimental treatment is removed so that improved behavior is continued beyond the treatment setting (Hersen & Barlow, 1976). Sometimes multiple-segment time-series designs are employed (e.g., ABABAB, . . . , AB) to study long-term changes in behavior following experimental treatment. Performance on the dependent variable may return to baseline level in the first few reversals and then carry-over effects may be evident in improved performance during subsequent baseline segments. Such multiple-segment designs may be costly or time-consuming, but are worthwhile efforts because short-term ABA studies may often obtain dramatic treatment effects with little or no carryover.

Baseline instability may threaten the internal validity of time-series designs. Instability could be the result of history, maturation, pretesting, regression, or instrumentation problems or of interactions among these factors. Also, the effects of these factors on the dependent variable may not be uniform with time and could, therefore, cause irregularities in the data that may be difficult to interpret. Of course, absolute stability of human behavior in a baseline segment can never be expected, so the real difficulty centers on determining how much variability should be tolerated in the baseline segment.

The external validity of time-series designs is sometimes cited as a problem by exponents of more traditional large-sample designs because of the small number of subjects used and the complications that may arise if multiple treatments are applied to subjects. Because time-series designs involve an in-depth analysis of behavior that is quite time-consuming, it is difficult to run them with large numbers of subjects. Critics of time-series designs believe that this may accentuate problems of the interaction of subject selection with the experimental treatment. Direct and systematic replications can often help to alleviate the external validity problem of subject selection. The problem of multiple-treatment interference is best alleviated by replications in which different treatments and treatment combinations are applied to individual subjects to assess their relative effectiveness.

The repeated testing done in time-series designs may be a reactive arrangement (Christensen, 1988) or may accentuate the interaction of pretesting with the experimental treatment, thereby limiting generalization to subjects who would normally undergo such repeated testing. This would not be a serious problem, however, if generalization were limited to subjects who were enrolled in relatively intensive or long-term treatment programs that would incorporate multiple testing as an integral part of treatment.

Time-series designs may be extended to include numerous combinations of experimental treatments and baseline segments that may become quite complicated. Readers who are interested in a more detailed discussion of these designs than could be presented within the limitations of this book are referred to Hersen and Barlow (1976), Cook and Campbell (1979), McReynolds and Kearns (1983), and Kratochwill and Levin (1992) for reviews of various time-series designs and comparisons of the relative merits of time-series and traditional experimental designs.

Meta-Analysis of Treatment Efficacy Research

In recent years, interest has developed in the possibilities for comparing treatment efficacy across various studies that have been published. The technique of cumulating research findings across various studies is called *meta-analysis* (Hunter, Schmidt, & Jackson, 1982), and it has been applied to a number of different kinds of research, including studies of treatment efficacy. In explaining the rationale for meta-analysis, Hunter et al. (1982, 26–27) stated:

> *What is needed are methods that will integrate results from existing studies to reveal patterns of relatively invariant underlying relations and causalities, the establishment of which will constitute general principles and cumulative knowledge. . . . At one time in the history of psychology and the social sciences, the pressing need was for more empirical studies examining the problem in question. In many areas of research, the need today is not additional empirical data but some means of making sense of the vast amounts of data that have accumulated. Given the increasing number of areas within psychology and the other social sciences in which the number of available studies is quite large and the importance to theory development and practical problem solving of integrating conflicting findings to establish general knowledge, it is likely that methods for doing this will attain increasing importance in the future.*

Hunter et al. (1982) have reviewed several different methods of meta-analysis, ranging from narrative review of studies to complex statistical comparison of the results of different studies that incorporate analyses of study characteristics, statistical corrections for factors such as test reliability, and weighting of the results of various studies according to their sample sizes. One important technique in meta-analysis of treatment studies is the evaluation of *effect size,* a method of standardizing across studies the measurement of the amount of pretreatment to posttreatment improvement. Effect size is often measured as the average pre–post difference in a dependent variable divided by the standard deviation of the pretreatment scores on the dependent variable. Calculating effect size in this way results in a reasonably comparable measure of improvement for all the studies that are compared. An effect size of zero indicates no improvement. An effect size of one indicates that the average of the posttest scores was one standard deviation higher than the average of the pretest scores. An effect size of two shows that the average posttest score increased two standard deviations above the average score on the dependent variable before therapy. In other words, the effect size allows the improvement results of all the studies to be expressed as a standard deviation relative to the pretreatment results.

Andrews, Guitar, and Howie (1980) published a meta-analysis of studies concerned with the effects of stuttering treatment. They analyzed effect sizes for 116 dependent variables that had been examined in forty-two studies of stuttering treatment that had included a total of 756 stutterers as subjects. The overall mean effect size for the 116 dependent variables was 1.3, indicating that stutterers had improved by 1.3 standard deviations relative to pretreatment measures on the average. Prolonged speech and gentle onset were the two treatment techniques that emerged with the best effect sizes from the meta-analysis.

There are a number of methodological problems in meta-analysis that must be assessed. First, there is the manner in which the author selects the studies for inclusion in the meta-analysis. Consideration must be given to factors such as the author's attempts to judge the internal and external validity of the original studies, the sample sizes used in the studies, whether the studies were published in refereed journals or in less-selective media, and the types of dependent variables used to measure improvement. Second, there are complex statistical issues that must be dealt with in trying to weigh the equivalence of different studies. Consideration must also be given to different study characteristics such as sample size, method of measurement of dependent variables, kinds of statistics used to report results, type and length of treatments, and selection criteria for including subjects in the studies. Hunter et al. (1982) have given extensive attention to a number of these and other problems in meta-analysis and provided an extensive bibliography of material relevant to meta-analysis. Andrews et al. (1980) have discussed some of these issues in relation to research on treatment efficacy in communicative disorders.

Ethics of Using Control Groups in Treatment Efficacy Research

In concluding this discussion of research designs for studying treatment efficacy, some comments are in order on the ethics of using control groups in therapy research. Some professionals have serious reservations about the ethics of withholding treatment from persons with speech, language, or hearing problems, whereas other professionals believe that control groups should be used to confirm treatment efficacy.

An exchange of letters in the *Journal of Speech and Hearing Disorders* illustrates this controversy. Kushnirecky and Weber (1978, p. 106), in commenting on the validity of evidence in a study of treatment efficacy stated:

> *Since matched control subjects were not used, the data have limited interpretive value. It is possible that a control group may have shown that these children may have improved without intervention. Even if the children's rate of gain of language*

development equaled that of nonlanguage-delayed children, in the absence of controls, any conclusions concerning the effectiveness of the method are at best conjectures.

Lee, Koenigsnecht, and Mulhern (1978, p. 107–108) replied that, in their opinion, the use of control groups:

is impossible on ethical grounds. Kushnirecky and Weber should be strongly advised not to embark on research that withholds treatment from children who need it. . . . It would be unconscionable to withhold clinical training for any period of time from any child who needs it and would be likely to gain from it. This precludes designs in which one group of children receives treatment while treatment is withheld from a comparable group in order to show that the treatment produced results.

An editor's note appended to these two letters indicated that communicative disorders specialists have an ethical obligation to provide treatment when possible but that they also have an ethical obligation to provide treatment that rests on "sound evidence" of its effectiveness. The editor's note also pointed out that control does not always mean withholding of treatment to a control group, as control can sometimes be accomplished with the use of multiple baselines (as in our discussion of time-series designs earlier in this chapter).

The major point illustrated by this exchange of letters is that a potential conflict of interest exists in our ethical obligations both to provide treatment and to demonstrate treatment efficacy when the latter obligation may sometimes require the withholding of treatment to a control group. This is a difficult argument to settle, but there are compromises available for its possible resolution.

The use of time-series designs is one obvious approach, and its potential for resolving this problem may be one of the reasons for the increased use of the time-series designs in recent years. Another possible solution lies in the use of waiting lists for construction of control groups. Many clinics have large case loads; therefore, staff clinicians often cannot accommodate all applicants immediately. Applicants for treatment could be randomly assigned to immediate treatment or to the waiting list and all applicants could be pretested at the time of application for treatment. At the end of the experiment, then, the control group on the waiting list could be used as the new experimental group in a direct or systematic replication of the study. This would be especially suitable when the experimental treatment can be accomplished in a relatively short time.

Despite these potential compromises, the issue of the ethics of withholding treatment from a control group remains controversial in a number of disciplines. Many professional and popular articles that have appeared in a number of journals and newspapers in recent years have presented a variety of opinions on these ethical issues. Cook and Campbell (1979) have discussed ethical concerns in withholding treatment from control groups and Hersen and Barlow (1976) have discussed ethical considerations in time-series designs. Readers who are interested in a more detailed discussion of these issues should consult the symposium on ethics and statistics in medical research that was published in the 18 November 1977 issue of *Science.* The whole topic of ethical responsibility in human research is controversial and widely written about; we expect that it will be some time before many of these issues are resolved to the satisfaction of the public and the professions alike.

Protection of Human Subjects in Research

A broader issue than the ethics of using control groups in treatment research also needs to be addressed: the protection of human subjects who participate in any research studies in communicative disorders. In recent decades,the scientific community and various governmental agencies have taken steps to safeguard the rights of human subjects participating in any kind of research. Past abuse of human research subjects is one reason for this concern, but even in the absence of actual abuse of human subjects, researchers and consumers of research need to be aware of the potential for physical or psychological harm to human subjects and of the need to protect the dignity and privacy of research participants. Maloney (1984) has provided a detailed account of the federal laws and regulations regarding the protection of human subjects in research.

The issue of protection of research subjects is complex, and federal regulations have been established to provide safeguards for human research subjects. These regulations are quite detailed, and a comprehensive coverage of them goes beyond the scope of this text. The consumer of research, however, should be aware of the general history of these regulations and how they are applied to human subjects in communicative disorders research.

The National Research Act of 1974 (Public Law 93-348) created the National Commission for the Protection of Human Subjects in Biomedical and Behavioral Research. This commission was given the responsibility to develop the basic principles that should underlie subject protection in biomedical and behavioral research and the methods to ensure compliance with those principles. After seven years of development, the final code of federal regulations was published in the *Federal Register* in 1981 under the title "Protection of Human Subjects," Title 45, Code of Federal Regulations, Part 46.

Since their introduction in 1981, the federal regulations for protection of human research subjects have undergone several revisions. For example, in 1983, Subpart D was added to the code, extending protection for children used in research, and in 1991 Subpart A of the code was amended to include all government agencies that conduct or sponsor research. This latter addition is known as the "Final Common Rule for Protection of Human Subjects." Also, on a regular basis the Office for Protection From Research Risks (OPRR), a division of the Department of Health and Human Services, issues recommendations to institutions conducting research that need to be considered in conjunction with the federal code of regulations.

The local Institutional Review Board (IRB) is the major component of the federal regulations for protection of human research subjects. Members of a local IRB are appointed by top officials of the administration at the institution. IRBs at institutions such as universities, hospitals, or school districts applying for federal research funding must provide written assurance that they will comply with the regulations. Federal funding will not be granted without these assurances. Each IRB must have a minimum of five members, and federal regulations require that one person on the board must have a nonscientific background (e.g., lawyers or members of the clergy) and one person must not be affiliated with the institution.

Local IRBs can reject research proposals if the potential benefits of the study in relation to the potential risks to the subject are great. IRBs must also ensure that potential subjects have been adequately informed about their participation in the study and that the subjects have signed informed consent documents. The informed consent document must include (a) statements about the purpose of the study, (b) description of potential benefits and risks to the subject, (c) disclosures of alternate procedures or treatments, if any, and (d) statements regarding how subject confidentiality will be maintained.

Interested consumers of research can obtain the current federal regulations by contacting National Institutes of Health, Office for Protection from Research Risks, 6100 Executive Boulevard, MSC 7507, Rockville, MD 20892-7507. In addition, animals are sometimes used in research that relates to communicative disorders and strict federal regulations govern the use of these animals. The current regulations for the humane care and use of laboratory animals can also be obtained by contacting OPPR at the given address. Finally, Metz and Folkins (1985) have provided an in depth review of the federal regulations for protection of human research subjects as they relate specifically to communicative disorders research.

Study Questions

1. Read the following article:

   Boberg, E., & Kully, D. (1994). Long-term results of an intensive treatment program for adults and adolescents who stutter. *Journal of Speech and Hearing Research, 37,* 1050–1059.

   a. What measures were taken to strengthen the potential internal validity threat of instrumentation?

   b. To what groups could you generalize these findings?

2. Discuss the reasons for the following points made by Campbell and Stanley (1966):

   a. efforts to increase internal validity may jeopardize external validity and vice versa;

   b. internal validity is the *sine qua non* of research; and

   c. the question of external validity can never be completely answered.

3. Read the following article:

   Brookshire, R. H. (1983). Subject description and the generality of results in experiments with aphasic adults. *Journal of Speech and Hearing Disorders, 48,* 342–346.

   What subject characteristics did Brookshire suggest should be reported in experiments with aphasics in order to determine the population to which results can be generalized?

4. Read the following article:

   Kelly, J. F., & Whitehead, R. L. (1983). Integrated spoken and written English instruction for the hearing impaired student. *Journal of Speech and Hearing Disorders, 48,* 415–422.

   a. What factors could jeopardize the internal validity of this kind of treatment study?

   b. What steps did the authors take to try to strengthen internal validity?

5. Read the following article:

   Yoder, P., & Davies, B. (1990). Do parental questions and topic continuations elicit replies from developmentally delayed children? A sequential analysis. *Journal of Speech and Hearing Research, 33,* 563–573.

   What are the authors' cautions regarding the generalizability of their findings?

6. Read the following article:

Lodge-Miller, K. A., & Elfenbein, J. L. (1994). Beginning signers' self-assessment of sign language skills. *Journal of Communication Disorders, 27,* 281–292.

a. What internal validity threats do the authors claim are controlled by the Solomon Randomized Four-Group Design?

b. How does the design also control external validity threats?

7. Read the following article:

Grievink, E., Peters, S., van Bon, W., & Schilder, A. (1993). The effects of early bilateral otitis media with effusion on language ability: A prospective cohort study. *Journal of Speech and Hearing Research, 36,* 1004–1012.

a. Is there a potential mortality problem in this study?

b. Explain your answer.

8. Read the following article:

Andrews, G., & Harvey, R. (1981). Regression to the mean in pretreatment measures of stuttering. *Journal of Speech and Hearing Disorders, 46,* 204–207.

Summarize Andrews and Harvey's findings regarding regression to the mean in stuttering measures and identify their implications for the design of stuttering treatment experiments.

References

Andrews, G., Guitar, B., & Howie, P. (1980). Meta-analysis of the effects of stuttering treatment. *Journal of Speech and Hearing Disorders, 45,* 287–387.

Bordens, K. S., & Abbott, B. B. (1988). *Research design and methods: A process approach.* Mountain View, CA: Mayfield Publishing Company.

Bracht, G. H., & Glass, G. V. (1968). The external validity of experiments. *American Educational Research Journal, 5,* 437–474.

Brookshire, R. H. (1967). Speech pathology and the experimental analysis of behavior. *Journal of Speech and Hearing Disorders, 32,* 215–227.

Brookshire, R. H. (1983). Subject description and generality of results in experiments with aphasic adults. *Journal of Speech and Hearing Disorders, 48,* 342–346.

Campbell, D. T., & Stanley, J. C. (1966). *Experimental and quasi-experimental designs for research.* Chicago, IL: Rand McNally.

Christensen, L. B. (1988). *Experimental methodology* (4th Ed.). Boston, MA: Allyn & Bacon.

Cook, T. D., & Campbell, D. T. (1979). *Quasi-experimentation.* Chicago, IL: Rand McNally.

Girardeau, F. L., & Spradlin, J. E. (1970). *A functional analysis approach to speech and language.* (ASHA Monograph No. 14). Washington, DC: American Speech-Language-Hearing Association.

Gow, M. L., & Ingham, R. J. (1992). Modifying electroglottograph-identified intervals of phonation: The effect on stuttering. *Journal of Speech and Hearing Research, 35,* 495–511.

Hersen, M., & Barlow, D. H. (1976). *Single case experimental designs: Strategies for studying behavior change.* New York: Pergamon.

Huck, S. W., Cormier, W. H., & Bounds, W. G. (1974). *Reading statistics and research.* New York: Harper & Row.

Hunter, J. E., Schmidt, F. L., & Jackson, G. B., (1982). *Meta-analysis: Cumulating research findings across studies.* Beverly Hills, CA: Sage Publications.

Ingham, R. J., (1984). *Stuttering and behavior therapy.* San Diego, CA: College Hill Press.

Isaac, S., & Michael, W. B. (1971). *Handbook in research and evaluation.* San Diego, CA: Edits.

Kratochwill, T. R., & Levin, J. R. (1992). *Single-case research design and analysis: New directions for psychology and education.* Hillsdale, NJ: Lawrence Erlbaum Associates.

Kushnirecky, W., & Weber, J. (1978). Comment on Lee's reply to Simon. *Journal of Speech and Hearing Disorders, 43,* 106–107.

Lee, L. L., Koenigsnecht, R. A., & Mulhern, S. T. (1978). Reply to Kushnirecky and Weber. *Journal of Speech and Hearing Disorders, 43,* 107–108.

Levine, S., & Elzey, F. F. (1976). *A programmed introduction to research.* Belmont, CA: Wadsworth.

Lloyd, L. L. (Ed.). (1976). *Communication assessment and intervention strategies.* Baltimore, MD: University Park Press.

Lodge-Miller, K. A., & Elfenbein, J. L. (1994). Beginning signers' self-assessment of sign language skills. *Journal of Communication Disorders, 27,* 281–292.

Maloney, D. M. (1984). *Protection of human research subjects: A practical guide to federal laws and regulations.* New York: Plenum Press.

McReynolds, L. V., & Kearns, K. P. (1983). *Single-subject experimental designs in communicative disorders.* Baltimore, MD: University Park Press.

Metz, D. E., & Folkins, J. W. (1985). Protection of human subjects in speech and hearing research. *Asha, 27,* 25–29.

Montgomery, A. A. (1994). Treatment efficacy in adult audiological rehabilitation. *Journal of the Academy of Rehabilitative Audiology, 27,* 317–336.

Olswang, L. B., Thompson, C. K., Warren, S. F., & Minghetti, N. J. (Eds.) (1990). *Treatment Efficacy in Communication Disorders.* Rockville Pike, MD: American Speech-Language-Hearing Foundation.

Parsons, H. M. (1974). What happened at Hawthorne? *Science, 183,* 922–932.

Pedhazur, E. J., & Schmelkin, L. P. (1991). *Measurement, design and analysis: An integrated approach.* Hillsdale, NJ: Lawrence Erlbaum Associates.

Proceedings of the NIDCD workshop on treatment efficacy research in stuttering. (1993). *Journal of Fluency Disorders, 18,* 121–361.

Sloane, H. N., & MacAulay, B. D. (Eds.). (1968). *Operant procedures in remedial speech and language training.* Boston, MA: Houghton Mifflin.

Starkweather, C. W. (1983). *Speech and language: Principles and processes of behavior change.* Englewood Cliffs, NJ: Prentice-Hall.

Webb, E. J., Campbell, D. T., Schwartz, R. D., & Sechrest, L. (1966). *Unobtrusive measures: Nonreactive research in the social sciences.* Chicago, IL: Rand McNally.

Chapter *6*

Organization and Analysis of Data

The purpose of this chapter is to describe some basic terms, concepts, and procedures used in the organization and analysis of data derived from communicative disorders research. Our intention is to explain some basic considerations that will help consumers of research to understand the meaning of research results. This chapter will *not* be concerned with extensive details about derivations, formulae, calculations, or other aspects of data analysis that are necessary for the producer of research. For more detailed treatments of statistical methods, consumers are referred to statistical textbooks such as those by Ferguson and Takane (1989), Guilford (1965), Hays (1973), Kirk (1990), Pedhazur and Schmelkin (1991), or Siegel (1956) included in the reference list at the end of this chapter. Also, readers are reminded that Chapter 9 provides many examples of data organization and analysis that have been excerpted from communicative disorders research articles.

Data organization and analysis techniques are statistical tools that assist the researcher in drawing conclusions and making inferences from a study. Experimental and descriptive studies both employ data organization or analysis procedures to aid in answering research questions by indicating how plausible certain conclusions are in light of the obtained data. Because many of the same statistical techniques may be used to analyze either experimental or descriptive data, the type of data organization or analysis used does not indicate whether a study is experimental or descriptive.

The organization and analysis techniques for empirical research are commonly referred to as *statistics* because they are derived from a branch of mathematics by that name. However, the term *statistics* also refers to the numeric descriptors of a *sample,* as opposed to the companion term *parameter,* which refers to the numeric descriptors of the *population* from which a sample is drawn. In this usage, then, the term *statistics* may be defined as computed estimates of parameters because it is only rarely that an entire population can be studied directly.

To illustrate, suppose that we wished to know the average number of articulation errors made by children at age five years. The average number of errors made by all five-year-old children (i.e., the population of interest) would be a parameter. We could never test all of the five-year-olds who speak English to get a direct measure of this population characteristic. So, we would select a sample of five-year-old speakers of English, say two hundred, and determine their average number of articulation errors. The average number of articulation errors made by this sample of five-year-olds would be a statistic and could be used in estimating the parameter. In other words, a statistic is a number describing a sample characteristic, and a parameter is a number describing a population characteristic.

Data Organization

Completion of data collection results in the amassing of a body of *raw* data. These unprocessed data have not been arranged or organized for viewing. The data need to be organized so that they can be interpreted in regard to the structure of the research design.

Data Distributions

Whenever measures on one or more variables are obtained in a research study, the obtained values form a *distribution.* The distribution is the frequency count of attributes of objects or events that fall into different categories for a nominal level measurement or the arrangement of relative attribute values in a rank order for an ordinal level measurement. For interval or ratio level measurements, the distribution will include a listing of the number of cases that occurred at each score value on the interval or ratio level measurement. The distributions of nominal and ordinal level measurements are relatively straightforward and usually are demonstrated in a table or figure that shows the category frequencies or the relative rankings. However, the distributions of interval and ratio level measurements often require more attention to determine their characteristics. Most of the following discussion, then, will concern the distribution of interval and ratio level measurements; for the most part, the issues in describing the distributions of interval and ratio level measurements are the same.

The distributions of interval and ratio level measurements have four characteristics that are usually described: *central tendency, variability, skewness,* and *kurtosis.* Before proceeding with the analysis of research results, the researcher usually ascertains these characteristics and presents information on at least the first two so that readers may examine the organized data to see the overall pattern of results. There are two ways to provide this information that we will discuss in the next two sections: (1) through graphic or tabular presentation and (2) through calculation of summary statistics.

Tabular and Graphic Presentation

Many researchers present the distribution of data in the form of a table or a figure for inspection before performing further data analysis. Tabular or graphic presentations have the advantage of showing the overall contour of the distribution so that the four characteristics of the distribution can be seen visually. Frequency tables, histograms, polygons, and cumulative frequency distributions are some of the more common means of tabular and graphic presentations.

To illustrate some of these basic data-organization techniques, a set of hypothetical data is shown in Table 6.1. The data for eighty subjects are first presented in raw form, just as they might appear in the researcher's notes. The data are then *grouped* in a frequency table so that, for each score value, the number of cases obtaining that score is shown in the frequency (*f*) column. The cumulative frequency (cum *f*) column shows, for each score value, the number of cases that obtained scores *at* or *below* that value. Thus, looking at the score of six, we note that sixteen subjects received scores of six and forty-nine subjects received scores at or below six.

In some instances, when the researcher is working with a fairly small number of values and wishes to keep individual subject data on a number of variables together, the use of *ungrouped* data is feasible. This type of organization would simply show the score values listed in order rather than showing the *f* and cum *f* columns. In addition, the mechanics of calculating some of the indices to be shown later would be altered somewhat from the examples given in this chapter.

Figure 6.1 shows how this hypothetical set of scores can be presented graphically. Figure 6.1*a* shows a histogram, or bar graph, of the scores. Note that the midpoint of each bar is directly above the score value on the horizontal axis of the graph. If we were to take these midpoints, record them on a graph, and connect these points with straight lines, the results would be the frequency polygon shown in Figure 6.1*b*. Figure 6.1*c* shows a cumulative frequency polygon. This is a graphic representation of the cumulative frequency (cum *f*) column rather than the frequency (*f*) column in Table 6.1. One distinctive characteristic of cumulative frequency polygons is that the graph is always ascending or stable; it never descends because it always represents the cumulation of scores so far in the distribution. In contrast, the frequency polygon ascends or descends to show the frequency with which cases occur at each possible score point.

TABLE 6.1   Hypothetical Example of Conversion of Raw Scores into a Frequency and Cumulative Frequency Table Using Grouped Data

Raw Scores								Grouped Scores — Score	Frequency — *f*	Cumulative Frequency — cum *f*
4	4	3	6	8	8	2	5	10	5	80
7	9	2	7	4	5	6	6	9	6	75
3	8	3	6	3	4	5	9	8	9	69
6	5	4	1	4	7	8	4	7	11	60
2	4	2	10	1	2	5	3	6	16	49
5	8	6	7	5	6	5	7	5	13	33
7	9	5	7	6	9	5	6	4	8	20
5	6	8	9	8	7	5	5	3	5	12
6	7	6	9	10	6	7	8	2	5	7
6	8	6	7	10	10	10	6	1	2	2
									N = 80	

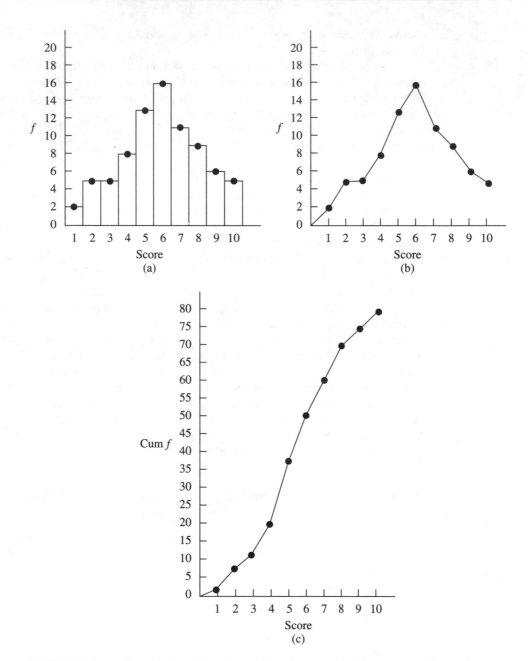

FIGURE 6.1   Graphic Presentation of Test Scores: *(a)* **Histogram of Scores,** *(b)* **Frequency Polygon of Scores,** *(c)* **Cumulative Frequency Polygon**

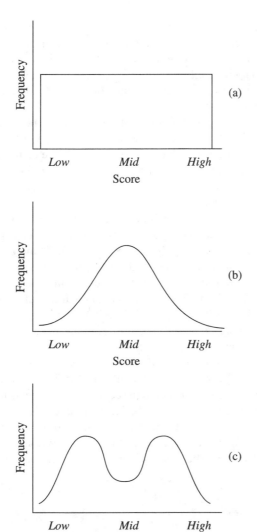

FIGURE 6.2
Three Distributions with Different
Shapes: *(a)* **Rectangular,** *(b)* **Normal,**
(c) **Bimodal**

The overall shape of the distribution and the four characteristics of data distributions listed can be visualized graphically through inspection of figures. Figure 6.2 shows three distributions with different shapes. Figure 6.2*a* is a rectangular-shaped distribution indicating the same frequency of occurrence of each score in the distribution. The distribution shown in Figure 6.2*b* is bell-shaped (the so-called "normal" distribution), indicating the higher frequency of occurrence of middle scores and lower frequency of both higher and lower scores in the distribution. The distribution shown in Figure 6.2*c* is bimodal, indicating two clusterings of high frequency of occurrence of scores within the distribution toward the high and low ends, rather than a single clustering of scores in the middle. The next four figures will graphically illustrate each of the four characteristics of data distributions listed previously.

Figure 6.3 illustrates three distributions with different *central tendencies*. The central tendency, or average, can be seen graphically by examining the concentration of scores toward the middle of the distribution. Figure 6.3*a* is the distribution with the lowest average, Figure 6.3*c* is the distribution with the highest average, and Figure 6.3*b* has an average between the other two. Calculation of various measures of central tendency is shown in Table 6.2 and discussed in the next section.

Figure 6.4 illustrates three distributions with different *variabilities*. The variability, or degree to which the scores spread out from the center of the distribution, can be seen graphically by examining the width of the distribution. Figure 6.4*a* is the distribution with the lowest variability, Figure 6.4*c* has the highest variability, and Figure 6.4*b* has a variability between the other two. Calculation of various measures of variability is shown in Table 6.3 and discussed in the next section.

Figure 6.5 illustrates three distributions with different *skewness*. The skewness, or lack of symmetry of the distribution, can also be visualized graphically by examining the form of the distribution. A symmetrical distribution (Figure 6.5*a*) looks the same on right and left sides; therefore, it is not skewed in one direction or the other. A negatively skewed distribution (Figure 6.5*b*) is one in which most scores cluster around a high value but a small number of scores spread out (or skew) into the very low score end at the left of the distribution. A positively skewed distribution (Figure 6.5*c*) is one in which most scores cluster around a low value but a small number of scores spread out (or skew) into the very high score end at the right of the distribution.

Figure 6.6 illustrates three distributions with different *kurtosis*. The kurtosis, or general form of concentration of scores around the center of the distribution, can be seen graphically by examining the center of the distribution to see if it is flat or peaked in shape. Kurtosis also affects the shape of the bend at the tails of the distribution. Kurtosis is often evaluated relative to the bell-shaped normal distribution (Figure 6.6*a*), which is called *mesokurtic* because of its medium shape between flat and peaked. A *leptokurtic* distribution (Figure 6.6*b*) is more peaked than normal and a *platykurtic* distribution (Figure 6.6*c*) is flatter than normal.

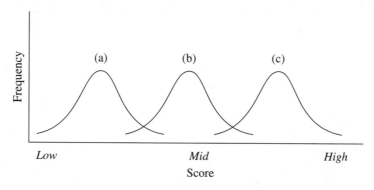

**FIGURE 6.3   Three Distributions with Different Central
Tendencies: *(a)* Low, *(b)* Medium, *(c)* High**

TABLE 6.2   Determining Measures of Central Tendency

Scores				Mean	$= \bar{X} = \dfrac{\Sigma f(X)}{N} = \dfrac{473}{80} = 5.91$
X	f	cum f	fX	Mode	= the most frequently occurring score is 6.0.
10	5	80	50	Median	= The score separating the upper half of the cases ($\frac{1}{2}$ N) from the lower half of the cases.
9	6	75	54		In this instance, it is the point separating the upper 40 cases from the lower 40 cases.
8	9	69	72		
7	11	60	77		
6	16	49	96		
5	13	33	65		Inspection of the cum f column shows that this point is somewhere between a score of 5 and 6.
4	8	20	32		
3	5	12	15		
2	5	7	10		The exact value, by interpolation, is 5.43.
1	2	2	2		
			$\Sigma fX - 473$		

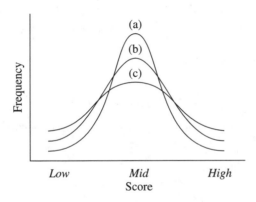

FIGURE 6.4
Three Distributions with Different Variabilities: *(a)* **Low,** *(b)* **Medium,** *(c)* **High**

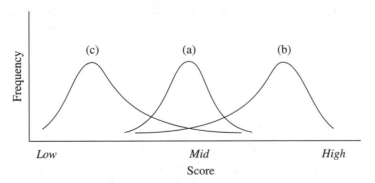

FIGURE 6.5   Three Distributions with Different Skewness:
(a) **Symmetrical,** *(b)* **Negatively Skewed,**
(c) **Positively Skewed**

TABLE 6.3   Determining Measures of Variability

X	f	cum f	fX	$X - \overline{X}$	$(X - \overline{X})^2$	$f(X - \overline{X})^2$
10	5	80	50	+4	16	80
9	6	75	54	+3	9	54
8	9	69	72	+2	4	36
7	11	60	77	+1	1	11
6	16	49	96	0	0	0
5	13	33	65	−1	1	13
4	8	20	32	−2	4	32
3	5	12	15	−3	9	45
2	5	7	10	−4	16	80
1	2	2	2	−5	25	50
			$\Sigma fX = 473$			$\Sigma f(X - \overline{X})^2 = 401$

$\overline{X}$ (from Table 6.2) = 5.91   median = 5.43   mode = 6.0

Statement of range = "the scores ranged from 1 to 10."

$$\text{Standard deviation} = SD = \sigma = \sqrt{\frac{\Sigma f(X - \overline{X})^2}{N}} = \sqrt{\frac{401}{80}}$$

$$= \sqrt{5.01} = 2.23$$

$$\text{Semi-interquartile range} = Q = \frac{P75 - P25}{2}.$$

P75 = (calculation not shown) the point separating the upper 25% of the cases from the lower 75% of the cases. For these data, P75 is 7.0.

P25 = (calculation not shown) the point separating the upper 75% of the cases from the lower 25% of the cases. For these data, P25 is 4.0.

Q = one-half the range of the middle 50% of scores

$$\frac{7.0 - 4.0}{2} = \frac{3.0}{2} = 1.5$$

---

[a]For convenience sake, the mean has been rounded to 6.0 for calculation of the deviation scores $(X - \overline{X})$.

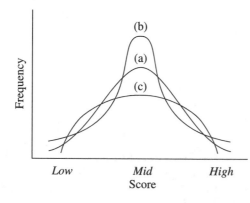

FIGURE 6.6
Three Distributions with Different Kurtosis: *(a)* Normal Mesokurtic, *(b)* Leptokurtic, *(c)* Platykurtic

Summary Statistics

The second way to organize research data is to summarize them in numerical form. Because summary statistics are the foundation on which most data-analysis techniques rest, the selection of appropriate summary statistics is critical to the clear reporting of research findings. These statistics describe the characteristics of the data by answering the following questions: "What is the average or typical value in the distribution?" and "How much variety or dispersion is there in the values represented by the distribution?" Although graphs and tables can provide a pictorial presentation of answers to these questions, the summary statistics present more precise quantitative information that is amenable to further data analysis. Summary statistics include measures of central tendency, variability, skewness, and kurtosis.

Measures of Central Tendency

There are three common measures of central tendency—the mode, the median, and the mean. The *mode* is the most frequently occurring score in a distribution. The *median,* or middlemost score, can be determined as long as the data can be ranked. The median describes the point in the distribution that separates the upper half of the data from the lower half. It is determined by counting how many scores there are and finding out which score is in the middle of the distribution. If the median is 40, then you know that one-half the scores in the distribution are below 40 and one-half are above 40. The last index of central tendency is the *mean,* or arithmetic average, of the values in a set of data. It is found by adding up all the values and dividing by the number of values there are in a set of data. Table 6.2 illustrates the calculation of these three measures of central tendency for the hypothetical set of grouped data presented in Table 6.1.

   Readers will note that Table 6.2 and other tables in this chapter contain statistical formulae and notation. These are presented for illustrative purposes for those readers who wish to examine the calculation of these statistics, and they were derived from two basic statistics texts (Guilford, 1965; Siegel, 1956). There are numerous alternate formulae and notation conventions for most statistical calculations; readers should not feel that one type of notation or one formula is inherently superior to other techniques for obtaining the same information.

Measures of Variability

The other major category of summary statistics includes those that indicate the amount of dispersion, spread, or variability in a set of data. Known as indices of variability, the major statistics in this category include: the range, the variance (σ^2), the standard deviation (SD or σ), and the semi-interquartile range *(Q).*

   The *range* is simply the spread from the lowest value to the highest value in a distribution of data. It can be expressed in several ways, including the following: "scores ranged from _____ to _____" and "the range was _____ points." The smaller the range, the less variability there is in a distribution; conversely, the larger the range, the more variability there is in a distribution.

   The *variance* is determined by finding the mean of the values in a distribution and determining how far each value in the distribution deviates from the mean. Then these deviation scores are each squared to deal with the fact that half of the deviation is negative (i.e., below the mean) and half is positive (i.e., above the mean). If these deviation scores were not squared, their sum would always be zero and, therefore, useless. Then the squared deviation scores are summed and averaged to compute the variance. The variance cannot be presented in the original units of measurement because of the squaring, so it is not usually used as an absolute index of how the data spread out from the mean. But, the variance has two particularly important uses in data organization and analysis.

First, the variance is a most important number that represents variability and is used in the calculation of some statistics that will be described later in this chapter. These statistics include the correlation coefficient for analyzing relationships among variables and the analysis of variance for analyzing differences between groups of subjects. Second, the square root of the variance is a useful measure of the average amount by which all of the scores deviate from the mean of a distribution, and it is presented in the original units of measurement. This average amount of dispersion of the scores in a distribution is called the *standard deviation* (SD) and is a most important statistic for organizing the data of a study. A small SD indicates that the scores in the distribution did not spread out from the mean very much; that is, the group was relatively homogeneous. A large SD, on the other hand, indicates a wide dispersion of scores from the mean of the distribution; that is, the group was more heterogeneous.

The interpretation of the SD depends on what statisticians call the normal curve model and assumes that the values in the distribution are symmetrically arranged on either side of the mean. The normal curve model and its uses will be discussed later. The last measure of variability, the *semi-interquartile range,* is used if the values in a distribution are *not* symmetrically arranged around the central tendency and it indicates one-half the range of the middle 50 percent of the scores in the distribution. Table 6.3 illustrates calculation of some measures of variability for the set of grouped data presented in Tables 6.1 and 6.2.

In general, if the SD is about one-fourth to one-sixth as large as the range, the sample is typical of that usually found in most statistical work. Likewise, if the SD is about one-and-one-half times as large as the semi-interquartile range, the distribution is not significantly skewed (Guilford, 1965).

Measures of Skewness

A skewness statistic (called *Sk*) is sometimes computed to indicate the degree of asymmetry of a distribution (Kirk, 1990, pp. 140–143). The Sk statistic is calculated from the third power of the deviations above and below the mean (rather than from the square of deviations as in the variance): an Sk of zero indicates a symmetrical distribution, a positive Sk indicates a positively skewed distribution, and a negative Sk indicates a negatively skewed distribution. Skewness can also be detected by comparing indices of central tendency, particularly the mean and median. Positive skewness inflates the mean and negative skewness deflates the mean, but neither type of skewness affects the median. Thus, if the mean is greater than the median, the distribution is positively skewed; if the mean is smaller than the median, the distribution is negatively skewed.

Measures of Kurtosis

A kurtosis statistic (called *Kur*) is sometimes computed to indicate the degree of kurtosis of a distribution (Kirk, 1990, pp. 140–143). The Kur statistic is calculated from the fourth power of the deviations above and below the mean: a Kur of zero indicates a normal or mesokurtic distribution, a positive Kur indicates a leptokurtic distribution, and a negative Kur indicates a platykurtic distribution.

The author of a research article should provide appropriate summary statistics to describe the data distribution. Usually the mean and standard deviation are reported for a normal distribution of interval or ratio level measurements. A distribution is considered normal if it is bell-shaped, mesokurtic, symmetrical on right and left sides (i.e., not skewed in either direction), with a concentration of scores in the middle and progressively fewer cases occurring at score values toward the extremes (tails) of the distribution. If the distribution is not normal, then the median and semi-interquartile range are often reported. Sometimes a comparison of mean and median or the measures of skewness and kurtosis are reported to document the lack of normality. Appropriate data organization is the prelude to data analysis and the characteristics of the data distribution, along with other factors such as the level of measurement and the specific research design employed, determine the type of statistical analysis procedure to be used.

Data Analysis

Basic Concepts of Data Analysis

Appropriate Methods

As indicated previously, selection and application of data-analysis techniques beyond summary statistics is determined partly by the research questions of a study and partly by the level of the data yielded by the research. Basically, analysis techniques may be either *correlational* or *inferential,* depending on whether they are used to describe existing *relationships* or *differences* among data. In addition, the choice of the exact analysis procedure also depends on the number of variables being examined, the size and characteristics of the samples used, and the type of research plan in effect. Techniques of data analysis seem to be amenable to classification and description by "families" based on their derivation and their methodological assumptions. Because this is not a statistics text, each member of the procedural "families" will not be discussed at length. Instead, a summary of which procedures fit into the various situations described appears in Table 6.18 (at the end of the chapter).

For our purposes, it is sufficient to indicate that the various families of data-analysis techniques are more or less powerful (able to detect trends or differences in data), more or less well known, and more or less respected. However, each has unique characteristics that set it apart from the others and make it particularly useful in the right circumstances. Later sections of this chapter will describe each of these techniques and give some examples of how they may be used in communicative disorders research.

The Normal Curve Model

We have previously referred to statistical procedures based on assumptions of the normal curve model, and it is appropriate to summarize the basic concepts of the model before proceeding.

The normal curve model is a construct based on the observation that measures of physical or psychological variables derived from large numbers of people (or animals) tend to form a characteristic type of distribution when graphed. This distribution is the familiar symmetrical, bell-shaped curve that shows a concentration of values in the middle of the distribution with fewer and fewer values as the extremes are approached (Figure 6.7). The generalizability of this curve and its mathematical properties were first described by Gauss, and it is sometimes known as a Gaussian curve. Because it is the kind of distribution that data typically resemble, it also became known as a "normal" curve.

Inspection of Figure 6.7 reveals the symmetry of a normal distribution. It can be seen that most cases fall in the middle of the distribution, with fewer cases seen at the lower and higher score values at the extreme right- and left-hand sides of the distribution. About two-thirds of the cases fall within plus-or-minus 1 SD of the mean; 95 percent of the cases fall within plus-or-minus 2 SDs of the mean; and 99 percent of the cases fall within plus-or-minus 3 SDs of the mean. Although a perfect Gaussian or normal distribution is never attained in practice, there is enough resemblance between it and the actual obtained-data distributions to warrant its adoption as a mathematical model for statistical procedures that are used to analyze relationships and differences. The extent to which actual data resemble the model determines the usefulness of the model and statistical procedures derived from it. If data do not approximate a normal distribution in the way they occur in a sample or population, then the normal curve model and the statistical procedures based on it are simply not applicable. Therein lies the necessity to ascertain whether the assumptions of the model and methods based on it fit the particular set of data to be analyzed. These considerations lead us to a discussion of statistics based on a normal curve model *(parametric statistics)* vs. statistics that are not based on a normal curve model *(nonparametric statistics)*.

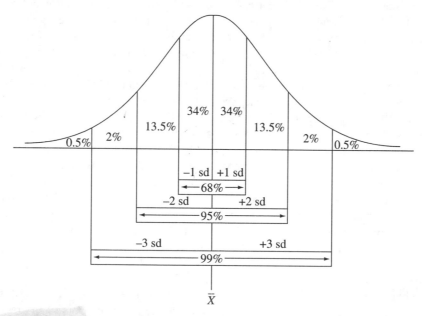

FIGURE 6.7   Normal Distribution with Percentages of Cases Falling within SD Bands

Parametric and Nonparametric Statistical Procedures

Parametric statistics are based on certain assumptions about the population from which the sample data were obtained. Because population quantities are often called parameters and sample quantities are often called statistics in statistical work, the term *parametric statistics* has been applied to data-analysis procedures that rest on certain assumptions about the population.

There are several assumptions about the population, and the sample drawn from it, that underlie the use of parametric statistics:

1. The population parameter should be normally distributed.
2. The level of measurement of the parameter in question should be interval or ratio.
3. When there are two or more distributions of data to be analyzed (e.g., two groups of subjects are tested or one group of subjects is tested under two different conditions) the *variances* of the data in the two different distributions should be about the same.
4. The sample should be fairly large. There is no agreed-on, absolute definition of "large," but most statisticians consider thirty subjects to be large enough (Hays, 1973).

When all of these assumptions can be met, parametric statistics are appropriate for data analysis. If one or more of these assumptions is seriously violated, parametric statistics may be inappropriate.

When assumptions about the populations cannot be met, researchers use nonparametric statistics. Nonparametric statistics are often called *distribution-free* statistics because they do not rest on assumptions about the distribution of the population parameter. Nonparametric statistics deal with data at the nominal or ordinal level of measurement. When a researcher has interval- or ratio-level data, but realizes that they are not normally distributed (or fail to meet one of the other assumptions listed), the data can be *transformed* from interval or ratio level to nominal or ordinal level in order to be used in a nonparametric test. For example, interval-level scores could be classified as "pass" or "fail" by using a cutoff score on the interval scale. Another alternative would be to rank-order all the subjects on the basis of their interval-scale scores and then use their ranks as the data for a nonparametric statistical analysis. Of course, if the original data were already nominal or ordinal, then a nonparametric statistical procedure would have to be used instead of a parametric procedure.

Although it may appear that the use of nonparametric alternatives to parametric statistical analysis is always the "safest" way to analyze data, this is not really true. Parametric statistics are more powerful (i.e., more sensitive to differences and relationships) than nonparametric tests; therefore, they are preferred when the assumptions listed can be met. Throughout the rest of this chapter, we generally will describe a parametric procedure for each particular kind of analysis and then consider nonparametric alternatives to each parametric statistic.

Testing a Null Hypothesis

Statistical analysis is concerned with making decisions about the existence vs. the nonexistence of differences between groups or relationships among variables. This is usually done by examining the plausibility of a *null hypothesis* in light of obtained data. A null hypothesis is a hypothesis that states that there is no difference between groups or no relationship among variables. A simple null hypothesis may state, for example, that there is no difference between the means of two groups of subjects (e.g., stutterers vs. nonstutterers) on some dependent variable. The mean of the sample of stutterers would be compared to the mean of the sample of nonstutterers to decide how plausible that null hypothesis is. If the means of the two groups are about the same, then it is plausible that the null hypothesis is true, and the researcher could accept it. If, however, the means of the two groups are quite different, it does not seem plausible that the null hypothesis is true, and the researcher could reject it. The concept of testing a null hypothesis is the basis for *statistical inference* and underlies all of the methods for testing differences to be discussed subsequently in this chapter. Inferential hypothesis testing can also be applied in analyzing relationships, as will be seen later.

Type I and Type II Errors

When a researcher makes a decision about a null hypothesis, one of four things can happen: the hypothesis can be true or false and the researcher can accept or reject it. Figure 6.8 illustrates the contingencies of this situation.

Inspection of Figure 6.8 reveals that there are two possible correct decisions that a researcher can make: accepting a true null hypothesis and rejecting a false null hypothesis. There are two possible incorrect decisions: rejecting a true null hypothesis (called a *Type I error*) and accepting a false null hypothesis (called a *Type II error*).

If a researcher concludes on the basis of the sample data that two groups are different, the decision will either be correct (if the groups are different) or a Type I error (if the groups are not different). If a researcher concludes on the basis of the sample data that the two groups are not different, the decision will either be correct (if the two groups are not different) or a Type II error (if the two groups are different). Statistical analysis helps the researcher to make the decision about a null hypothesis by indicating the probability that a decision to reject a null hypothesis is a Type I error. Statistical analysis can also help a researcher to make a decision to accept a null hypothesis by indicating the probability of making a Type II error. Unfortunately, the probability of making a Type II error is not as easily determined as the probability of making a Type I error. Consumers of research are more likely to find analyses of the probability of making a Type I error in articles that report group differences and are less likely to find analyses of the

H_0
Status of null hypothesis

		Null hypothesis is true	Null hypothesis is false
Researcher's decision	Accept null hypothesis	Correct decision	Type II error
	Reject null hypothesis	Type I error	Correct decision

FIGURE 6.8   Contingencies Involved in Making a Decision about a Null Hypothesis

probability of committing a Type II error in articles reporting no differences between groups or conditions.

The Level of Significance

The probability of making a Type I error is called the *level of significance*. When a researcher decides to reject a null hypothesis and conclude that there is a difference between two sets of data, he or she does so because the statistical test comparing the two sets of data indicates that the probability of making a Type I error in rejecting the null hypothesis is quite small. This probability is expressed by stating the level of significance (sometimes called *alpha*) associated with the comparison. Stating the level of significance indicates the degree of confidence that the researcher has that the difference seen in the sample data would not have occurred by chance alone. In fact, the level of significance is sometimes called the *level of confidence* for the comparison. The comparison of two data sets may be a between-subjects comparison such as the comparison of the means on some dependent variable for stutterers vs. nonstutterers. It may also be a within-subjects comparison such as the comparison of the means on some dependent variable of stutterers tested under two different experimental conditions.

If the statistical analysis shows that it is highly improbable that an obtained sample difference would have occurred if the null hypothesis were true, then the researcher will reject the null hypothesis because the probability of committing a Type I error is small. If, however, the statistical analysis shows that it is not improbable that an obtained sample difference would have occurred if the null hypothesis were true, the researcher will not reject the null hypothesis because the probability of committing a Type I error is not small enough. How small must the probability of committing a Type I error be for a researcher to reject the null hypothesis? In other words, what must the level of significance be for a comparison of sample groups of data for a researcher to conclude that the groups of data are different?

Although there is no absolute answer to the question of what level of significance should be adopted, there are conventional preferences that have evolved. The most frequently used levels of significance are 0.05 and 0.01. These figures mean that the probability of committing a Type I error is 0.05 (five chances in one hundred) or 0.01 (one chance in one hundred). In other words, if the level of significance yielded by a statistical analysis indicates that the difference between the data sets could have resulted by chance (if null hypothesis were true) only five times out of one hundred, then, the null hypothesis will be rejected and the difference will be called "significant at the 0.05 level." Sometimes the level of significance is indicated by using the letter p (for probability) and then stating the value of the probability of committing the Type I error. For example, a researcher might state: "The difference between the two groups was significant ($p = 0.05$)." Selection of the 0.05 vs. the 0.01 level of significance by an investigator is arbitrary. Because the 0.01 level of significance indicates less chance of a Type I error than the 0.05 level, it is stricter or more conservative than the 0.05 level of significance. In other words, other things being equal, a larger difference between two sets of sample data must be found to reach the 0.01 level of significance than to reach the 0.05 level of significance.

The selection of a level of significance is a complicated process, a discussion of which is beyond the scope of this chapter. In general, however, if the study is in a previously unexplored domain or is one in which the researcher is trying to identify possibilities for further study at a later time, then a more lenient level of significance may be reasonable. If, on the other hand, the researcher is examining well-developed hypotheses or replicating a study, a stricter level of significance may be desired.

Two final remarks about significance levels are in order. First, many consumers of research interpret the term *significant* to mean a result that has clinical relevance or theoretical meaning. This is not necessarily true. A very small difference between groups that has little or no clinical relevance or theoretical meaning may be statistically significant in the sense that it is highly improbable to occur if the null hypothesis were true. Perhaps in that sense the term *significant* is inappropriate and the term *level of confidence* is a better one because it simply indicates the confidence that the researcher has that the result did not simply occur by chance. Whether a statistically significant difference between two groups of data also has theoretical or clinical significance is a rational matter that is more often treated by an author in a discussion section of an article than in the results section. Second, it should be pointed out that there are many researchers who prefer not to analyze results with statistical-significance testing procedures. Proponents of this point of view prefer to rely on replication studies and stronger rational examination of the meaning of their research results. Carver (1978) presented this perspective in a lengthy criticism of statistical-significance testing. Consumers of research should realize, then, that not all research articles will include statistical-significance tests and that the absence of such tests does not necessarily mean that the results are not clinically or theoretically significant or that the researcher has been faulty in the data analysis. It may simply mean that the particular researcher is in Carver's camp in opposition to statistical-significance testing. Young (1993; 1994) has raised similar issues regarding statistical-significance testing in communicative disorders research.

One- and Two-Tailed Tests

Another important consideration in evaluating the results of data analysis is whether the researcher has chosen a one-tailed (directional) test or a two-tailed (nondirectional) test. This decision is made in relation to the questions or hypotheses posed in the study. If the researcher has made a directional hypothesis, he or she applies one-tailed tests. Examples of statements calling for one-tailed tests include: "Scores of group X will be higher than scores of group Y," "Scores will be significantly below average," and "There will be more persons in the X category than in the Y category." If the researcher is considering questions or hypotheses that are nondirectional, she or he applies two-tailed tests. Examples of statements calling for two-tailed tests include: "There will be a difference in scores between group X and group Y," "Scores will be significantly different from the average," and "There will be different number of persons in the X category than in the Y category."

Consumers of research should be aware that two-tailed tests are more strict or conservative than one-tailed tests. That is to say, a greater difference between groups must be found to call the difference significant when using a two-tailed test. A somewhat smaller difference may not be significant with a two-tailed test but may be significant when analyzed with a one-tailed test. Typically, one-tailed tests are used when the researcher has some reason to suspect in advance that the difference between groups or conditions should be in one direction. There is some controversy about when it is appropriate to select the more liberal one-tailed test, and more conservative statisticians and researchers generally recommend the more stringent two-tailed tests. For example, Cohen (1988) strongly advises researchers to avoid one-tailed tests. Consumers should expect to find both one-tailed and two-tailed tests in the literature, however, and they should realize that significant differences found with two-tailed tests are, in a sense, more significant than those found with one-tailed tests.

Degrees of Freedom

The importance of sample size in the selection and application of a particular analysis procedure is highlighted by the concept of degrees of freedom. To interpret the results of a given statistical procedure, the researcher must know the degrees of freedom *(df)* in the data before tables of statistical significance can be used. In a most basic sense, *df* indicate the number of values in a set of data that are free to vary once certain characteristics of the data are known. Generally, if the mean or the sum of a set of scores is known, then the *df* are equal to the number of scores in each distribution minus 1 *(df = n − 1)*.

The formula for determining the number of the *df* varies according to the procedure employed for analysis, and the number of the *df* should always be reported when analyses are described and interpreted. In a table or in the text of the results section of an article, the *df* are usually listed as an accompaniment to the outcome of the particular data-analysis procedure that was used. A discussion of the techniques for calculating *df* for all the various analysis procedures is beyond the scope of this text. Consumers of research, however, should be aware that each analysis procedure must take into account the correct number of *df* in determining statistical significance. Authors usually show *df* in the results section to demonstrate to the editors and to readers more familiar with statistical analysis that the *df* were correctly accounted for in the analysis.

The following sections will examine how some of the commonly used parametric and nonparametric analysis procedures are used in communicative disorders studies. Procedures are grouped under two major headings: (1) methods for analyzing relationships and (2) methods for describing differences. The reader will find it useful to refer frequently to Table 6.18 while reading these sections because this table summarizes these analysis procedures regarding: (1) the level of measurement for which each is appropriate, (2) whether the procedure analyzes differences or relationships, and (3) whether the procedure is parametric or nonparametric. Although this table is not a complete list of all statistical methods used in communicative disorders research, it does give an organized overview of those common procedures considered in this chapter.

Methods for Analyzing Relationships

Often the researcher wishes to determine the strength and direction of relationships that exist in a set of data or simply whether some overall association occurs among variables in a given sample or population. To do this, two or more sets of scores or ranks or classifications are derived from a particular sample and subjected to analysis.

The relationship between two variables can be described graphically using a scattergram or scatterplot. Each subject has a pair of scores or ranks on the variables, and these are plotted on a bivariate graph with the axes representing the variables under study. Table 6.4 shows three sets of score pairs for ten subjects. The corresponding scatterplots for these data sets appear in Figure 6.9.

Examination of the scatterplot will reveal the *direction* of the relationship. If the scores on one variable tend to *increase* as the other variable *increases,* the relationship is

TABLE 6.4 Score Pairs for Three Sets of Ten Subjects

	Illustration A			Illustration B			Illustration C	
Subjects' Initials	Score on First Variable	Score on Second Variable	Subjects' Initials	Score on First Variable	Score on Second Variable	Subjects' Initials	Score on First Variable	Score on Second Variable
RB	4	16	CJ	21	8	DS	21	2
CS	6	14	DD	53	5	BC	83	1
JD	8	17	NS	14	9	WD	45	7
WM	3	13	IV	67	6	MC	17	4
SV	2	11	TY	82	4	HC	62	8
BP	7	18	BH	98	1	DR	91	3
BD	1	12	GS	34	10	AT	37	9
TM	5	15	JF	47	7	JN	99	6
FD	10	19	RF	94	2	RP	72	5
MC	9	20	TD	76	3	JF	56	10

positive (Figure 6.9*a*). If one variable *decreases* as the other variable *increases,* the relationship is *negative* (Figure 6.9*b*). These relationships are shown by the direction in which the plot moves across the graph as in Figure 6.9*(a–c)*. Moreover, the density with which the data points on the plot are clustered together reveals the *strength* of the relationship. Figures 6.9*a* and *b* show points tightly clustered, indicating a strong relationship whereas Figure 6.9*c* shows a wide dispersal of points, indicating a weak relationship.

Although scatterplots are useful, they do not give a precise index of association between variables. For this reason, most relationships are reported as *correlation coefficients.* Many types of coefficients exist, depending on the methods used to obtain them, but the two most common ones are the *Pearson Product-Moment Correlation Coefficient* (a parametric index) and the *Spearman Rank-Order Correlation Coefficient* (a nonparametric index). Occasionally, a partial, multiple, biserial, point biserial, tetrachoric, or phi correlation may be cited, but these indices are interpreted in essentially the same way as the Pearson and Spearman indices.

Correlation coefficients have two components: a sign and a numeric value. The sign indicates the *direction* of the relationship (– is a negative or inverse relationship; + is a positive relationship). The numeric value indicates the strength of the relationship and may take on an absolute value ranging from 0.00 (no relationship) to 1.00 (a perfect relationship). Thus correlation coefficients can range from –1.00 (a perfect negative relationship) to +1.00 (a perfect positive relationship), as shown in the interpretive guide in Figure 6.10.

One point of confusion in interpreting these indices lies in the fact that the strength and direction of the coefficient are independent. Commonly, we think of negative numbers as being less desirable or significant than positive numbers; this is not true of correlation. For instance, if we were given the two correlation coefficients:

$$r_{ab} = -0.79$$
$$r_{ac} = +0.63$$

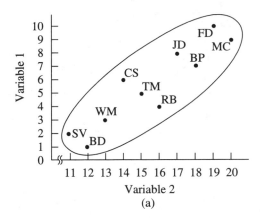

(a)

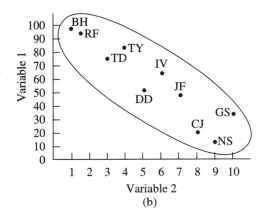

(b)

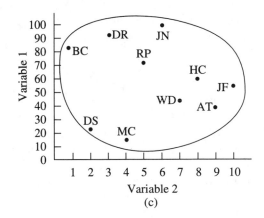

(c)

FIGURE 6.9
Graphic Presentation of Relationships:
(a) **Scatterplot for Data in Illustration A (Table 6.4),** *(b)* **Scatterplot for Data in Illustration B (Table 6.4),**
(c) **Scatterplot for Data in Illustration C (Table 6.4)**

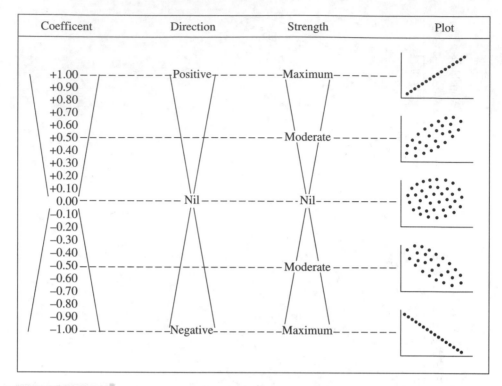

FIGURE 6.10 Interpretive Guide for Correlation Coefficients

and asked which describes a *stronger* relationship, the answer is $r_{ab} = -0.79$, even though it is a negative coefficient. Incidentally, the subscripts *ab* and *ac* are a statistical convention for telling the reader which variables are being correlated; in this case r_{ab} is the correlation between two variables, *a* and *b,* whereas r_{ac} is the correlation between two variables *a* and *c.*

Moreover, the coefficients

$$r_{ad} = -0.43$$
$$r_{bc} = +0.43$$

indicate relationships of the *same* strength, even though the relationship between variable *a* and variable *d* is inverse and the relationship between variables *b* and *c* is positive.

The Pearson Product-Moment Correlation Coefficient uses actual scores in the calculation, whereas the Spearman Rank-Order Correlation Coefficient requires that ranks or scores converted to ranks be used in the calculation. Generally, the Pearson coefficient applies to sample sizes of twenty-five or more with data at the interval or ratio levels, whereas the Spearman is used for ordinal data or when the sample size is less than twenty-five. No matter which of these or the other methods listed earlier is used, the researcher

TABLE 6.5   Correlation Coefficients for Data of Illustrations A, B, and C Listed in Table 6.4 and Graphed in Figure 6.9

Data Set	Pearson r	Spearman Rho
A	+0.91	+0.92 (Very strong positive correlation)
B	−0.93	−0.93 (Very strong negative correlation)
C	−0.10	−0.13 (Very weak correlation)

should clearly specify the procedure selected for analyzing particular sets of data. For purpose of illustration, both the Pearson and Spearman indices have been computed (Table 6.5) for the illustrative data sets in Table 6.6.

Rather than reporting entire lists of correlation coefficients showing relationships between variable pairs in a multivariate study, many researchers present these data in a *table of intercorrelations* or in a *correlation matrix*. This way, the reader can, by locating the desired variable pairs in the row and column headings, find the correlation between those two variables. Table 6.6 shows a correlation matrix for five variables. By consulting the table, the reader can see that the correlation of variable *b* with variable *d* is −0.60, and so forth. Note that the entries in the table are duplicated below the underlined diagonal values. For that reason, the shaded portion often does not appear in research reports. In addition, the underlined diagonal values represent the correlation of each variable with itself and, therefore, equal +1.00, a perfect positive correlation.

When correlation coefficients are reported, the researcher may accompany this with some statement of the *statistical* significance of the index, that is, whether the correlation coefficient is *significantly different from zero*. Because statistical significance may be obtained for very small correlations if the sample is large enough, small correlation coefficients should be interpreted cautiously. For example, for a sample size of two hundred, a correlation of plus or minus 0.14 is considered statistically significant (Guilford, 1965, p. 581). However, the *practical* usefulness of this index is limited because it is, at best, a modest correlation.

TABLE 6.6   A Hypothetical Correlation Matrix

Variable	a	b	c	d	e
a	1.00	0.64	0.14	−0.39	0.04
b	0.64	1.00	0.79	−0.60	0.43
c	0.14	0.79	1.00	0.98	0.16
d	−0.39	−0.60	0.98	1.00	−0.37
e	0.04	0.43	0.16	−0.37	1.00

To evaluate the practical meaning of a correlation coefficient of a given magnitude, a statistic known as the Index of Determination is often used. This index, commonly known as r^2, is the square of the correlation coefficient, and it gives an indication of the actual amount of overlap between two variables in terms of shared variance. For example, a correlation, r_{de} = +0.50 indicates that there is actually only a 25 percent (0.50^2) overlap between the variables d and e in terms of variance accounted for. This is illustrated by Figure 6.11, which shows two variable domains—domain G and domain H. If the correlation between the two variables (G and H) is r_{gh} = +0.60, then this indicates that 36 percent (0.60^2) of the two domains actually overlap, leaving a full 64 percent of the domain variability unaccounted for. Figure 6.11 also illustrates the Indices of Determination for cor-

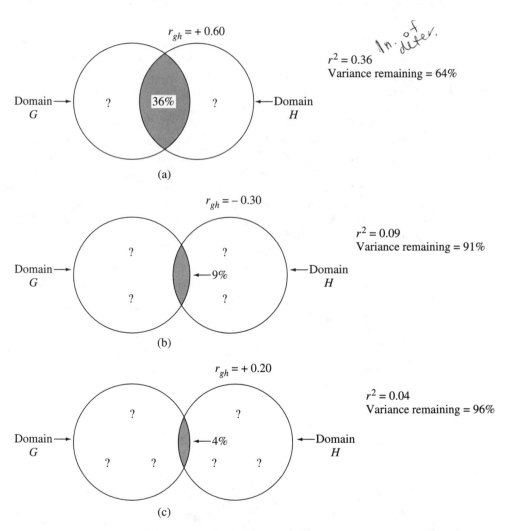

FIGURE 6.11   The Index of Determination as an Indication of the Variance Shared by Two Variables

relations of –0.30 and +0.20. The shaded areas represent the amount of variance that overlaps or is shared by the two variables; the white areas with question marks indicate the variance that is not accounted for by the correlation. The reader can readily see that the statistical significance of a correlation is only one indication of its quality and that the r^2 value can be a more pragmatically useful index for judging the meaning of the correlation.

Another consideration necessary for proper interpretation of correlation coefficients is that correlation does *not* imply that a cause–effect relationship exists between the variables being correlated. Thus, if variable *a* and variable *b* are correlated, this should be interpreted to mean that they *co*-relate, or vary together in some describable way so that as one variable moves in one direction, the other *tends* to move in the same direction (for a positive relationship) or the opposite direction (for a negative relationship). One does not necessarily *cause* the other to vary.

In addition to ascribing causality to correlations, there exists another common *mis*interpretation of correlation coefficients. This is the direct translation of a coefficient into a percentage or proportion. Often, students tend to think that if we knew the correlation between two variables was +0.58 and had data for one of these variables, we would correctly predict what the data for the other would be 58 percent of the time. This is *not* correct, and researchers who make these kinds of statements are being inaccurate. Instead, a +0.58 correlation indicates that there is a moderately positive relationship between two variables so that, in general, the individuals who had high scores or rankings on one variable would probably tend to have high scores or rankings on the other. Note the qualifiers: "in general," "probably," and "tend to" in the preceding statement. These indicate the tentative nature of interpretation of correlation coefficients and the possibility that, unless the relationship is *perfect,* there will be some cases in any sample or population that do not behave in the same way as the majority.

In addition to allowing researchers to understand the relationships among variables, correlational analysis allows researchers to make predictions of the value of one variable from knowledge of the values of other variables. For example, a research study may be concerned with prediction of some criterion performance such as degree of success in a treatment program (designated a dependent variable) from knowledge of factors such as subject characteristics, pretreatment test scores, prognostic indicators, or severity of disorder (designated as independent variables). To accomplish this, the researcher assembles data for a sample of subjects and correlates all of the independent variables with the dependent variables. Often, the independent variables are termed *predictor* variables and the dependent variables are termed *predicted* variables because of the direction of the prediction. The relationships, expressed as correlation coefficients, can be presented in tables of intercorrelations showing how each variable relates to each other variable and to the criterion. In rare instances, a single factor emerges as having such a strong relationship with the criterion that it can be used as the sole predictor in a regression equation. Most of the time, however, the array of correlations indicates that several variables should be used in combination to predict the criterion more closely than any single variable could.

The researcher then sets out to find the best linear combination of predictors, that is, one that acknowledges the unique relationship of each predictor with the criterion, minimizes the overlap (correlation) among predictors, and maximizes the combined strength of the predictors. Rather than attempt this task of finding the optimal combination of predictors through trial and error, the researcher uses a statistical technique known as multiple-regression analysis. In brief, this technique mathematically enables the researcher to determine the *order* in which predictor variables should be entered in a prediction equation to maximize prediction; assigns a *weight* to each predictor variable entered into the equation; and (in a stepwise multiple regression) indicates the *contribution* of each new added variable to the predictive validity of the equation. By the use of these methods, the researcher may initially examine the relationships among each of twenty variables themselves. The researcher may then conclude the analysis by specifying three or four variables that can be combined in a given order and with given weights in a regression equation to best predict the criterion.

The success and meaning of multiple regression analysis depends on a number of factors the researcher must consider. These factors include: (1) care in selection of the initial variables for the analysis, (2) the reliability and validity with which the variables are measured, (3) the size and representativeness of the sample used for study, (4) the reliability and validity of the criterion measure, and (5) the practicality of gathering all of the predictor data appearing in the equation. Multiple-regression analysis is a popular and appealing data-manipulation procedure. Unfortunately, the attractiveness of this procedure often results in its misuse.

The correlation and regression methods discussed previously give quantitative descriptions of the strength and direction of association among variables that can be assigned ranks or score values. Occasionally, however, the researcher is faced with the task of ascertaining whether there is an association between two or more variables when at least one of them is a nominal variable. This is especially pertinent to studies using questionnaire or demographic data that can be reported as frequencies in categories but cannot satisfactorily be expressed in ordinal or interval scales.

To organize such nominal-level data, the researcher may present them in *contingency tables*. The categories used for one variable are listed across one axis of the table, whereas those for a second variable are listed along the other axis. Contingency tables can also be generated for more than two variables, but they are somewhat awkward and are not found as often in the research literature. The entries in the table are the frequencies with which subjects had that particular combination of values. Table 6.7 shows a contingency table having two rows and two columns, which is therefore known as a 2×2 contingency table.

TABLE 6.7   A 2×2 Contingency Table Illustrating Data from Hypothetical Performance of Speakers with and without Cleft Palate on Some Categorical Performance Measure

	Cleft Palate	Normal Palate
Passed	3	17
Failed	13	6

$$X^2 = 9.39$$
$$C = 0.44$$

Hypothetical data on pass–fail performance of speakers with normal palate and cleft palate are entered in the cells of Table 6.7.

Although contingency tables are useful on their own, they are usually accompanied by further data analysis that enables the researcher to determine whether significant relationships exist among the variables. Two common analysis techniques that may be applied to such data are the chi square (χ^2) and the contingency coefficient *(C)*.

Application of chi square to the data in the contingency table discussed previously yields a value of 9.39. Consulting a table of chi square values required for the 0.01 level of statistical significance shows that the required value for this set of data having 1 *df* is 6.64 (Siegel, 1956, p. 249). Thus, this chi square would be statistically significant beyond the 0.01 level, indicating that there is a relationship between the two categorical variables that could only have occurred by chance less than one time in one hundred.

Briefly, a chi square analysis requires that the actual observed *(O)* frequencies listed in the contingency table be compared to expected *(E)* frequencies generated during the analysis or postulated by the researcher earlier on the basis of some theory or prior experience with similar data. If the discrepancy between what was actually observed in the study and the estimates given by the expected values is large enough, the resulting chi square value will reach statistical significance. The reader will note that the outcome of the analysis must be evaluated by consulting statistical tables of significance using the *df* determined from the data. These significance tables give the minimal values of the chi square statistic needed with various *df* to permit the conclusion that there is a statistically significant relationship between or among the variables in question. The chi square analysis does *not* indicate the strength of any relationship that exists nor the direction of that relationship. Chi square indicates only the extent to which the relationship is outside the realm of chance or normal probability. The contingency coefficient is used to measure the extent or strength of the relationship and can be computed by a formula that employs the chi square value. The contingency coefficient for the data in Table 6.7 is *C* = 0.44 and this coefficient would be interpreted in much the same way as the other correlation coefficients discussed earlier except that the upper limit for *C* for a 2 × 2 table is 0.707, not 1.0.

The upper limit of *C* is a function of the number of categories under examination in the contingency table (Siegel, 1956). When the number of rows *(r)* and columns *(c)* of the contingency table are the same (as in Table 6.7), the upper limit of *C* is computed as follows:

$$C = \sqrt{\frac{r-1}{c}}$$

Thus, for the 2 × 2 contingency table, the upper limit of *C* is $\sqrt{1/2}$ = 0.707. For a 3 × 3 contingency table, the upper limit of *C* is $\sqrt{2/3}$ = 0.816.

Although chi square is often used for ascertaining the presence of significant bivariate relationships, it can be extended to multivariate situations as long as a subject's data can be classified within one value or category in each variable. Thus, chi square can be used for a 2 × 3 × 5 contingency table or a 3 × 6 × 2 × 7 contingency table. The only difficulties lie in finding a way to present these data and interpret the meaning of three-way and four-way relationships.

Although chi square is used to determine the presence of relationships in nominal-level data, it is an extremely flexible procedure that can also be used as a method for analyzing *differences* in groups. In this sense, the method provides a link between procedures that show relationships and those that describe differences. The major difference among the applications of this procedure lies in the nature of the questions or hypotheses examined, as we will see in the next section.

Methods for Analyzing Differences

Many research problems in communicative disorders concern differences between (or among) groups of subjects. For example, a researcher might ask if there is a difference between normal-hearing and hearing-impaired children on a particular language measure. Other problems concern differences between (or among) conditions for the same group of subjects. For example, a researcher might ask if there is a difference between hearing-impaired subjects' speech-discrimination scores before and after auditory training. In other words, researchers are concerned about the analysis of between-subjects differences and within-subjects differences. In analyzing the between-subjects and within-subjects differences, researchers want to determine whether the differences are large enough in the sample data to rule out the probability that they could be attributed to chance or sampling error. The procedures of statistical inference are used to make such an analysis for determining the statistical significance of differences between-subjects and within-subjects. In other words, the researcher will examine the probability of making a Type I error in concluding that there is a between-subjects or a within-subjects difference.

Table 6.18 (at the end of this chapter) summarizes many of the common analysis procedures and the situations in which they are applicable. The table indicates the level of measurement for which each procedure is applicable and shows which procedures are parametric and which are nonparametric. Also indicated is whether the procedure is applicable to between-subjects comparisons (i.e., independent samples tests) or within-subjects comparisons (i.e., related samples tests). Some of the statistical tests are also identified as appropriate for comparing only two samples or for comparing more than two samples of data.

We will first consider statistical methods that are used to ascertain the significance of the difference between *two groups of data* on a *single dependent variable.* These procedures could be used to compare two different groups of subjects, such as stutterers vs. nonstutterers, or to compare one group of subjects under two different conditions, such as stutterers speaking in quiet vs. noise. In other words, these procedures can be used to make between-subjects comparisons (i.e., to compare independent or uncorrelated samples) or to make within-subjects comparisons (i.e., to compare related or correlated samples).

In the two-group one-variable analysis situation described previously, the basic parametric procedures for determining the significance of differences are the *z*-ratio and the *t*-test. The *z*-ratio is used when the samples are large (thirty or more) and the *t*-test is applicable for smaller samples. Basically, both of these methods (and their various subroutines) examine a theoretical distribution of *differences* in means to determine how the observed differences derived from a particular study compare to the average differences in a theoretical distribution. If the observed difference departs markedly from the average difference in the theoretical distribution, it is judged significant at a given level of significance (usually the 0.05 or 0.01 level, as described earlier). This is accomplished through the use of established formulae and tables available in statistical texts.

In the case of the z-ratio, the values required for statistical significance are 1.96 (0.05 level) and 2.58 (0.01 level) for two-tailed tests and 1.65 (0.05 level) and 2.33 (0.01 level) for one-tailed tests. With the t-test, the values required for statistical significance vary according to the number of degrees of freedom available for the data and require the consultation of a table showing significant t-values for different degrees of freedom. The researcher who uses these procedures should cite both the z-ratio or t-value obtained for the data in the study and the z-ratio or t-value required for statistical significance at the level chosen for the study.

Table 6.8 shows examples of the application of the z-ratio to compare means from two different groups and to compare the pretreatment and posttreatment means from a single

TABLE 6.8   Summary Table for z-Ratio

Illustration Different Groups			Illustration Same (Correlated) Groups		
$H_0 : M_1 = M_2$ $H_1 : M_1 \neq M_2$			$H_0 : M_1 = M_2$ $H_1 : M_1 \neq M_2$		
Group 1		*Group 2*	*Testing 1*		*Testing 2*
N 35		41	N 40		40
M^* 29.5		31.2	M 53.1		55.4
σ 5.3		4.8	σ 7.9		8.1
σ_M 0.91		1.76	$r_{M_1 M_2}{}^\dagger$ —	0.80	—
σ_{D_M} —	1.18	—	σ_M 1.3		1.3
			σ_{D_M} —	0.83	—

(handwritten: nondir. hypoth. 2-tailed; df = 78)

Formula for z-ratio: $z = \dfrac{D_M}{\sigma_{D_M}}$

$$(\text{where } D_M = M_2 - M_1) = \frac{31.2 - 29.5}{1.18}$$
$$= 1.44$$

Formula for z-ratio: $z = \dfrac{D_M}{\sigma_{D_M}}$

$$(\text{where } D_M = M_2 - M_1) = \frac{55.4 - 53.1}{0.83}$$
$$= 2.77$$

The z-ratio of 1.44 is less than that required for statistical significance at the 0.05 level (1.96) for a two-tailed test. Therefore, the difference in the two means is not significant and could have occurred by chance more than 5 times in 100.

Decision: accept H_0.

The z-ratio of 2.77 exceeds that required for statistical significance at the 0.01 level for the two-tailed test (2.58). Therefore, the difference in means between the two testings is statistically significant and could have occurred by chance less than 1 time in 100.

Decision: reject H_0; accept H_1. *(handwritten: significant diff. btwn groups)*

*Either M or $\bar{X}$ can be used to represent the mean score.
$\dagger$Correlation between testing 1 and testing 2 derived during prior analysis and used in calculating σ_{D_M}.

[handwritten: Btwn. Subj. Design]

[handwritten: mean]

TABLE 6.9   Summary Table for *t*-Test (Uncorrelated Groups)

[handwritten: Null Hyp.]

[handwritten: directional Exp. Hyp.]

$$H_0 = \overline{X}_1 = \overline{X}_2$$
$$H_1 = \overline{X}_1 > X_2$$

Directional hypotheses; call for one-tailed test.

[handwritten: deg. of freedom 42]

	Group 1		Group 2
N	21		23
$\overline{X}$	15.7		13.5
σ	3.7		3.9
*Σx^2	287		349
$X_1 - \overline{X}_2$		2.2	

Formula for *t* (difference between uncorrelated means):
$$\frac{\overline{X}_1 - \overline{X}_2}{\sqrt{\left(\frac{\Sigma x^2_1 + \Sigma x^2_2}{N_1 + N_2 - 2}\right)\left(\frac{N_1 + N_2}{N_1 N_2}\right)}}$$

[handwritten: greater than table value]

[handwritten: so reject null hypoth.]

t for these data = 1.88 *df* for these data = 42

t required for 42 *df* one-tailed test = 1.68 (0.05 level)

The *t*-value of 1.88 exceeds that required for statistical significance at the 0.05 level for a one-tailed test with 42 *df*. Therefore, the difference in means between the two groups is statistically significant and would have occurred by chance less than 5 times in 100. The mean of Group 1 is significantly larger than the mean of Group 2.

[handwritten: ✳] Decision: reject H_0; accept H_1.

*Information derived during analysis; calculations not shown.

group. Similar examples for the *t*-test appear in Tables 6.9 and 6.10. In the examples in Tables 6.8 and 6.9, it is the *mean* of the group or groups that is examined rather than individual subject values. The *t*-test for correlated groups shown in Table 6.10 uses mean pair differences and deviations of pair differences in the calculations.

Also listed in these tables are the null hypotheses (H_0) and their alternates (H_1, H_2, etc.) that are tested with each statistical procedure. Each statistical procedure considers the probability of the hypothesis (H_0) that there are no differences between the groups of scores. If the obtained statistic indicates that this null hypothesis is highly improbable (i.e., the statistic reaches the significance level), then the H_0 is rejected in favor of one of the alternate hypotheses listed.

When the assumptions required for the use of parametric methods cannot be met (e.g., the data are not in interval or ratio scales or sample sizes are extremely small), the researcher would apply analogous nonparametric procedures to the data. Among them are the Wilcoxon Matched-Pairs Signed-Ranks Test for changes within a group over time and the Mann–Whitney *U* Test that examines differences between groups. The values reached by use of these procedures must be compared with values in appropriate tables. As with

TABLE 6.10   Summary Table for *t*-Test (Correlated Groups)

[handwritten margin: w/in subj. design]

$$H_0 = \bar{X}_1 = \bar{X}_2$$
$$H_1 = \bar{X}_1 \neq \bar{X}_2$$

[handwritten: nondirectional 2-tailed test]

Note: This procedure tests for differences in score pairs rather than means.

Raw Data for 18 Subjects

[handwritten: $N = 18$ $\bar{X}_1 = 21.8$ $\bar{X}_2 = 22.7$]
[handwritten: $df = n-1$ $df = 17$]

Subject	Pretest	Posttest	Subject	Pretest	Posttest
a	23	28	j	28	27
b	24	22	k	27	27
c	16	18	l	18	15
d	15	16	m	21	23
e	18	23	n	26	27
f	16	18	o	19	25
g	21	20	p	21	19
h	25	23	l	26	26
i	26	28	r	23	24

Information derived from these data during analysis includes:

$$M_d = 1.0 \quad \Sigma x^2_d = 110$$

$$t\text{-test formula}: \quad t = \frac{M_d}{\sqrt{\Sigma x^2_d / N(N-1)}}$$

t for these data = 1.69

t required for statistical significance (two-tailed test; *df* = 17)
    2.1 (at the 0.05 level);
    2.9 (at the 0.01 level).

The *t*-value of 1.69 is less than that required for statistical significance with 17 *df* at the 0.05 level for a two-tailed test. Therefore, the difference in the scores received on pretest and posttest is not statistically significant and could have occurred by chance variation more than 5 times in 100.

 Decision: accept H_0.

---

the *z*-ratio and *t*-test, both the observed and the required values should be reported. Examples of the Wilcoxon and the Mann–Whitney procedures are found in Tables 6.11 and 6.12. A more detailed description of nonparametric methods for describing differences is found in Siegel (1956).

We will now consider situations in which there are *more than two groups* for comparison and *more than two conditions* under which each group is tested. The parametric statistical procedure used for these situations in most studies is the *analysis of variance* (usually abbreviated ANOVA). The statistic calculated in ANOVA is called the *F-ratio,* and the outcome of the analysis is usually reported in the form of a summary table. Interpretation of an *F*-ratio requires consultation of special significance tables. However,

TABLE 6.11   Summary of Wilcoxon Matched-Pairs Signed-Ranks Test *(T)*

$$H_0 = \Sigma Ranks_1 = \Sigma Ranks_2$$
$$H_1 = \Sigma Ranks_1 \neq \Sigma Ranks_2$$

Subject	Score before Treatment X_1	Score after Treatment X_2
a	14	16
b	17	17
c	18	23
d	15	20
e	16	14
f	12	11
g	16	18

This procedure determines an index known as *T* for the data and compares this value to those required for statistical significance at various levels.

The value of *T* for these data = 6.

T required = 2 (0.05 level); 0 (0.02 level).

Note: In this procedure observed *T* must be *smaller* than the required value to be significant.

The observed *T* is larger than that required for statistical significance at the 0.05 level. Therefore, the shift in scores between pretesting and posttesting is not significant and could have occurred by chance more than 5 times in 100.

Decision: accept H_0.

the summary table should present the value of *F* required for significance (or the *p* value of each reported *F*) and the appropriate number of *df* for each comparison.

We cannot provide a detailed explanation of the assumptions underlying ANOVA and the procedures for calculating *F*-ratios. However, we will try to present the overall logic of ANOVA as a test for differences among several means. If there is a difference among a set of group means, the variance *between the groups* will be significantly larger than the variance *within each of the groups*. The variance between the groups can be thought of as the variance of the group means around the *grand mean* of all the scores.

For instance, a researcher might ask if children of different ages would differ in their performance on some language task. Using a cross-sectional developmental approach, the researcher assembles four age groups (5-, 6-, 7-, and 8-year-olds), with one hundred children in each group, and assesses the performance of these four hundred children using a one-way ANOVA design (see Table 6.13). This ANOVA is called a one-way ANOVA because there is only one independent (classification) variable. In other words, the structure of an ANOVA, or the number of "ways" it tests for mean differences, is determined by the structure of the independent variables in the research study.

TABLE 6.12   Summary of Mann–Whitney *U* Test (*U*)

$$H_0 = \text{Ranks}_1 = \text{Ranks}_2$$
$$H_1 = \text{Ranks}_1 \neq \text{Ranks}_2$$

Hypothetical raw data for two samples of 10 subjects on a vocabulary test.

Group 1	Group 2
10	25
25	23
20	14
16	12
14	20
12	20
15	15
23	17
16	18
12	22

The *U* value for these data = 34.5.

The required value of *U* at the 0.05 level = 23;
0.01 level = 19.

Note: The observed value of *U* must be *smaller* than the required value to be statistically significant at that level.

The observed *U* is larger than that required for statistical significance at the 0.05 level. Therefore, the difference between Groups 1 and 2 is not statistically significant and may have occurred by chance more than 5 times in 100.

Decision: accept H_0.

TABLE 6.13   Representation of a One-Way ANOVA Design for Comparing the Means of Four Age Groups

	Independent (Classification) Variable = Age			
	Group A (5-year-olds)	*Group B* (6-year-olds)	*Group C* (7-year-olds)	*Group D* (8-year-olds)
Dependent (criterion) variable	$\bar{X}_a$ σ_a $N_a = 100$	$\bar{X}_b$ σ_b $N_b = 100$	$\bar{X}_c$ σ_c $N_c = 100$	$\bar{X}_d$ σ_d $N_d = 100$

H_0 = there are no differences in the means of the four groups.
H_1 = there is a difference among the means of the four groups.

Within each age group, there will be some variation among the one hundred children tested so that there will be an age-group mean and an age-group variance for each of the four age groups. If the variance *between the age-group means* (relative to the grand mean) is much larger than the variance *within each age group,* then there will be a significant difference among the age groups as shown by the *F*-ratio. The *F*-ratio that results from such an ANOVA is the ratio of the between-groups variance (called Mean Square between groups or MS between) to the within-groups variance (called MS within). When the between-groups variance is much larger than the within-groups variance, the *F*-ratio is large and reaches statistical significance when it is large enough for the appropriate number of *df* and alpha level. When the between-groups variance is not larger than the within-groups variance, the *F*-ratio is small and does not reach statistical significance. A table summarizing a possible ANOVA for the hypothetical cross-sectional study discussed previously is shown in Table 6.14.

If there is only one independent or classification variable in a study (i.e., age or clinical diagnosis), then the data form a one-way classification problem, and a one-way ANOVA is performed with the resulting *F*-ratio reported, as in the example in Table 6.14. The *F*-ratio is the ratio of a between-groups value called the mean square (MS between) to the within-groups mean-square (MS within) value, which are calculated during the analysis.

Let us now proceed to a more complex situation that takes the basic problem outlined previously one step further. Suppose our researcher felt that the children's gender was also a factor involved in language performance. The research design would then be constructed so that in addition to the four age categories, each age group would be divided into a group of males and a group of females. The researcher now has a 4 by 2 design (often abbreviated 4×2), and the resulting data would be analyzed using a two-way ANOVA in which one variable of interest is age and the other is gender. Hypothetical data for a 4×2 design are shown in Table 6.15 with a list of the statistical hypotheses that would be evaluated. The researcher is, then, asking more than one question in the analysis, namely:

1. Is there a difference in language performance among children of different ages?
2. Is there a difference in language performance among children of different genders?

Both of these questions concern so-called *main effects* in the ANOVA. In addition, another question has been implicitly introduced: Is there an *interaction* of age and gender with respect to language performance? Thus, might males and females show a different pattern of language performance across ages? Therefore, ANOVA has to examine three sources of variance in this problem—variance across age (MS age), variance across genders (MS gender), and variance owing to the interaction of age and gender (MS age $\times$ gender)—and compare each of these three sources of variance with the variance within the eight groups (MS within groups). There will then be three *F*-ratios calculated: the *F*-ratio for age, the *F*-ratio for gender; and the *F*-ratio for the interaction. Any, all, or none of these might be statistically significant. The summary table for the example we have discussed is shown in Table 6.16. The information in the table that is most pertinent to the consumer of research is in the far-right column where the *F*-ratios appear. These can be compared with the required values given below the body of the table to determine their statistical

TABLE 6.14   Summary Table for One-Way ANOVA (Using Example from Text)

Components	Sum of Squares	Degrees of Freedom (*df*)	Mean Squares	*F*-Ratio
Between groups (ages)	53.19	3	17.73	3.1
Within groups	2265.12	396	5.72	
Total	2318.31	399		

$$F = \frac{\text{MS between}}{\text{MS within}} = \frac{17.73}{5.72} = 3.1$$

F_{required} (3/396 *df*) = 2.62 (*p* = 0.05)
3.83 (*p* = 0.01)

The observed *F*-ratio of 3.1 falls between that required at the 0.05 level and that required at the 0.01 level. Therefore, there is a statistically significant difference among the four groups. This difference could occur by chance less than 5 times in 100 but more than 1 time in 100.

Decision: reject H_0; accept H_1.

TABLE 6.15   Representation of a 2 × 4 Design Suitable for a Two-Way ANOVA

	Independent (Classification) Variable Age of Subjects			
	Group A (5-year-olds)	*Group B (6-year-olds)*	*Group C (7-year-olds)*	*Group D (8-year-olds)*
Males	$\bar{X}_{ma}$ σ_{ma} $N_{ma} = 50$	$\bar{X}_{mb}$ σ_{mb} $N_{mb} = 50$	$\bar{X}_{mc}$ σ_{mc} $N_{mc} = 50$	$\bar{X}_{md}$ σ_{md} $N_{md} = 50$
Females	$\bar{X}_{fa}$ σ_{fa} $N_{fa} = 50$	$\bar{X}_{fb}$ σ_{fb} $N_{fb} = 50$	$\bar{X}_{tc}$ σ_{fc} $N_{fc} = 50$	$\bar{X}_{fd}$ σ_{fd} $N_{fd} = 50$

H_0 (for main effect of gender): there are no differences between the means of the male and female groups.

H_1 (for main effect of gender): there are differences between the means of the male and female groups.

H_0 and H_1 for main effect of age take the same form as above.

H_0 (for age by gender interaction): there are no differences between the means of various ages by gender groups.

H_1 (for age by gender interaction): there are differences between the means of various ages by gender groups.

TABLE 6.16   Summary Table for Two-Way ANOVA (Using Example from Text)

Components	Sum of Squares	Degrees of Freedom (df)	Mean Squares	F-Ratios
Between groups (ages)	54.00	3	18	5.8**
Between groups (genders)	12.10	1	12.1	3.9*
Interaction of age × gender	38.10	3	12.7	4.1**
Within groups	1215.20	392	3.1	
Total	1319.40	399		

$*p < .05$
$**p < .01$

Calculation of F-Ratios		Required F-Ratios for Significance		
F for age	$= \dfrac{0.18}{3.1} = 5.8$	2.62	3.83	$(df = 3,392)$
F for gender	$= \dfrac{12.1}{3.1} = 3.9$	3.86	6.70	$(df = 1,392)$
F for age × gender interaction	$= \dfrac{12.7}{3.1} = 4.1$	2.62	3.83	$(df = 3,392)$
		0.05	0.01	
		Level of significance		

The obtained F-ratios can be evaluated as follows:
   F for main effect of age indicates significant differences among ages
   F for main effect of gender indicates significant differences between genders
   F for interaction of age and gender indicates significant interaction effect

significance. In addition, a frequent notation for indicating level of significance appears in the table: the use of the single asterisk (*) to denote statistical significance at the 0.05 level, and the use of the double asterisk (**) to denote statistical significance at the 0.01 level.

We should now return to the notion of interaction and deal with it in a bit more detail. We have seen that once the researcher moves away from designs having a single independent or classification variable to designs having several independent or classification variables, concern for the main effects of each of these variables is supplemented by consideration of the interaction between or among the variables. These interactions are aptly named because interaction variations are not attributable to any of the main effects acting *alone* but rather to the *joint action* of two or more variables. Sometimes, interactions are called crossover effects because of the way they show up in graphic representations of data. In the hypothetical example used earlier, gender and age showed a significant interaction. This is illustrated in Table 6.17 and Figure 6.12 that show the

TABLE 6.17   Hypothetical Row and Column Means Illustrating Main Effects of Age and Gender on Language Performance and Interaction of Age and Gender

Gender of Subjects	Group A (5-year-olds)	Group B (6-year-olds)	Group C (7-year-olds)	Group D (8-year-olds)	Ages Combined
Males	12.0	16.0	21.0	24.0	18.25
Females	17.0	20.0	23.0	23.0	20.75
Genders combined	14.50	18.00	22.00	23.50	

Age of Subjects spans Groups A–D.

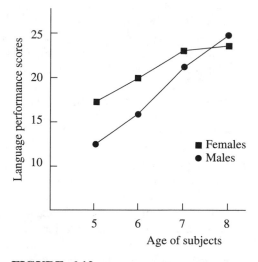

FIGURE 6.12
Graphic Plot for Visualizing Interaction of Two Independent (Classification) Variables in a Hypothetical Two-Way (4 × 2) ANOVA Problem

performances for the various ages and genders. Note that the plots for gender and age are *not* parallel; although females *generally* have a higher performance than males, the female performance advantage is not the same at each age, and by age eight, male and female scores are essentially equivalent. That is to say, the performance difference between males and females decreases as the subjects' ages increase to eight years when males catch up to females.

Every field of research has identified and studied variables that tend to interact. In our hypothetical example we have considered a so-called two-way interaction. In a design using three variables, both two-way and three-way interactions must be examined. For instance, a communicative disorders study might look at the effects of gender, clinical classification, and length of time in treatment on some outcome variable. The ANOVA for this situation would consider the following main effects and interactions:

1. Gender *(G)*
2. Clinical classification *(C)*
3. Length of time in treatment *(T)*
4. $G \times C$ interaction
5. $G \times T$ interaction
6. $C \times T$ interaction
7. $G \times C \times T$ interaction

From a practical standpoint, most studies do not involve interactions of more than three variables. Not only are more complex interactions difficult to interpret but also the sample size and other design considerations required for such studies present difficulties for the researcher. Moreover, interaction effects should be carefully evaluated when reporting research results. In fact, in some research studies, interaction effects may be more important than main effects. Often ANOVA will show both significant main effects and significant interaction effects.

Once a researcher has, through application of ANOVA procedures, shown that a significant difference occurs among the groups in the study, further analyses may be conducted to ascertain the location of the significant differences among the groups. Historically, *t*-tests were used to compare pairs of means following determination of a significant *F*-ratio. However, newer procedures are often used instead of *t*-tests for various mathematical and logical reasons. Among these are the Tukey, Duncan, Newman-Keuls, and Sheffé procedures. The reader may often find that research reports contain references to these analyses following ANOVA in order to identify specific significant differences.

The application of nonparametric methods to designs that lend themselves to ANOVA procedures is found in communicative disorders research when data are in the form of nominal or ordinal scales, making use of such methods imperative. As noted in Table 6.18, the nonparametric procedures that more or less parallel the parametric ANOVA are the Kruskal-Wallis One-Way ANOVA by Ranks (H), the Friedman Two-Way ANOVA by Ranks (X_r^2), the Cochran Q test, and a chi square test for independent samples. Discussion of each of these methods can be found in Siegel (1956). H and X_r^2 both test the hypothesis that a number of samples (groups) have been drawn from the same population and, hence, have similar average values in rank. Cochran's Q tests whether frequencies or proportions from correlated groups (or repeated measures on a single set of subjects) differ across occasions. The chi square test for independent samples tests the hypothesis that different samples come from the same population; it is useful for data that can be presented as frequencies.

This overview of methods for describing differences will close with a very brief description of still another variety of analysis included here because it may be mistakenly confused with ANOVA. It is Analysis of *Co*variance (or ANCOVA for short), and it is used in studies in which one of the independent or classification variables is related inextricably to the dependent variable. The analysis itself controls for the *co*-relation of the two

TABLE 6.18   Summary of Selected Analysis Procedures

Inferential stats

Level of Measurement		Methods of Analyzing Relationships	Methods for Analyzing Differences		
			Related Samples *Within Group*		*Btwn Gr.* Independent Samples
Nominal	Nonparametric methods	Contingency Coefficient *(C)* Chi Square *(X²)*	Cochran *Q* Test		Chi Square Test for Independent Samples *(X²)*
Ordinal		Spearman Rank-Order Correlation Coefficient (Rho)	Two Samples	Wilcoxon Matched-Pairs Signed-Ranks Test *(T)*	Mann–Whitney *U* Test
			More than Two Samples	Friedman Two-Way ANOVA	Kruskal-Wallis One-Way ANOVA
Interval or ratio	Parametric methods	Pearson Product-Moment Correlation Coefficient *(r)*	Two Samples *pretest & posttest*	*t*-Test for Correlated Groups *z*-Ratio	*t*-Test for Independent Groups *z*-Ratio
		Multiple-Regression Analysis	More than Two Samples	ANOVA *(F)* ANCOVA *(F)*	ANOVA *(F)* ANCOVA *(F)*

variables by virtue of the method used to compute the *F*-ratios and the outcome is interpreted in the same manner as ANOVA results. An example of a situation requiring the use of ANCOVA would be one in which subjects' verbal aptitude is an independent classification variable and vocabulary scores are a dependent variable in a study of the comparative effects of training programs for language-disordered children. Because verbal aptitude is significantly related to vocabulary scores, the ANCOVA would control for this relationship in determining whether significant differences in vocabulary scores existed as a function of the program independent of verbal aptitude.

Study Questions

1. Read pages 18–22, 30–34 in Chapter 3 of Siegel, S. (1956). *Nonparametric statistics for the behavioral sciences.* New York: McGraw-Hill.

   Write a brief summary of Siegel's discussion of statistical models and parametric and nonparametric statistical tests.

2. a. Which measures of central tendency and variability are usually reported when the distribution of data is normal?

   b. Which measures are usually reported when the distribution is skewed?

3. Examine the data in each of the following tables:

   Table 1 in: Gravel, J. S., & Wallace, I. F. (1992). Listening and language at 4 years of age: Effects of early otitis media. *Journal of Speech and Hearing Research, 35,* 588–595.

   Table 1 in: DePaul, R., & Brooks, B. R. (1993). Multiple orofacial indices in amyotrophic lateral sclerosis. *Journal of Speech and Hearing Research, 36,* 1158–1167.

   Which measures of central tendency and variability were used in each table to summarize the distribution of the data?

4. Examine the data in each of the following figures:

   Figure 4 in: Weismer, S. E., Murray-Branch, J., & Miller, J. F. (1994). A prospective longitudinal study of language development in late talkers. *Journal of Speech and Hearing Research, 37,* 852–867.

   Figure 1 in: Onslow, M., Hayes, B., Hutchins, L., & Newman, D. (1992). Speech naturalness and prolonged speech treatments for stuttering: Further variables and data. *Journal of Speech and Hearing Research, 35,* 274–282.

   a. How are the means displayed in each of these figures?

   b. Summarize, in your own words, what differences among the means are displayed in these figures.

5. a. Describe what is meant by the strength and direction of a relationship between two variables.

   b. How are these two aspects of a relationship demonstrated in a scattergram?

   c. How are they demonstrated in a correlation coefficient?

6. Examine the data in the following table:

   Table 7 in: Shriberg, L. D., Gruber, F. A., & Kwiatkowski, J. (1994). Developmental phonological disorders III: Long-term speech-sound normalization. *Journal of Speech and Hearing Research, 37,* 1151–1177.

   a. Which correlation coefficient was used to analyze the relationships among the variables listed in this table?

   b. Which correlations were significantly different from zero at the 0.05 level? At the 0.01 level?

   c. Which pair of variables showed the strongest relationship? Which pair showed the weakest relationship?

7. Examine the data in the following table and the analysis in the accompanying paragraph:

   Table 2 in: Conrad, R. (1973). Some correlates of speech coding in the short-term memory of the deaf. *Journal of Speech and Hearing Research, 16,* 375–384.

   a. What technique was used to analyze the relationships among the variables?

   b. Which pairs of variables showed significant relationships?

   c. Which pairs of variables did not show significant relationships?

8. a. What are Type I and Type II errors?

   b. Is it possible to make *both* types of error at the same time in reaching a decision about the plausibility of a null hypothesis? Why or why not?

References

Carver, R. P. (1978). The case against statistical significance testing. *Harvard Educational Review, 48,* 378–399.

Cohen, J. (1988). *Statistical power analysis for the behavioral sciences* (2nd ed.). Hillsdale, NJ: Lawrence Erlbaum Associates.

Ferguson, G. A., & Takane, Y. (1989). *Statistical analysis in psychology and education.* New York: McGraw-Hill.

Guilford, J. P. (1965). *Fundamental statistics in psychology and education.* New York: McGraw-Hill.

Hays, W. L. (1973). *Statistics.* New York: Holt, Rinehart & Winston.

Kirk, R. E. (1990). *Statistics: An introduction.* New York: Holt, Rinehart & Winston.

Pedhazur, E. J., & Schmelkin, L. P. (1991). *Measurement, design, and analysis.* Hillsdale, NJ: Lawrence Erlbaum Associates.

Siegel, S. (1956). *Nonparametric statistics for the behavioral sciences.* New York: McGraw-Hill.

Young, M. A. (1993). Supplementing tests of statistical significance: Variation accounted for. *Journal of Speech and Hearing Research, 36,* 644–656.

Young, M. A. (1994). Evaluating differences between stuttering and nonstuttering speakers: The group difference design. *Journal of Speech and Hearing Research, 37,* 522–534.

Part *II*

Evaluation of the Components of a Research Article

Overview

The main purpose of Part II is to show how the principles discussed in Part I can be applied to the evaluation of research. Part ll provides specific guidelines for analyzing and critically evaluating the four basic parts of the research article.

The four chapters of Part II cover the Introduction, Method, Results, and Discussion sections of a research article. The journals published by the American Speech-Language-Hearing Association (ASHA)—as well as many other journals of interest in communicative disorders—follow the style specified in the current edition of the *Publication Manual of the American Psychological Association*. The manual states (American Psychological Association [APA], 1994, p. 4–5):

> *Journal articles are usually reports of empirical studies, review articles, or theoretical articles. Reports of empirical studies are reports of original research. They typically consist of distinct sections that reflect the stages in the research process and that appear in the sequence of these stages:*
>
> - introduction: *development of the problem under investigation and statement of the purpose of investigation;*
> - method: *description of the method used to conduct the investigation;*
> - results: *report of the results that were found; and*
> - discussion: *interpretation and discussion of the implications of the results.*

Thus, we will follow the APA style suggestions in outlining the various parts of a research article in this part of the book.

Although much has been written about methods and statistical analyses in a number of texts, relatively little attention has been devoted to the evaluation of the research problem itself. Chapter 7 presents some guidelines for evaluating the introductory part of the research article. Emphasis here is placed on assessing the adequacy of the rationale for the study, on deciding if the literature citations support the need for the study, and on evaluating the research questions or hypotheses. Numerous examples, drawn from the communicative disorders literature, are used throughout this chapter and the chapters that follow. The chapter concludes, as do the other chapters in this part, with an Evaluation Checklist.

A brief word is necessary here about the Evaluation Checklists. Our intention in presenting the Checklists is to help the reader *focus* on those *key* elements of an article that deserve careful attention. We recognize that it is unlikely that most consumers of research will conduct the type of intensive analysis suggested by the Checklists, at least not in ordinary circumstances. We also recognize that because of the variety of research designs found in the literature, not all items on the Checklists will be applicable to all research reports. This is especially true for the Method Checklist. Nevertheless, the Checklists represent a didactic device that should be useful to the consumer, the would-be researcher, the researcher preparing a report of his or her study, and editorial consultants.

Chapter 8 deals with the Method section of the research article. It is in this section of the article that threats to internal and external validity are identified; thus, the Method section is of vital importance to the critical evaluator. Chapter 8 is divided into the three typical components of a Method section: subjects, materials, and procedures. The reader is urged to pay careful heed to how subjects are selected, how they are assigned to treatment groups, the reliability and validity of measurements used in the research, the research design employed, and whether the design reduces confounding threats to internal and external validity.

The next chapter is concerned with the results section of an article. Nothing is introduced in Chapter 9 that has not already been treated in Chapter 6. The whole point of this chapter is simply to illustrate the concepts and principles detailed earlier. The chapter deals with the adequacy of figures and tables, with the appropriateness of the statistical treatment, and with the interpretation of the data analysis.

The final chapter of Part II outlines criteria to be used in evaluating the Discussion and Conclusions section of the research article. Here, as in the Introduction section of an article, remarkably few guidelines are available to the critical evaluator. Yet, the Discussion and Conclusions section represents the culmination of a particular research effort and frequently is of considerable interest to the practitioner because of the possible implications for clinical practice. Some of the questions that are addressed in this chapter include: Are the conclusions fairly and accurately drawn from the results? Are the limitations of the study identified? Are there implications for future research, theory, or application and do these implications stem from the data? Are comparisons with previous research fair and objective?

Reference

American Psychological Association. (1994). *Publication manual of the American Psychological Association* (4th ed.). Washington, DC: American Psychological Association.

Chapter 7

The Introduction Section of the Research Article

We have emphasized previously the importance of the problem in initiating and designing a research study. The Introduction section of the research article is of the utmost importance to the critical reader of the research literature. It is in this section that the researcher presents the rationale for doing the research. If the author fails in this task, the remainder of the article may founder as well. It cannot be emphasized too strongly that the research problem, as described in the introduction to the article, is the thread that ties together the Method, the Results, and the Discussion sections. In essence, the good introduction is very much like a legal brief. Just as a legal brief is designed to convince the judge or jury, so, too, is the introduction designed to convince the reader of the need and the value of the study being proposed.

The various components of the introduction to a research article are the following:

1. Title
2. Abstract
3. General statement of the problem
4. Rationale for the study
5. Review of the literature
6. Specific purposes, research questions, or hypotheses

These six components do not always appear as separate entities in this order in every research article. Different authors have different writing styles and preferences for the organization of the introduction. Each of these components is identified in one form or another in the *APA Publication Manual* (APA, 1994, pp. 7–19) as a key part in writing the introduction to a research article. Therefore, we will identify, describe, and exemplify each of these six components of the introduction in this chapter.

Title of the Article

The introduction to a research article actually begins with the title of the article. The title is important because it is the first thing the reader sees. It alerts the reader to an article that may be of professional interest. The title should identify the general problem area, including the specification of independent and dependent variables and the target population.

The *APA Publication Manual* (APA, 1994, p. 7) states that the "title should summarize the main idea of the paper" and that it should be "fully explanatory when standing alone" because a title has two main functions. The title informs readers about the article and is used as the basis for indexing the article in the journal's index and in the various abstracting services and journals.

Three examples of research article titles are shown in Excerpts 7.1, 7.2, and 7.3.

EXCERPT 7.1

Effects of Stimulus Repetition Rate and Frequency on the Auditory Brainstem Response in Normal, Cochlear-impaired, and VIII Nerve/Brainstem-impaired Subjects.

From C. G. Fowler and D. Noffsinger, 1983, *Journal of Speech and Hearing Research, 26,* pp. 560–567.

Copyright 1983 by the American Speech-Language-Hearing Association. Reprinted with permission.

The title shown in Excerpt 7.1 is long, but complete. It identifies the independent variables (stimulus repetition rate and frequency), the dependent variable (auditory brainstem response), and the target populations (normal, cochlear-impaired, and VIII nerve/brainstem-impaired subjects). The reader should have no difficulty in knowing what the article is about, and the article can be indexed quite well from the title alone.

EXCERPT 7.2

Speaking fundamental frequency changes over time in women: A longitudinal study.

From A. Russell, L. Penny, and C. Pemberton, 1995, *Journal of Speech and Hearing Research, 38,* pp. 101–109.

Copyright 1995 by the American Speech-Language-Hearing Association. Reprinted with permission.

The title shown in Excerpt 7.2 is shorter, but it still conveys the essence of the study. The article examined changes in women's vocal fundamental frequency over time. The title also clearly states that the research design was longitudinal.

EXCERPT 7.3

Acoustic Patterns of Apraxia of Speech.

From R. D. Kent and J. C. Rosenbeck, 1983, *Journal of Speech and Hearing Research, 26,* pp. 231–249.

Even a very short title can fully inform the reader about the nature of a study. In the six words of Excerpt 7.3, Kent and Rosenbeck have told us what their study is about. A reader would know immediately if the article is of interest and an abstracting service could do a reasonable job of indexing the article from the title.

In summary, the title of an article should capture the essence of the topic that was investigated. It should be concise and well written, and should identify the variables studied and the target population.

The Abstract

Many journals require a short abstract that briefly summarizes the major points of the article. The *APA Publication Manual* (APA, 1994, pp. 8–11) suggests that an empirical research article should contain an abstract of 100 to 150 words that describes the problem, the subjects, the method, the findings, and the conclusions. The manual further states that the abstract should be accurate, self-contained, concise, specific, comprehensive, and readable. It should be aimed at increasing the audience and the future retrievability of the article. Abstracts are not easy to write. Important, precise information must be packed into a small space. But the importance of the abstract is highlighted by the following statement (APA, 1994, p. 8):

> *A well prepared abstract can be the most important paragraph in your article. . . . Readers frequently decide on the basis of the abstract whether to read the entire article; this is true whether the reader is at a computer or is thumbing through a journal. The abstract needs to be dense with information but also readable, well organized, brief, and self-contained.*

The abstract shown in Excerpt 7.4 is an example of an abstract that covers considerable ground in a small space. The first sentence states the purpose and identifies the subjects. The next few sentences describe the method and results; the last sentence deals with implications of the findings.

EXCERPT 7.4

The purpose of this study was to compare deaf speakers' ($n = 4$) laryngeal behavior during voiced and voiceless consonant productions to that of normal hearing subjects ($n = 4$). Laryngeal behavior

Continued

EXCERPT 7.4 *Continued*

during these two speaker groups' productions of six word-initial stop plosives (/b d g p t k/) and fricatives (/v z ð f s θ/) was visually observed by means of a flexible fiberoptic nasolaryngoscope (fiberscope). The visualizations and their acoustic correlates were audiovisually recorded. The audiovisual recordings were analyzed by means of both frame-by-frame categorical judgments of laryngeal behavior and broad phonetic transcriptions of the accuracy/inaccuracy of consonantal voicing. Results indicated that deaf speakers' laryngeal behavior during production of those consonants perceived as *accurately* voiced was comparable to that of normal speakers, whereas deaf speakers'

laryngeal behavior during production of consonants perceived as *inaccurately* voiced generally differed in various ways from normal. Findings seem to suggest that some aspects of deaf speakers' atypical laryngeal behavior associated with inaccurately voiced consonants may be due to an aberrant linguistic system while other aspects may be due to inadequate laryngeal motor control.

The abstract shown in Excerpt 7.5 also deals concisely and clearly with the study reported thereafter. The purpose of the study is described, subjects and method are briefly treated, and the results are summarized.

EXCERPT 7.5

The purpose of this study was to evaluate the effectiveness of several acoustic measures in predicting breathiness ratings. Recordings were made of eight normal men and seven normal women producing normally phonated, moderately breathy, and very breathy sustained vowels. Twenty listeners rated the degree of breathiness using a direct magnitude estimation procedure. Acoustic measures were made of: (a) signal periodicity, (b) first harmonic amplitude, and (c) spectral tilt. Periodicity measures provided the most accurate predictions of perceived breathi-

ness, accounting for approximately 80% of the variance in breathiness ratings. The relative amplitude of the first harmonic correlated moderately with breathiness ratings, and two measures of spectral tilt correlated weakly with perceived breathiness.

A word of caution: the adequacy of a research article cannot be evaluated simply by reading the abstract. The purpose of the abstract is to provide an overview of the article so that the reader can determine quickly if the article should be read. What may seem on the basis of the abstract to be an exciting and original contribution to the literature may on closer inspection of the article itself turn out to be a poor study, both conceptually and methodologically. The only way to determine the quality of a research study is to read the whole article.

General Statement of the Problem

We have identified four major components in the text of the introduction to a research article. Although these components are frequently woven together in the introduction and may not receive separate subheadings to help the reader identify them, the evaluation process is facilitated if the reader can identify these components for the purpose of analysis.

The first component is the general statement of the problem. Here the author sets forth the topic of the article, including the major variables and the target population. The problem can be described in a variety of ways and different authors have different preferences and styles.

The general statement of the problem lends perspective to the specific empirical operations of a research article. It provides a context for the specific purpose, method, and results to make the conclusions meaningful. The general problem statement may be a short first paragraph or it may run through a few initial paragraphs, including references to previous research, to help establish the context of the research.

A simple, straightforward general problem statement is shown in Excerpt 7.6. In a short paragraph, the author clearly states what general issues will be addressed. The concept of speech intelligibility will be analyzed, the variables that influence it will be identified, and their relative importance will be considered. Later in the article, the author describes a study of the influence of specific syntactic and phonologic variables in the oral speech intelligibility of deaf children.

EXCERPT 7.6

The oral speech intelligibility of hearing-impaired individuals has long been the fulcrum of the discussion on how they should be educated, and yet it is a concept that is difficult to define and about which there are many questions, both unanswered and unposed. Because the oral speech intelligibility of hearing-impaired children is likely to remain an important issue, it is worthwhile to try to analyze the concept in great detail, to pinpoint the many factors which influence it, and to understand the extent to which they do so.

From "The Oral Speech Intelligibility of Hearing-Impaired Talkers," by R. B. Monsen, 1983, *Journal of Speech and Hearing Disorders, 48,* pp. 286–296. Copyright 1983 by the American Speech-Language-Hearing Association. Reprinted with permission.

The example shown in Excerpt 7.7 regards the external validity issue of generalizability. The general problem statement includes a concise rationale for the replication of a previous research study. The concluding sentence of Excerpt 7.7 states what the authors hope to accomplish through such a replication.

EXCERPT 7.7

The veracity of a self-assessment inventory is enhanced when its psychometric properties can be replicated across a variety of settings beyond the one in which it was developed. The sources and magnitude of measurement error can vary from one facility to another because of differences, for instance, in demographic composition and clinical operating procedures (Demorest & Walden, 1984). Cox and Gilmore (1990) developed a self-report questionnaire to quantify the performance of hearing aid users in communicative and environmental situations typically encountered in daily life. These researchers designated their inventory the Profile of Hearing Aid Performance (PHAP), and a salient feature of their study was to establish test-retest reliability and criti-

cal difference values for the PHAP scales and subscales. The purpose of the present study was to replicate the test-retest reliability and critical difference components of the Cox and Gilmore (1990) investigation. Repeating the Cox and Gilmore (1990) study with a different group of subjects in a different setting would serve to assess the generalizability of the PHAP test-retest reliability data and critical difference values reported by the original investigators.

From "Test–Retest Reliability of the Profile of Hearing Aid Performance," by C. T. Nelson and C. V. Palmer, 1994, *Journal of Speech and Hearing Research, 37*, pp. 1211–1215. Copyright 1994 by the American Speech-Language-Hearing Association. Reprinted with permission.

Excerpt 7.8 shows the first three paragraphs of a study of developmental disfluency and emerging grammar. The first paragraph identifies the relationship under investigation, the second paragraph shows the lack of knowledge of this relationship, and the third paragraph sets forth the general plan for studying the problem.

EXCERPT 7.8

Young children in the process of learning to talk display varying degrees of disfluent speech (Adams, 1932; Branscom, Hughes, & Oxtoby, 1955; Davis, 1939, 1940a, 1940b; Egland, 1955; Johnson, 1955; Métraux, 1950; Silverman, 1971, 1972a, 1972b, 1973). As language learning and the development of fluent speech co-occur during the preschool years, a question exists as to what extent observed disfluent behavior in nonstuttering children is related to their emerging language.

Parental reports of the existence of disfluency from the moment children begin to use two-word phrases during the second year of life are common, but few systematic explorations of this period of developmental disfluency have been made. Several investigators have reported on group data with preschool children, using the 2-year-old child as the lower limit of their population (Davis, 1939; Johnson, 1955; Métraux, 1950; Hughes, Note 1). There are no published studies that describe either the frequency of disfluency types used by 2-year-

old children or subsequent changes in the distribution of disfluency types with development. No studies have used longitudinal data to investigate variation in individual patterns of disfluency observed during early language acquisition.

The purpose of this longitudinal study was to describe the characteristics of developmental disfluency in the spontaneous speech of four nonstuttering children as language developed from single words through early multiword utterances. In a related study, the same data were examined to determine if developmental disfluency covaried over time with the emergence of specific semantic-syntactic structures in each child's speech during the early acquisition of grammar.

From "Developmental Disfluency and Emerging Grammar: I. Disfluency Characteristics in Early Syntactic Utterances," by N. Colburn and E. D. Mysak, 1982. *Journal of Speech and Hearing Research, 25*, pp. 414–420. Copyright 1982 by the American Speech-Language-Hearing Association. Reprinted with permission.

In all of these introductory statements, the essence of the general problem area is defined along with an implicit or explicit statement of the importance of the problem. Literature citations are used, if necessary, to buttress the authors' position. As we will see later, the reader's substantive background in the area investigated plays a critical role in the evaluation of the introductory section. Familiarity with the theory and data concerning a particular topic is necessary for the reader to evaluate the arguments developed in an introduction. Even the novice reader, however, should be able to follow the *logic* of the arguments presented and should understand the importance of the general problem.

The Rationale for the Study

The rationale for the study constitutes the second component of the text of the introduction and should stem from the general statement of the problem. The rationale presents the reasons for doing the particular study. It is here that the author justifies the selection of the particular independent and dependent variables studied with the specific population. Because it is impossible to investigate all aspects of the general problem in one research study, the rationale presents the case for studying selected aspects of the problem and may identify limitations imposed on the study.

The major question that the critical reader needs to ask about the rationale is whether the reasons for doing the study are clearly and explicitly stated and documented with literature citations. A variety of reasons are offered by investigators to support the importance and need for the study. The author may cite and attempt to document the inadequacy of previous research in the area under investigation. Another reason for doing the research is to follow up on previous research or to resolve conflicting or inconclusive results reported by other investigators. Still another reason offered by researchers is to provide empirical data related to theoretical aspects of the phenomenon under question. Finally, the rationale may be based on the paucity or absence of previous research in a given area. Any one or combination of these reasons might be used to develop a need for the study.

Excerpt 7.9 is from a study concerning the potential causes underlying the difficulty some elderly persons experience understanding speech in noise. Grose, Poth, and Peters (1994) speculate that impaired central binaural auditory processing capacity could potentially contribute to such speech understanding difficulties. The authors further point out, however, that degraded information from the periphery could contribute to diminished binaural processing. To rule out the possibility that degraded information from the periphery is diminishing binaural processing, the authors use elderly persons who have relatively normal audiograms to test their hypothesis.

EXCERPT 7.9

Many elderly listeners experience some difficulty understanding speech in noise. Age-related, or presbycusic, changes of the auditory system include both a reduced speech understanding in noise and a high-frequency sensorineural hearing loss (cf. Marshall, 1981; Working Group on Speech Understanding and Aging, 1988). Both aspects of hearing impairment tend to worsen with advancing age (Davis, 1989;

Continued

EXCERPT 7.9 *Continued*

Gilad & Glorig, 1979; van Rooij, Plomp, & Orlebeke, 1989). It is therefore not surprising that the reduction in speech understanding appears to be largely attributed to a loss in sensitivity (Humes & Roberts, 1990). However, it is likely that factors other than sensitivity loss also contribute to speech understanding difficulties in noise among the elderly (Abel, Krever, & Alberti, 1990; Bergman, 1971; Helfer & Wilber, 1990; Jerger 1992; Lutman, 1991; Marshall, 1981, 1985; Noble, 1978; Plomp, 1986; Ventry & Weinstein, 1983).

One factor that could potentially contribute to speech understanding difficulties in noise is impaired binaural auditory processing. In typical competitive listening situations, listeners with normal hearing are able to use binaural cues to their advantage in facilitating speech understanding in noise. The binaural cues are based largely on the interaural time and level differences arising from the spatial separations of the target speech and competing noise sources (Durlach, Thompson, & Colburn, 1981; Green & Yost, 1976). Impaired binaural processing would be expected to result in a diminished binaural advantage for distinguishing between spatially separated target speech and noise sources (Warren, Wagner, & Herman, 1978). It is the intent of this study to examine the status of binaural processing in elderly listeners.

Reduced binaural processing in the elderly might be due to a combination of two factors. First, the "bin-aural processor" itself might be impaired. Physiological and anatomical studies have highlighted changes due to aging throughout the auditory system (Bredberg, 1990; Hinchcliffe, 1991; Marshall, 1981; von Wedel, von Wedel, & Streppel, 1991). It is reasonable, therefore, to expect some change in the central aspects of auditory processing in elderly listeners. The second factor that might contribute to reduced binaural processing in the elderly listener is a degradation of the input to the "binaural processor" from the auditory periphery (Roush, 1985). Corruptions in the coding of time and level cues in the periphery would be expected to diminish binaural performance. In an effort to distinguish between these two factors, the present study examined binaural processing in elderly listeners whose peripheral sensitivity was normal, or near-normal. By measuring binaural effects in elderly listeners in the absence of presbycusic sensitivity loss, any changes in binaural processing that might be observed could be more strongly attributed to changes at a central level.

From "Masking Level Differences for Tones and Speech in Elderly Listeners with Relatively Normal Audiograms," by J. H. Grose, E. E. Poth, and R. W. Peters, 1994, *Journal of Speech and Hearing Research, 37,* pp. 422–428. Copyright 1994 by the American Speech-Language-Hearing Association. Reprinted with permission.

The introductory paragraphs shown in Excerpt 7.10 present the general and specific rationales from a study of airflow characteristics of normal and hearing-impaired speakers' fricative productions. The first paragraph presents a general rationale for studying speech physiology in order to understand better the speech production problems of hearing-impaired speakers. The subsequent paragraphs review some of the important literature on speech physiology with the hearing impaired. The fourth and fifth paragraphs present a more specific rationale for studying the aerodynamics of fricative production. Both basic considerations about the nature of aberrant speech production and applied considerations about remediation of the speech of hearing-impaired persons are entertained in this rationale.

EXCERPT 7.10

Identification of the factors which contribute to the reduced speech intelligibility of some hearing-impaired persons has been addressed primarily from an acoustic and/or descriptive frame of reference. Findings have included errors or disorders in prosody (phrasing and intonation), articulation, vowel duration, breath control, timing, tension/harshness, nasality, breathiness/weakness, pitch control, pitch register, and rate of syllable articulation (Boone, 1966; Hudgins, 1934; Hudgins & Numbers, 1942; Markides, 1970; Miller, 1946; Monsen, 1974; Silverman, 1960; Stevens, Nickerson, & Rollins, 1983; Subtelny, 1976). The descriptions of the speech errors of the hearing impaired are generally consistent, but fail to identify the underlying nature of the reduced speech intelligibility. The study of speech physiology, however, can provide insights relative to the fundamental properties of speech production. Zimmermann and Rettaliata (1981) have suggested that analyses of the physiological parameters of speech produced by hearing-impaired persons are important because they may lead to a better understanding of the speech errors which reduce intelligibility and may assist in the development of remediation procedures designed to modify aberrant physiological patterns.

Early investigations into the physiology of speech produced by the hearing impaired appear to have focused primarily on the respiratory mechanism. Authors such as Hudgins (1934, 1937) and Rawlings (1936) reported that many of the speech and voice deficits exhibited by the hearing impaired were directly correlated with aberrant respiratory characteristics. Hudgins and Numbers (1942), however, concluded that the intelligibility of hearing-impaired speakers depended not only on respiratory behaviors but also on proper coordination between respiratory and articulatory mechanisms.

Recent physiological investigations regarding the speech of the hearing-impaired have included measures of respiratory kinematics (Forner & Hixon, 1977; Whitehead, 1983), laryngeal dynamics (Mahshie, 1980; Metz & Whitehead, Note 1), and interarticulatory timing (Huntington, Harris, & Sholer, 1968; McGarr & Harris, 1983; McGarr & Löfqvist, 1982; Rothman, 1977). These investigations have focused primarily on one physiological component of the speech mechanism and have utilized relatively small numbers of subjects, usually because of the invasive and/or highly sophisticated nature of the data collection procedures. Despite the limitations, there is mounting evidence from these investigations that some hearing-impaired speakers significantly mismanage and fail to coordinate the biomechanical aspects of speech properly. The data from many of these investigations also suggest that a relationship exists between aberrant biomechanical functioning and the degree of speech intelligibility exhibited by the hearing-impaired individual.

Data regarding the aerodynamic components of speech produced by the hearing impaired also have been reported (Gilbert, 1974; Hutchinson, Kornhauser, Beasley, & Beasley, 1978; Hutchinson & Smith, 1976; Whitehead & Barefoot, 1980). The study of speech aerodynamics in the hearing impaired is critical because measures of airflow and/or air pressure are a direct reflection of the management of the entire physiological process for speech. Furthermore, the specific measure of airflow during speech production is accomplished with a noninvasive procedure which allows for data collection on a large number of subjects with relative ease. Gilbert (1974) and Hutchinson and Smith (1976) have reported both differences and similarities between hearing-impaired and normally hearing speakers for measures of airflow and/or air pressure during production of plosive consonants. Because of the large variability in speech production skills within the hearing-impaired population, Whitehead and Barefoot (1980) categorized hearing-impaired

Continued

EXCERPT 7.10   *Continued*

adults on the basis of overall speech intelligibility and degree of hearing loss. These authors reported consistent similarities in measures of airflow for plosive consonants between normally hearing and intelligible hearing-impaired speakers and consistent differences between semi-intelligible hearing-impaired speakers and both the normally hearing and intelligible hearing-impaired groups.

Presently, there appear to be very few data regarding the aerodynamics of fricative consonants produced by hearing-impaired adults (Hutchinson & Smith, 1976). Such information is necessary in order to gain a better understanding of the dynam-

ics regarding the physiological management of speech by hearing-impaired persons. The purpose of the present study, therefore, was to investigate the patterns of airflow for fricative consonants produced by hearing-impaired young adults categorized according to speech intelligibility and degree of hearing loss.

From "Airflow Characteristics of Fricative Consonants Produced by Normally Hearing and Hearing-Impaired Speakers," by R. L. Whitehead and S. M. Barefoot, 1983. *Journal of Speech and Hearing Research, 26,* pp. 185–194. Copyright 1983 by the American Speech-Language-Hearing Association. Reprinted with permission.

In the example shown in Excerpt 7.11, Young developed a rationale for studying articulation effort. His rationale was based on a careful review of previous research studies and a critical analysis of their results and limitations. His first two paragraphs review the previous studies and point to their discrepancies and the third paragraph describes some procedural problems with such studies. Finally, in the fourth paragraph, he states his goals as a consequence of his review and analysis.

EXCERPT 7.11

Recent studies by Locke (1972) and Parnell and Amerman (1977) have shown that judgments of articulation effort are associated with phonological acquisition, frequency of occurrence of sounds in English, and pattern of children's substitutions. An earlier study by Malecot (1955) was concerned with force of articulation as a factor in the lenis-fortis distinction.

Although all three studies employed similar paired-comparisons procedures to rank selected consonants on an articulation effort dimension, the results were greatly discrepant. Parnell and Amerman (1977) and Malecot (1955) used a VCV context and had observers voice each stimulus. A correlation (tau) between the 12 consonants com-

mon to both studies generated a nonsignificant index of .15. (Malecot's study is described in a brief paragraph and the procedures must be inferred.) Locke (1972) employed a CV stimulus and had observers whisper. In comparison with the 13 consonants in common ranked by Parnell and Amerman's whispered task, Locke's ranks generated a correlation (tau) of −.18, also nonsignificant. Daniloff (1973) and Parnell and Amerman (1977) have suggested how important procedural differences among the three studies may have accounted for the disagreement in results.

Apart from procedural differences, the three studies used certain nonstandard design and analysis methods which may have contributed to some of

Continued

EXCERPT 7.11   *Continued*

the disaccord in results. All three had observers underline on typed lists which member of the consonant pair was harder to say or required the most effort. The consequences of this procedure were that (1) the order of the pairs was the same for all observers or for groups of observers, (2) there was no systematic control of the space effect—a consonant was always in the same position in a pair, and (3) the observers could review previous judgments. In Locke's study, moreover, the observers performed the task in groups of 11, and there was no check on whether observers actually whispered aloud or made their judgments on some other basis. With respect to the mode of analysis, Locke (1972) and Parnell and Amerman (1977) ranked the consonants by summing judgments across observers; Malecot probably did the same since he appears to refer to Guilford's Composite Standard Method of Scaling (Guilford, 1954, p. 169). A limitation to ranking the consonants by summing across observers is that a rank order can be achieved even when observers cannot perform the task or when observers disagree with each other. None of the studies provided data to show that observers could

actually perform the discriminations reliably or that they agreed with each other if they could.

The validity of a construct such as articulation effort needs to be established before it can have any useful explanatory or predictive potential, especially when the construct reflects a perceptual continuum likely to be multidimensional. Determining the physiological or acoustical correlates of such a continuum may be desirable, but to do so requires the prior demonstration that the dimension shows some perceptual reality. I have examined in detail this position in previous articles (Young, 1969a, 1969b, 1975; Young & Downs, 1968). The goals of the present study, therefore, were to repeat the paired-comparison task without the design limitations of the earlier studies, and to comment on the validity or reality of the articulation effort construct.

From "Articulation Effort: Transitivity and Observer Agreement," by M. A. Young, 1981, *Journal of Speech and Hearing Research, 24,* pp. 224–232. Copyright 1981 by the American Speech-Language-Hearing Association. Reprinted with permission.

Excerpt 7.12 shows the first two introductory paragraphs of an article regarding the evaluation of a computer-assisted speech training system, the IBM SpeechViewer. The first paragraph develops the recent increased usage of technological devices in speech training. The second paragraph focuses specifically on the IBM SpeechViewer with a brief discussion of the system and then raises the issue of whether the system can provide any demonstrable benefits beyond what the clinician can provide independently of the system.

EXCERPT 7.12

In recent years there has been a substantial increase in the development and use of technological devices for the treatment of speech production of individuals with hearing impairment. Many mechanical and electronic devices have been designed to provide hearing-impaired speakers with an awareness of

speech production events not readily available to them through their visual and reduced auditory channels (Fletcher, 1989; Fletcher & Hasegawa, 1983; McGarr, Youdelman, & Head, 1989).

Although the treatment success with these technologies has been mixed, the approaches have

Continued

EXCERPT 7.12   *Continued*

expanded and progressed into the area of computer-based systems (Osberger, Moeller, Kroese, & Lippmann, 1981; Povel & Wansink, 1986; Watson, Reed, Kewley-Port, & Maki, 1989). The IBM SpeechViewer system is a recent addition to this area, although it was not developed specifically for use with hearing-impaired persons. The system consists of 12 modules or programs that provide various types of visual and auditory feedback based on certain acoustic parameters of speech. The visual feedback of the different modules appears to be salient, and, as such, the system has a great deal of face validity for the treatment of hearing-impaired children, as well as other clinical populations that benefit from additional visual cues. Nonetheless, the IBM SpeechViewer's modules have been largely untested. Bernstein (1989) as well as Watson and Kewley-Port (1989) have suggested that clinical trials are necessary for the appropriate use of computer-based speech training aids. It is not known whether the system provides any benefit beyond what clinicians already con-

tribute. It is also unknown which clients are likely to show gains with the different modules when minimum or no supervision is provided. This issue is critical for clinicians with large caseloads. In the case of hearing-impaired children, for whom substantive progress in speech production often requires long-term and extensive treatment, the addition of an effective computer-based system could greatly expand the overall treatment time for children. In addition, if computer systems can effectively direct certain aspects of therapy, individuals with minimal training (such as classroom aides and parents) could supervise some of the speech training.

From "The Efficacy of Using the IBM SpeechViewer Vowel Accuracy Module to Treat Young Children with Hearing Impairment," by S. R. Pratt, A. T. Heintzelman, and S. E. Deming, 1993, *Journal of Speech and Hearing Research, 36,* pp. 1063–1074. Copyright 1993 by the American Speech-Language-Hearing Association. Reprinted with permission.

The rationale shown in Excerpt 7.13 takes a somewhat different approach. This argument is not based so much on a review of discrepant results or the need to compare measurements for accuracy but rather on a logical development of the implications of the nature of different relationships among variables. The relationships among acoustic variables and fluency enhancement have both theoretical implications regarding the process of speech motor control and practical implications regarding the enhancement of fluency through therapy. Notice how the article introduces these notions with a brief literature review in the first paragraph and then develops the argument logically in the next two paragraphs.

EXCERPT 7.13

In the decade following Wingate's seminal articles (1969, 1970) on artificially induced fluency, considerable research effort was directed toward identifying underlying conditions related to fluency enhancement among stutterers. The emphasis of

much of this research was on isolating acoustic speech parameters of stutterers' fluent speech that varied concomitantly with stuttering frequency. For example, the relationships among changes in vocal sound pressure level (Adams & Hutchinson, 1974;

Continued

EXCERPT 7.13   *Continued*

Adams & Moore, 1972; Conture, 1974), vocal fundamental frequency, and vowel duration and the growth of fluency associated with stutterers' speaking in the presence of loud noise and speaking in accordance with a rhythmic stimulus (Brayton & Conture, 1978) were investigated. Attention was paid to the relationships among changes in vowel duration, continuity of phonation, and vocal sound pressure level and the growth of fluency associated with stutterers' singing (Colcord & Adams, 1979; Healey, Mallard, & Adams, 1976) and choral speaking (Adams & Ramig, 1980). Additionally, it is clear from both perceptual (Runyan & Adams, 1978) and acoustic studies (Metz, Onufrak, & Ogburn, 1979) that stuttering therapy can alter certain acoustic properties of the stutterer's fluent speech.

These and other related studies have advanced our knowledge regarding which acoustic variables associated with the fluent speech of stutterers change concomitantly with the growth of fluency. However, these studies are based on group data and consequently provide limited information about the nature of the relationships between acoustic variable changes and fluency enhancement. Furthermore, there is no a priori reason to assume that all systematic changes in the acoustic properties of stutterers' speech are necessarily related to fluency enhancement. Some of these alterations may reflect changes in the operation of the motor control processes that underlie fluency enhancement, whereas others may be systematic by-products of the particular fluency-enhancing condition. That is, a given fluency-enhancing condition (or therapy procedure) may have two types of effects on a stutterer's speech: (a) one that imposes changes in speech that directly enhance fluency, and which are

reflected in certain acoustic changes and whose occurrence is probably common, to greater or lesser degrees, to all fluency-enhancing conditions; and (b) one that imposes changes in speech that do not directly enhance fluency, and which are also reflected in certain acoustic changes but whose occurrence is probably an idiosyncratic result of ancillary aspects of the particular fluency-enhancing condition. By examining the relationship between stuttering frequency and various acoustic features of stutterers' speech across individuals (in addition to examining group data), we may obtain some clues regarding those variables that are most closely related to changes in stuttering frequency. Although correlation does not necessarily imply causation, acoustic variables closely related to stuttering frequency more likely reflect control processes underlying fluency than variables that are statistically independent of the stuttering frequency dimension within the population of stutterers.

In the present study we explored such relationships in more detail. Specifically, we examined several acoustic variables measured from a single group of stutterers. These measurements included both traditional and previously unexplored acoustic properties of stutterers' fluent speech production. Furthermore, we examined the relationship between these acoustic variables and fluency within a group of mild-to-severe stutterers both prior to and after a concentrated program of stuttering therapy.

From "Acoustic Analysis of Stutterers' Fluent Speech before and after Therapy," by D. E. Metz, V. J. Samar, and P. R. Sacco, 1983, *Journal of Speech and Hearing Research, 26,* pp. 531–536. Copyright 1983 by the American Speech-Language-Hearing Association. Reprinted with permission.

As these examples have shown, a major part of the introduction to a research article spells out the reasons for doing the particular study. The rationale describes the need for the research. The logic of the arguments presented, with appropriate citations from the literature, should convince the reader of the value of the investigation. The rationale may take different forms, depending on the nature of the study. Some introductions stress the practical nature of a study such as the need to assess the accuracy of a measurement. Others stress the need to resolve conflicting results or conclusions from previous studies. Many studies develop their rationales on the basis of the importance of the research for theoretical or practical applications. In any case, the rationale for the study is an important component of the text of the introduction.

Review of the Literature

The third component of the text of an introduction is the review of literature. The literature review is not really a separate part of an introduction, but it is the fabric from which the statement of the problem and rationale are woven. The literature citations not only serve to document the need for the study, but they also help to put the research into context or historical perspective. Through the use of appropriate references, the researcher identifies how the investigation reported fits into the general theme of research in the same problem area. In a sense, the literature citations pay tribute to those who have gone before. In another sense, the literature citations allow the reader to examine the sources used by the author to make the case for the study. Thus, the reader has an opportunity to evaluate directly the adequacy of the literature citations and to determine whether, in fact, the citations used justify the research reported.

The literature review, then, should be evaluated in regard to (1) the degree to which it helps to place the general problem into perspective and (2) the degree to which it helps to develop the rationale for the study. Different authors have different styles and preferences for the way they use the literature review in relation to the other components of the text of the introduction. For example Colburn and Mysak in Excerpt 7.8 use the literature review mainly to place the general problem in perspective, whereas Young, in Excerpt 7.11, uses the literature review to develop his rationale. Whitehead and Barefoot in Excerpt 7.10 use the literature review throughout the introduction to develop the general problem and the rationale for the study. Also, some others make a general summary point and then cite a string of references as Grose et al. did in Excerpt 7.9.

Sometimes the literature review does stand on its own, especially if the author's intent is to review new literature or literature from areas that are probably unfamiliar to most readers of a particular journal. An example of this can be seen in Excerpt 7.14 where literature from the areas of gerontology and nursing is briefly reviewed. This literature is likely to be unfamiliar to most speech pathologists and audiologists and needs to be summarized on its own before the development of a general problem statement and rationale.

EXCERPT 7.14

The fastest growing age group in the United States are those persons 65 years of age and older (Brotman, 1977), and thus, by the year 2000, 12%
of our population will be elderly. As we age, our special needs multiply. Many of the elderly require supportive services to meet their housing, food,

Continued

EXCERPT 7.14   *Continued*

health care, financial and social needs. While a majority of the aged can function independently or with community support, at least 5% become institutionalized. In 1975 there were over one million people 65 years old and above residing in 23,000 long-term care settings (Health Resources Statistics, 1976). This number represents a dramatic increase from the previous decade, and we can expect even more elderly people will become institutionalized in the next 25 years.

Relocation to a long-term care setting, such as a nursing home or chronic disease hospital, generates a series of personal and social problems for the older person. Social gerontologists have investigated the effects of institutionalization on the elderly (Ainsworth, 1977; Bennett, 1963; Kahana, 1971; Lieberman & Lakin, 1963; Wessen, 1964), the criteria for adjustment to long-term care (Bennett & Nahemow, 1965; Havighurst, 1968;

Lowenthal & Haven, 1968), and the social interaction and organization of such settings (Lawton, 1968; Rosow, 1967; Weinstock & Bennett, 1968). An underlying and recurrent theme in this literature is that communication is a factor in the integration and adjustment of older people to institutional life. Similarly, the nursing literature emphasizes the strong relationship between staff-patient communication and effective nursing care (Collins, 1977; Lewis, 1973; Meyers, 1964; Shipper & Leonard, 1965). Collins (1977) states that communication is the core of the nurse-patient relationship.

From "Perception of Spoken Communication by Elderly Chronically Ill Patients in an Institutional Setting," by R. Lubinski, E. B. Morrison, and S. Rigrodsky, 1981, *Journal of Speech and Hearing Disorders, 46,* pp. 405–412. Copyright 1981 by the American Speech-Language-Hearing Association. Reprinted with permission.

There are several important questions for the critical evaluator of research to ask about the review of literature in the introduction to a research article. Most of these questions assume some knowledge of the topic on the part of the reader of the article.

First, how thorough is the literature review? Are there important omissions that might change the nature of the rationale or the perspective of the problem? Space limitations in a journal obviously place some constraints on the scope of any literature review. It is simply impossible to cite all the pertinent literature without running into objections by a journal editor who is interested in conserving valuable space. Nonetheless, the key references should be cited to substantiate the need for the study. Despite the apparent thoroughness of a particular literature review, the reader must still determine if key references have been omitted. It is here that the reader's background and expertise in the particular topic of an article play a crucial role in the evaluation process. It is extremely difficult to judge the thoroughness of the literature review without familiarity with the relevant literature.

How recent are the literature citations? Has the author overlooked recent work in reviewing the literature? This does not mean that older references should not be cited. Some older references are classics in a field and have had such a germinal influence on so many studies since their publication that they are constantly referred to. See, for example, Excerpt 7.10 where Whitehead and Barefoot refer to the classic work of Hudgins and Numbers that was published in 1942. It is not surprising that this reference is cited because it is a classic study on speech of the deaf. The point is that the author has an obligation to cite the relevant work, new and old, that is necessary to place the problem in perspective and develop a convincing rationale. It may be that there is no recent literature on a given topic because the article represents renewed interest in a topic that received considerable attention twenty or thirty years ago but little attention in the last five or ten years. Here the researcher may be justified in citing only older studies to make the case for a new study. However, when recent literature on a particular topic exists and is relevant, it should be cited.

A third point is whether the review is critical of previous literature and whether the criticism is objective, unbiased, and justified. Have the data of the previous studies been accurately reported and interpreted? Were the conclusions of the previous research criticized fairly? These are not easy questions to answer because they require the reader to refer to the original studies to determine if the criticisms were justified.

The next question is whether the literature citations are relevant to the purpose and to the need for the study. Once again, the ideal way to evaluate the relevancy of the literature review is to be knowledgeable about the subject matter under investigation. We raise the question of relevancy but we cannot answer it for the reader. There is no easy way of evaluating relevancy without some in-depth familiarity with the topic.

Finally, the careful evaluator of research should be alert to the overuse of unpublished research, citations from obscure references, frequent reference to materials appearing in publications that are inaccessible. The major problem is that the reader cannot consult the original sources to determine whether the researcher has cited them correctly, drawn appropriate conclusions from them, and so forth. The researcher's use of these citations may also suggest research that is out of the mainstream, idiosyncratic, or unimportant.

In summary, the literature review is at the heart of the introduction to the research report. It is of fundamental importance for the critical reader of research to evaluate carefully the adequacy of the literature citations. Special attention should be given to the extent and thoroughness of the review, the recency and relevance of the citations, the objectivity and accuracy of the criticism of previous research. In the final analysis, the reader of the research report must bring expertise, experience, and knowledge to the evaluation of the literature citations. And, if need be, the reader must return to the cited sources to fully appreciate, understand, and evaluate this aspect of the introduction.

Statement of Purpose, Research Questions, and Hypotheses

The introduction of a research article usually concludes with a specific statement of the purpose of the research, with one or more research questions, or with testable hypotheses. Whichever form is used, this section represents the logical culmination of the general problem statement and rationale. As such, the specific purpose, question, or hypothesis should relate directly to what has preceded it. It is important that the statement be clear and precise. If possible, the statement should allow the reader to identify the independent and dependent variables and the type of research strategy used to study them.

Excerpt 7.15 shows the statement of purpose from a study that compared normal and apraxic speakers on a number of acoustical measures. The statement is broken down into five specific objectives for description of segmental and prosodic characteristics of apraxia. These specific objectives followed quite naturally from the literature review that stressed the need to define and quantify terms used to describe apraxia of speech. The results of the study are later presented in an orderly fashion that follows the outline shown in this statement of specific objectives.

EXCERPT 7.15

This study sought to determine:

1. if the utterances of apraxic subjects are lengthened in comparison to the utterances of normal-speaking subjects

and, if so:

2. whether differential lengthening effects exist as a function of the segmental properties or the syllabic length of utterances
3. whether apraxic and normal speech are distinguished by nondurational aspects of prosody, such as relative syllable intensity or F_o-frequency contour
4. if spectrograms show evidence of phonetic (subphonemic) errors in apraxic speech

5. the degree to which acoustic patterns of apraxic speech confirm perceptually based descriptions of the disorder.

These five objectives were selected because they are within the scope of an acoustic study and because they should lead to a refined description of the segmental and prosodic features of the disorder.

From "Acoustic Patterns of Apraxia of Speech," by R. D. Kent and J. C. Rosenbeck, 1983, *Journal of Speech and Hearing Research, 26,* pp. 231–249. Copyright 1983 by the American Speech-Language-Hearing Association. Reprinted with permission.

The statement of purpose and specific research questions shown in Excerpt 7.16 come from a longitudinal study of the language development of hearing children of deaf parents. The two specific purposes of the study are stated first, and then the specific questions and subquestions to be answered are spelled out in detail. The reader can see from the purposes that the study is developmental in nature and that it also includes a comparison of the children's language when talking with their deaf mothers and with a hearing adult. The dependent variables to be examined developmentally are clearly identified. The purposes of the study stem quite naturally from the rationale developed in the introduction and the results section of the article is broken down according to the sequence of the research questions listed in the excerpt. Readers should have no problem in following the presentation of the results, given the outlining of the specific research questions in the introduction.

EXCERPT 7.16

The purpose of this study was (1) to compare the language development of five two-year-old hearing children of deaf parents with the language development of normal children reported in the develop-

mental literature described above; and (2) to study the discourse interactions of these children with their mothers and with a hearing adult to determine the effect of the mothers' defective speech on the

Continued

EXCERPT 7.16 *Continued*

children's ability to process and learn from the mothers' oral language. The specific questions to be answered by this study are as follows:

1. Is the proportional distribution of the semantic-syntactic relations encoded in these children's utterances similar to that found in the messages of children from hearing environments?
2. Are the forms these children use to code the semantic relations different from those used by children from hearing environments in terms of the following:

   - the ordering of subject-verb-object relationships?
   - the sequence of development of Brown's 14 grammatical morphemes?
   - the predominant use of pronominal or nominal references for linguistic representation?

3. Are the oral discourse patterns of these children similar to those of children from hearing environments, and do they vary according to whether the recipient is hearing or deaf in terms of the following:

   - imitations?
   - categories of contingent speech?

4. Does the mothers' speech contain grammatical morphemes and systematic ordering of constituents?

From "The Influence of Deviant Maternal Input on the Development of Language During the Preschool Years," by N. B. Schiff, 1979, *Journal of Speech and Hearing Research, 22,* pp. 581–603. Copyright 1979 by the American Speech-Language-Hearing Association. Reprinted with permission.

The example shown in Excerpt 7.17 shows two specific research questions stated in the form of hypotheses. Excerpt 7.17 is from a study that investigated how laryngeal reaction times (LRT) differed (a) when mild and severe stutterers and nonstutterers were given various lengths of time to prepare to respond to a stimulus, and (b) when the complexity of the required response varied. It should be pointed out that this is *not* the null hypothesis tested by a statistical significance test. Although it used to be common for authors to list the various null hypotheses tested, this is relatively uncommon now because the null hypothesis is usually implied by the statement of a specific purpose or question.

EXCERPT 7.17

There were two hypotheses. (a) Stutterers vary as a function of severity in their ability to use a preparation facilitating stimulus presentation condition to reduce LRT. Specifically, nonstutterers and mild stutterers may reduce LRT in a preparation facilitating stimulus condition, whereas severe stutterers are unlikely to do so. (b) All subjects produce shorter LRTs in an isolated vowel response condition than in a VCV condition, but the magnitude of latency difference between response conditions varies as a function of stutterer severity. Specifically, within groups, severe stutterers increase LRT more than mild stutterers or nonstutterers as a function of increased response complexity, with consequently greater between-group differences in the VCV response condition than in the vowel response condition.

From "Preparation and Response Complexity Effects of Stutterers' and Nonstutterers' Acoustic LRT," by J. Dembowski and B. C. Watson, 1991, *Journal of Speech and Hearing Research, 34,* pp. 49–59. Copyright 1991 by the American Speech-Language-Hearing Association. Reprinted with permission.

Excerpt 7.18 shows the statement of the specific purpose from an experiment on the effect of segment and pause manipulations on the identification of treated stutterers. The statement begins with a brief rationale for the particular manipulations used to change tape-recorded speech samples for presentation to listeners and, then, states what effect will be studied. It is clear that rate is the independent variable to be manipulated and that labeling behavior of listeners is the dependent variable that may change as a result of manipulation of the independent variable. The rationale for this specific purpose is clearly developed in the introduction through a review of previous literature on the speech characteristics of treated stutterers and on the ability of listeners to discriminate between treated stutterers and normal speakers.

EXCERPT 7.18

If listeners use rate as their primary criterion for identifying treated stutterers, it should be possible to demonstrate this experimentally and to alter their judgments by manipulating rate. Specifically, if the difference in rate between a pair of talkers can be changed instrumentally from a substantial value to a minimum value, then the labelling behavior of listeners who judge both the original and altered samples should change. The purpose of the present study was to match instrumentally the rates used by a sample of nonstutterers and treated stutterers who were known to be perceptually distinguishable in order to determine the effect of this manipulation on listener judgments.

From "Effects of Segment and Pause Manipulations on the Identification of Treated Stutterers," by R. A. Prosek and C. M. Runyan, 1983, *Journal of Speech and Hearing Research, 26,* pp. 510–516. Copyright 1983 by the American Speech-Language-Hearing Association. Reprinted with permission.

The final example, shown in Excerpt 7.19, is from a study of vocal fundamental frequency of hearing-impaired speakers. The author first explains briefly why vocal fundamental frequency (F_o) should be compared for oral reading vs. spontaneous speech in hearing-impaired speakers and then states what will be studied. Two independent variables will be examined: normal hearing vs. hard-of-hearing (classification variable) and oral reading vs. spontaneous speech. The dependent variable is fundamental frequency. The results that follow show the means and standard deviations of the fundamental frequencies specifically broken down according to the two independent variables. Again, the author has clearly stated his purpose so that the reader will know exactly what to expect in examining the results of the study.

EXCERPT 7.19

Voice characteristics of deaf and hard-of-hearing individuals during spontaneous or impromptu speech need to be investigated because spontaneous speech is a speaking condition of primary interest. In addition, knowledge of differences (or lack of them) in voice characteristics between oral reading and spontaneous speech should be useful in estimating spontaneous oral performance of hard-of-hearing individuals from their oral reading performance. For normal-hearing individuals, there is some evidence that f_o distributional characteristics are different between oral reading and spontaneous speech.

Continued

EXCERPT 7.19   *Continued*

Snidecor (1943), for example, found that oral reading conditions produced both greater means and standard deviations of fundamental frequency. It was the purpose of the present study to investigate f_o distributional characteristics of hard-of-hearing individuals during spontaneous speech and oral reading, and to test whether or not f_o relationships, similar to those found in normal-hearing individuals, exist between the two speaking conditions.

From "Some Voice Fundamental Frequency Characteristics of Oral Reading and Spontaneous Speech in Hard-of-Hearing Young Women," by Y. Horii, 1982, *Journal of Speech and Hearing Research, 25,* pp. 608–610. Copyright 1982 by the American Speech-Language-Hearing Association. Reprinted with permission.

A number of factors lead researchers to use one form or another to state the specific purpose of a study. The specific manner of stating the purpose or question or hypothesis is not as important as the clarity with which it is stated. The important point is that the author should capture the nature of the study in a brief paragraph or so and specify the independent and dependent variables. The reader should move from the statement of specific purpose with a clear idea of what to expect in the results section of the article. Whichever form is used, the statement should be well written, explicit, and related to the preceding rationale.

Miscellaneous Considerations

Two final issues need to be addressed with respect to the introduction. First, the reader should be alert to the need for, or the use of, definitions of terms that the author employs throughout the study. Many terms have different meaning for different people. The author has the responsibility of indicating, in the introduction, how those terms are defined in the article. This is accomplished by either defining the term in the introduction or, more commonly, by appropriate citation of other sources that have already defined the term. The reader must remember, however, that the researcher frequently writes for a specific audience, that is, for other researchers working in the same area or for clinicians who presumably are familiar with the subject (and the terminology) under investigation. Thus, terms that the naive reader would like to see defined may not be. Nonetheless, idiosyncratic usage or the use of terms about which there may be differences of opinion as to their meaning require the specific attention of the author and should be defined in the introduction.

Second, the researcher may spell out some of the limitations of the study about to be reported. There are two types of limitations that might be noted. The first is a limitation that is beyond the investigator's control. An example of this extrinsic limitation is the situation in which a researcher may want to include both males and females in a study but must collect data in a setting in which males predominate. The second type of limitation is an intrinsic one, that is, a limitation self-imposed by the investigator in recognition of the fact that all aspects of a problem area simply cannot be investigated in a single study. Longitudinal studies have to end, despite the researcher's desire to continue to study a child's language development beyond the data-collection period. The investigator who is studying hearing loss in a geriatric population may want to include a number of auditory tests but, because of the nature of the population, limits the study to a selected few procedures.

The limitations of the study, as expressed by the researcher, are important and deserve careful consideration by the reader. Because of the limitations, a study may turn out to be of no consequence. The limitations may suggest that the author should have, at the very least, delayed submitting the research report until the limitations were overcome. The fact that an author recognizes and states the limitations in the introduction does not necessarily relieve the author of the responsibility of dealing with these limitations later in the Discussion section. Because most limitations are, in fact, detailed in the final section of the article, we will have more to say about evaluating author-stated limitations in Chapter 10.

Finally, it goes without saying that the introduction should be well written, clear, and logically organized.

The Evaluation Checklist that follows summarizes the important points made in the chapter and is designed to facilitate the critical evaluation of the Introduction section of the article.

EVALUATION CHECKLIST

Instructions: The four-category scale at the end of this checklist may be used to rate the Introduction section of an article. The *Evaluation Items* help identify those topics that should be considered in arriving at the rating. Comments on these topics entered as *Evaluation Notes* should serve as the basis for the overall rating.

Evaluation Items   *Evaluation Notes*

1. Title identified target population and variables under study.

2. Purpose, procedures, important findings, and implications were summarized in the abstract.

3. A clear statement of the general problem was given.

4. There was a logical and convincing rationale.

5. There was a current, thorough, and accurate review of literature.

6. The purpose, questions, or hypotheses were logical extensions of the rationale.

7. The introduction was clearly written
   and well organized.

8. General Comments.

Overall Rating (Introduction):

Poor	Fair	Good	Excellent

Reference

American Psychological Association. (1994). *Publication manual of the American Psychological Association* (4th ed.). Washington, DC: American Psychological Association.

Chapter 8

The Method Section

If the Introduction section can be considered the foundation of the research article, then the Method section can be considered its structural framework. Understanding this framework is crucial to the critical evaluation of the Results and Discussion sections that follow. It is in the Method section that the author describes the subjects used in the study, the materials employed, and how those materials are used with the subjects; that is, the procedures. In addition, the Method section helps the reader to identify the research strategy being reported and the specific research design incorporated in the study. Finally, it is in the Method section that the careful reader can identify how the author dealt with threats to internal and external validity.

The Method section stems directly from the rationale and the purpose of the study stated in the introduction. As such, the first major concern of the critical evaluator is whether the Method section, viewed in its entirety, is related to what has preceded and whether the methods chosen are appropriate to the problem posed in the introduction. The second concern, and one that we seek to answer in this chapter, is whether the methods chosen by the investigator are adequate in and of themselves.

Subjects

We have noted in Part I that subject selection can pose a threat to the internal and external validity of both experimental and descriptive research. The careful reader of a research article must determine, therefore, if the subject-selection procedure reported and the type of subjects used compromise the adequacy of the research. Before we present some evaluative guidelines, one general guideline needs to be emphasized with respect to the description of the subjects (as well as the description of materials and procedures). This guideline is simply, but importantly, that sufficient description be provided to allow the reader to *replicate* the study reported, at least in its important aspects. Researchers must resist the blue pencil of the cost-conscious editor, and the reader must insist on adequate detail or, at the very least, references to previous research that contain the detailed description of procedures.

The important point, again, is that the description of methods must be sufficiently complete to allow for replication.

Sample Size

The diversity of research in communicative disorders is reflected, in a sense, in the different sample sizes employed in different studies. Sample sizes range from $N = 1$ to $N =$ thousands. Thus, one of the first questions that must be asked by readers (and doers) of research is whether the size of the sample is adequate for the purposes of the study. Unfortunately, there is no simple answer to this question. For example, Pedhazur and Schmelkin (1991, p. 336) state that "decision regarding sample size is a complex one subject to a host of concerns. These include, . . . sampling strategy, types of estimators, practical and economic concerns . . . Type I and Type II errors." Additionally, the purpose of the investigation, previous research, the concern about generalizability, the variability found for the attribute under study, and the research design itself all play a role in deciding whether the number of subjects used is appropriate. For instance, in within-subjects designs, in which there are many repeated observations and many data points, small samples have been used and are quite adequate. This type of small sample study is found, for example, in the language-acquisition literature and the psychoacoustic literature. Test standardization and survey research require large samples of subjects. Between-subjects designs usually require larger samples than within-subjects designs. If one wishes to generalize data to the majority of children who have articulatory disorders, then, a large number of subjects will have to be used. If the experimental treatment is expected to produce only small group differences, large samples may have to be employed to demonstrate statistically significant differences. It has to be acknowledged, of course, that small statistically significant differences obtained on a large sample of subjects may have little clinical meaning or value. On the other hand, if large treatment differences are anticipated, on the basis of either pilot data or previous research, then a small sample may be adequate.

Excerpts 8.1 through 8.4 illustrate the broad range of sample sizes found in the communicative disorders literature. The four articles from which the excerpts were selected reflect different purposes, previous sample-size traditions, different research designs, expected variability of the data, and statistical analysis. Each of these considerations may have been more or less responsible for the sample sizes chosen.

Excerpt 8.1 illustrates the use of a large sample of randomly selected subjects. We have mentioned previously that consumers of research can have more confidence in the generalization of results when a large number of subjects have been randomly selected from the population of interest. Most studies, however, do not incorporate random selection of subjects from the total population of interest. The most common reasons are that the universe of subjects of interest is not available to the researcher and the cost of such random sampling procedures may be prohibitive. For practical reasons, then, most studies in communicative disorders do not use large random samples of subjects. The exceptions are usually large-scale descriptive studies such as the one by Quigley, Smith, and Wilbur (Excerpt 8.1). Great care was taken to randomly select a large sample of subjects stratified according to the type of school, age, gender, and geographical region. As the authors noted in the reference to external validity in the last sentence, the generalization of the results of this study should be remarkably good.

EXCERPT 8.1   Subjects

Subjects for the total research program were 450 prelingually and profoundly deaf students, 25 males and 25 females in each of nine age groups ranging from 10 to 18 years, selected from 10 residential and six day programs for deaf students in the United States. All educational programs with 100 or more deaf students were stratified on the basis of geographical region (as categorized by the U.S. Bureau of the Census) and type of program (day or residential). One day and one residential program were then selected randomly from each of the nine geographical regions. Only six day programs were included since three of the geographical regions, New England, East South Central, and Mountain, did not contain day programs with 100 or more deaf students. A 10th residential school was added to provide a sampling of residential students from an oral school. When the 16 educational programs had been selected, 25 male and 25 female subjects were chosen at random from each of the nine age levels, with the number of subjects selected in each geo-

graphical region being proportionate to the total number of deaf students in the region and to their distribution in day and residential programs. Also, subjects were selected only from among those students who (1) had sensorineural hearing impairment of not less than 90 dB (ANSI, 1969) at 500, 1000, and 2000 Hz; (2) had suffered hearing impairment before the age of two years; (3) had an IQ of at least 80 on the performance scale of the WISC or WAIS, or some comparable test; and (4) had (in the judgment of school personnel) no apparent disability other than hearing impairment. The stratified, random sampling procedures used for the total research program permit generalization of the results to all deaf students in the United States meeting the criteria established for the study.

From "Comprehension of Relativized Sentences by Deaf Students," by S. P. Quigley, N. L. Smith, and R. B. Wilbur, 1974, *Journal of Speech and Hearing Research, 17,* pp. 325–341. Copyright 1974 by the American Speech-Language-Hearing Association. Reprinted with permission.

The next excerpt (8.2) describes the selection and group assignment of 84 subjects in a study of fricative discrimination in infants. Although this sample is not as large as the one reported previously and was not randomly selected, it still represents a relatively large sample of subjects. Also, the purpose and design of this study are different from the Quigley et al. study. The more important point in the Eilers and Minifie study is that subjects were randomly *assigned* to experimental and control groups in this between-subjects experiment, a procedure that we indicated earlier is the best method for equating experimental and control groups. In other words, method of group assignment is more important than random selection and sample size in this study. More will be said about procedures for group assignment later in this chapter when we present excerpts dealing with procedures in between-subjects experiments.

EXCERPT 8.2   Subjects

The subjects were 84 infants between four and 17 weeks old identified by parental response to mail solicitation. Twenty-four infants completed Experiment I (16 in the experimental group where order of stimulus presentation was counterbalanced

and eight in the control group where no change in stimulus occurred following habituation) and 30 infants each completed Experiments II and III (20 in each experimental group and 10 in each control). Infants were excluded if they failed to suck (chewed

Continued

EXCERPT 8.2   Subjects   *Continued*

on nipple), failed to suck following the second habituation minute, cried persistently, or if termination was requested by the parent. Approximately 60% of the infant subjects completed the session in each of the three experiments. Infants were randomly assigned to either experimental or control groups. Approximately equal numbers of infants were excluded from the experimental and control groups in Experiments I, II, and III because they failed one or more of the inclusion criteria. The age range and median age, respectively of the subjects for each experiment were as follows: Experiment I, 4 to 15 weeks and 8.3 weeks; Experiment II, 4 to 17 weeks and 10 weeks; and Experiment III, 8 to 17 weeks and 12.4 weeks.

From "Fricative Discrimination in Early Infancy," by R. E. Eilers and F. D. Minifie, 1975, *Journal of Speech and Hearing Research, 18,* pp. 158–167. Copyright 1975 by the American Speech-Language-Hearing Association. Reprinted with permission.

In some types of communicative disorders research, listeners or raters are considered subjects in the same manner as speakers. Excerpt 8.3 is an example from a study that compared listener ratings of speech naturalness obtained from two different procedures: equal appearing interval ratings (EAI) and direct magnitude estimation procedures (DME). In an effort to minimize the effects of extraneous variables, listeners were randomly assigned to use either the EAI or the DME procedure to judge speech naturalness.

EXCERPT 8.3

Raters

The raters were 40 undergraduate college students enrolled in an introductory course in communication disorders. The raters had no academic or clinical experience with stuttering. None of the raters evidenced a significant speech, language, vision, or hearing problem.

Procedures

Half of the raters were randomly assigned to use the EAI rating procedure and the other half to use the DME procedure for the psychophysical scaling of speech naturalness from the audiovisual recordings.

From "Psychophysical Analysis of Audiovisual Judgments of Speech Naturalness of Nonstutterers and Stutterers, by N. Schiavetti, R. R. Martin, S. K. Haroldson, and D. E. Metz, 1994, *Journal of Speech and Hearing Research, 37,* pp. 46–52. Copyright 1994 by the American Speech-Language-Hearing Association. Reprinted with permission.

In some speech and hearing studies, the sample size and method of subject selection are less important than the instrumentation and procedures and, thus, become almost incidental. This is often true in basic physiologic and psychoacoustic research where the variability of the data is quite small and numerous repeated measurements are made in a within-subjects design. Take, for example, the study by Barlow and Muller on force generation produced by muscles in the perioral system. In Experiment 2, three subjects from the pool of thirty subjects in Experiment 1 volunteered to accept hook-wire electromyography electrodes. The subject selection section is reprinted in its entirety in Excerpt 8.4. Is this an adequate description of the three volunteer subjects? Does it matter? Simply put, the nature and purpose of the research were such that any three adults without a history of neurologic disorder or speech disorder could probably have been used without significantly affecting the data or modifying the conclusions. In this study, the instrumentation and procedures used to measure muscle force were more important than the subjects used. Similar examples could easily be cited. Once again the adequacy of the size of the subject sample and the way the subjects are selected depend to a very large extent on the basic purpose of the study, the nature of the research design, and the variability of the data.

EXCERPT 8.4   Subjects

Fifteen men, 21 to 48 years of age ($M = 32.3$, $SD = 7.32$), and 15 women 22 to 45 years of age ($M = 31.8$, $SD = 7.19$), served as experimental subjects for Experiment 1. Three of these subjects, who consented to accept hookwire intramuscular EMG electrodes, participated in Experiment 2. No subject had a prior history of neurologic disorder and all were free of speech impairments.

From "The Relation between Interangle Span and In Vivo Resultant Force in Perioral Musculature," by S. M. Barlow and E. M. Muller, 1991, *Journal of Speech and Hearing Research, 34*, pp. 252–259. Copyright 1991 by the American Speech-Language-Hearing Association. Reprinted with permission.

Criteria for Subject Selection

As we have mentioned throughout, much of the descriptive research in communicative disorders deals with differences and attempts to answer such questions as: Are stutterers different from nonstutterers? Do people with Ménière's disease differ from people with noise-induced hearing loss? Is test *A* more sensitive than test *B* in differentiating aphasics from other brain-injured people? In any study involving group differences (between-subjects designs), it is absolutely essential that the researcher describe and perhaps even defend the criteria used in forming the groups. Inadequate group composition, overlapping groups, and indefensible selection criteria all pose important threats to the internal and external validity of both experimental and descriptive research.

The example shown in Excerpt 8.5 is taken from an article by Orlikoff on the relationship of age and cardiovascular health on certain acoustic characteristics of voice production. The purpose of the study was to assess the stability of vocal fundamental frequency and amplitude during sustained vowel productions among groups of healthy young men, healthy elderly men, and elderly men who had been diagnosed with chronic atherosclerosis. The first part of the section details subject exclusion criteria and then goes on to describe the general characteristics of the three subject groups. Next, care was taken to ensure that extraneous variables were controlled that could affect subject performance. Table 1 is used to provide pertinent age and physiological information about the subjects.

EXCERPT 8.5   Subjects

Eighteen nonsmoking, vocally untrained men, with no history of speech, respiratory, or neuromuscular pathology or drug or alcohol abuse, were selected as subjects for this study. All were judged to have normal speech and voice quality by two certified speech pathologists. Subjects were separated into three experimental groups of equal number: (1) young, healthy, normotensive men; (2) elderly, healthy, normotensive men; and (3) elderly men with medically diagnosed chronic atherosclerosis in the absence of other systemic ailments such as diabetes or renal dysfunction. None of the subjects were taking medication likely to interfere with autonomic nervous system activity, gave evidence of bradycardia, or exhibited laryngeal or respiratory symptoms due to illness or allergy at the time of testing. Subject characteristics are shown in Table 1. Blood pressures were measured by standard auscultatory method; resting heart rate was measured by positive zero-crossings of the Q-R segment of a digitized (14.5k samples/s) Lead II electrocardiogram.

TABLE 1   Subject characteristics

Group		Age (years)	Resting Heart Rate (bpm)	Systolic Blood Pressure (mmHg)	Diastolic Blood Pressure (mmHg)
Healthy young men	*Mean*	30.0	62.4	127.5	70.5
	SD	2.3	3.9	3.8	4.2
	range	26–33	55–68	120–130	65–78
Healthy elderly men	*Mean*	73.3	66.9	132.0	77.2
	SD	3.7	13.2	8.8	3.7
	range	68–80	49–86	120–142	70–80
Atherosclerotic elderly men	*Mean*	70.3	74.5	172.0	92.7
	SD	6.5	13.2	6.8	8.3
	range	60–79	59–95	160–180	85–110

From "The Relationship of Age and Cardiovascular Health to Certain Acoustic Characteristics of Male Voices," by R. F. Orlifkoff, 1990, *Journal of Speech and Hearing Research, 33,* pp. 450–457. Copyright 1990 by the American Speech-Language-Hearing Association. Reprinted with permission.

Because subject-selection procedures are so important in between-groups studies in communicative disorders, we have chosen another illustration. Excerpt 8.6 is from a study by Anderson-Yockel and Haynes that compared communication strategies between working-class African American and white mother-child dyads during joint book-reading experiences. The primary research question being addressed by this study regarded differences between white and African American mother-toddler dyads communications during joint bookreading. In an attempt to equate the two groups, subjects were matched on the basis of child age, family income, parent educational level, and occupational status. Tables 1 and 2 provide specific information about the subjects' family income and occupational status. The authors acknowledge that their matching procedure was not precise, but it did allow for the exclusion of families from the upper-middle classes that were not of interest in this investigation.

EXCERPT 8.6 Subjects

The subjects were 20 working-class mother-toddler dyads (10 white/10 African American). They ranged in age from 18 to 30 months. The mean age for the African American children was 23.6 months (range 18 to 30), and the mean age of the white children was 24.3 months (range 18 to 30). Both groups were generally comparable in terms of family income, parent education level, and overall occupational status. This information was obtained by having all adult subjects complete a questionnaire on income and occupation. The goal was to assemble two groups that would be perceived by most observers as "blue-collar" or "working-class."

Subjects were asked about their education levels and occupations before completing the questionnaire so that families that clearly were upper-middle class or above would be eliminated. Although this procedure did not make for precise matches between the two groups on all variables, examination of the demographic data suggests the groups were roughly comparable on all variables. Tables 1 and 2 provide demographic data on each group. All African American caregivers were speakers of Black English, and white caregivers were speakers of Southern English Dialect.

TABLE 1 Mean income and educational levels of African American and white caregiver groups

| | African American | | White | |
Variable	*M*	*SD*	*M*	*SD*
Annual family income	24,000	11,300	23,200	8,200
Years of education	13.2	1.69	13.8	1.82

TABLE 2 Occupational status of African American and white caregiver groups (both parental occupations included)

| African American Group | | White Group | |
Maternal Occupations	*Paternal Occupations*	*Maternal Occupations*	*Paternal Occupations*
Homemaker	Unknown	Teacher assistant	Supply clerk
Homemaker	Production operator	Clerical worker	Computer operator
Teacher assistant	Telephone operator	Homemaker	Cemetery worker
Secretary/cashier	Forensic scientist	Waitress	Landscaper
Restaurant worker	Plant worker	Secretary	Truck driver
Office worker	Unknown	Office assistant	Welder
Industrial planner	Building inspector	Part-time teacher	Unemployed
Salesperson	City worker	Teacher	Unknown
Student	Student	Homemaker	Salesman
City inspector	Carpenter	Waitress	Bartender

Another aspect of subject selection that directly affects internal validity is whether subjects were selected on the basis of extreme scores. We pointed out in Part I that selecting subjects because of their extreme scores may produce regression effects. That is, apparent changes in posttreatment scores may merely reflect the tendency for extreme scores to become less extreme (regress toward the mean) rather than reflecting true treatment effects. The critical reader should be especially alert to regression effects in studies of treatment programs.

Excerpt 8.7 is taken from the Discussion section of a study by Andrews and Harvey of regression to the mean in stuttering measures. They measured regression during a pre-treatment waiting period and compared their findings to previous studies. Although the amount of regression they found was small, note their suggestions for incorporating a correction for regression in pretest-posttest studies of the effects of stuttering treatment. Note their comments about measures of speech attitude and reaction to speech situations, as well as the actual speech measures of fluency. Similar studies with other speech disorders would help to improve the design of treatment experiments.

EXCERPT 8.7

The six studies in the literature that have measured stutterers at two or three points in time prior to treatment have all reported a statistically nonsignificant improvement trend. This improvement may be evidence that stutterers come for treatment when their stuttering is worst and spontaneously improve a little with time. Although it is difficult to aggregate data from this small set of studies, examination of the time of the improvement, as reflected by the effect-size statistic, shows that the improvement can be evident as early as three months after initial contact.

The present study of 132 subjects showed that many stutterers waiting for treatment did improve significantly. This may be evidence of regression in the severity of their stuttering to a previously established mean level. Analysis of the present data by the time subjects spent on the waiting list showed that the improvement occurred within the first three months and that no further improvement occurred thereafter.

Regression to the mean appears an effect that could confound estimates of the improvement due to therapy in pre-post treatment outcome designs. There are two ways of allowing for the effect. First, stutterers could be held on a waiting list for three months or until a stable baseline is demonstrated so that the effects of treatment will not be confounded by regression to the mean. Second, if subjects receive treatment immediately after they apply for treatment, a small but definable part of the improvement following treatment will be due to spontaneous regression to the mean, and the treatment results should be corrected accordingly.

Aggregating the data from the six reports in the literature and from the present study suggests that the magnitude of this effect is small; mean effect size = 0.21 (SE 0.04). Subtracting this amount from the pre-post effect size would approximate the actual treatment-related improvement. In practical terms, a group of adult stutterers of mean severity 17%SS when first seen will spontaneously improve to a mean of 14%SS three months later, and improvement beyond this point following treatment is likely to be due to the effects of treatment.

Self-report measures of speech attitude and reaction to speech situations also showed improvement trends, but in both Gregory (1972) and the present study, the changes were of much smaller magnitude than those of speech measures. This improvement trend is so small that it can be disregarded when using self-report measures to calculate the improvement produced by therapy.

The relevant questions about subject-selection criteria that need to be asked for between-group studies can be summarized as follows: (1) Are the criteria for group composition clearly defined and defensible? (2) Is there overlap between groups on the variable that distinguishes the groups? (3) Are exclusion criteria defined and defensible? (4) Are the groups comparable on important extraneous variables? and (5) Have subjects been selected on the basis of extreme scores? These questions deal primarily with the issue of internal validity. Regarding external validity, the question is: Are the subjects comparable, on important dimensions, to the population to which the author wishes to generalize?

One final point deserves brief attention. The author of a research article should indicate if subjects were volunteers and whether they were paid (or unpaid) to participate in the study. A complete discussion of the effects of the volunteer subject on the outcomes of research is beyond the scope of this book. (The interested reader should consult Rosenthal and Rosnow [1975].) Suffice it to say that volunteer subjects, whether paid or unpaid, may be different in important respects from the population to whom the investigator wishes to generalize, thus affecting external validity.

Materials

The materials part of the research article is a key component of the Method section. The reason for its importance is that it is in this section that researchers identify the materials that have been used to measure or generate the variables under study, and it is here that the critical consumer of research can identify instrumentation threats to internal validity. Underscoring the importance of such threats is the fact emphasized in Chapter 5 that instrumentation threats to internal validity transcend type of research or research design.

There are two basic evaluation questions that need to be asked by the consumer: (1) Were there adequate selection and measurement of the independent (classification, predictor) variable? and (2) Were there adequate selection and measurement of the dependent (criterion, predicted) variable? Although the researcher's rationale for the selection of variables may appear either in the Introduction or the Method section (and this rationale requires careful scrutiny on the part of the reader), the measurement of variables will almost always be described either in the Materials or Procedures section. Our purpose here, then, is to lay down some general guidelines that can be used by the critical reader to evaluate possible instrumentation (i.e., materials) threats to the internal validity of both experimental and descriptive research.

Hardware Instrumentation and Calibration

Instrumentation

Hardware instrumentation plays an important role in research in communicative disorders, especially in speech and hearing science. Much of what we know about normal (and disordered) processes is due, in large part, to technological advances that have made possible the measuring, recording, and analyzing systems that are found in speech and hearing laboratories throughout the country. This is not to say that all research is dependent on or requires sophisticated electronic instrumentation. The exciting advances made in understanding how children acquire language have not required much more than an audio-tape recorder or a relatively simple videotape recording system. It is to say, however, that the critical reader of research is often required to read research articles that are heavily weighted in instrumentation. The critical evaluation of such material can be an exceedingly difficult task, especially for the student who has minimal course work or experience in electronics or instrumentation.

Although instrumentation can be complex, the purposes to which the instruments are put are reasonably straightforward. Instruments are used to produce signals (e.g., an audio-frequency oscillator), to measure the signal (e.g., a sound-level meter), to store the signal (e.g., a tape recorder or a computer disk), to control the signal (e.g., an electronic switch), to modify the signal (e.g., a band-pass filter), and to analyze the signal (e.g., a sound spectrograph). The reasons for using an instrument are equally straightforward. The researcher (or clinician) uses an instrument to standardize data-acquisition procedures, to help acquire data under known conditions, and to provide a permanent record of the data. Most important, instruments allow the measurement of events that are not directly observable by the senses (Plutchik, 1974). There is nothing inherently mysterious about instrumentation. What is mysterious, perhaps, is why so little attention is paid to laboratory instrumentation in many master's-level communicative disorders training programs. This may very well be the reason that many consumers of research approach the apparatus section of an article with fear and trepidation. Another point to keep in mind is that instruments, like statistics, are tools. The instrument itself, with few exceptions, is not the reason for the research. Thus, again like statistics, a sophisticated instrumental array cannot improve an inadequate research problem and cannot modify a poor research design.

Several guidelines can be used by the practitioner or student while reading the instrumentation section of an article. First, and at the very least, the principal components of the system should be identified by manufacturer and model number. This enables the interested reader to duplicate the system using the same or comparable equipment. It also allows the reader to determine if the components are reasonably standard pieces that have been manufactured by reputable companies. If a new instrument has been developed for a particular study, enough information should be provided to allow the reader to reconstruct the piece. Circuit diagrams, photographs, line drawings, and the like should be included for this purpose. The point here is that there should be sufficient detail for replication purposes and to permit the reader to determine if the components are standard pieces of equipment likely to be found in a well-equipped speech and hearing laboratory. A block diagram showing the interrelationships among components is a useful device for describing the instrumentation array.

Another criterion is whether the same or a similar instrumental array has been used by the investigator in a previously reported study or has been used by other investigators studying the same phenomenon. References to previous research can be of considerable value in assessing the adequacy of instrumentation. The absence of such references, especially when confronted with a custom-built instrument, should alert the reader to the possibility of instrumental error.

Some basic characteristics of the instrumentation used may also be reported in the instrumentation section and may be of value to the reader in helping to assess whether the instrumentation was appropriate to the task at hand. The frequency response characteristics of the earphones, the linearity of attenuators, and the intensity range of an amplifier are just three examples of the kind of descriptive information that might be provided in the instrumentation section.

Excerpts 8.8 and 8.9 represent two somewhat different instrumentation descriptions. Excerpt 8.8 is from a study that compared the reliability of the Speech Perception Test in Noise (SPIN) and the Dichotic Sentence Identification (DSI) test. Both tests are used commonly to evaluate speech-recognition capabilities of elderly persons. The Apparatus section provides all the information the reader would need to replicate this study. The source of each test is identified, and each piece of equipment is identified by the manufacturer and the model number. The exact test comparison procedures (not shown here) are detailed in a later section of the article.

EXCERPT 8.8   Apparatus

The tapes of the revised SPIN test were provided by Dr. Robert Bilger at the University of Illinois. The DSI tapes were provided by Auditec of St. Louis. Tapes were played through a two-channel cassette-tape deck (Sansui, D-W9). For the SPIN test, the output of one channel of the tape deck was routed to an attenuator and then to one channel of a two-channel amplifier (McIntosh, C24), and was mixed with the output of the other channel of the tape deck. Amplifier output was delivered to earphones of a network of matched TDH-39 earphones mounted in MX-41/AR cushions. All presentation levels were verified using an NBS-9A 6-cm³ coupler. The outputs of both channels were calibrated electrically prior to each test administration using a voltmeter.

From "Reliability of Two Measures of Speech Recognition in Elderly Persons," by C. G. Cokely and L. E. Humes, 1992, *Journal of Speech and Hearing Research, 35,* pp. 654–660. Copyright 1992 by the American Speech-Language-Hearing Association. Reprinted with permission.

The next excerpt (8.9) is from a study of laryngeal airway resistance in older men and women. Clearly, the equipment description provided by the authors would permit replication. However, the adequacy of the equipment array could probably best be evaluated by individuals who are familiar with equipment used to measure laryngeal airway dynamics. Many communicative disorders specialists would simply not have the background to allow a critical evaluation of this section in the Holmes, Leeper, and Nicholson article.

EXCERPT 8.9   Instrumentation

Air pressure, airflow, and the acoustic voice signal were collected simultaneously employing commercially available instrumentation. Oral air pressure was collected and transmitted to a differential pressure transducer using a rigid walled vinyl pitot tube (1.0 mm i.d.) with the proximal end situated behind the lower incisors at right angles to the first bicuspid. The distal end of the tube was joined in series to a differential pressure transducer (Statham, Model PM-6); the output was then amplified (Honeywell, Accudata, Model 113), low-pass fil-tered at 100 Hz (Krohn-Hite, Model 3202), and transmitted to one channel of an analog-to-digital converter, digitized, and displayed on a microcomputer (Zenith, Model 158 PC) using a commercial software package (Computerscope-PHY, ISC-16 Computerscope System Software, [RC Electronics, Inc., 5386 Hollister Avenue, Santa Barbara, CA 93111]).

Calibration of the air pressure system was performed weekly, employing a U-tube manometer for static measures from 1 to 10 cmH20. Zero balancing

Continued

EXCERPT 8.9   Instrumentation   *Continued*

of the transducer-amplifier system was performed prior to each subject's data collection to ensure a stable baseline.

Airflow data were collected simultaneously by directing flow from a face mask and associated pneumotachograph (Sanborn, Model A-9595) to a differential pressure transducer (Statham, Model PM15E). The output was amplified (Honeywell Accudata, Model 143), low-pass filtered at 100 Hz (Krohn-Hite, Model 3202), and fed to another channel of an analog-to-digital converter, and displayed on the screen of the computer terminal employing the Computerscope-PHY software package. Airflow calibration was obtained over a 100–1000 cc/sec range using a Rotometer (Fisher & Porter Company Core Flowrator, Model 10A1027) supplied by a tank of compressed nitrogen. Zero balancing of the transducer-amplifier system was performed prior to each subject's data collection to ensure a stable baseline.

The acoustic signal was transmitted from an ElectroVoice, Model 664, dynamic, directional microphone placed 15 cm anterior to the subject's mouth when positioned in the facemask, and amplified (Bruel & Kjaer, Model 2608) before transmission to a third channel of the Computer-

PHY system. The acoustic signal was used to display onset, duration, and offset of the vowel within the experimental syllable /pi/ utterance. The aerodynamic and acoustic data were displayed on the monitor of the same microcomputer, and employed the same software package used for data collection.

Sound pressure level (SPL) of phonation was determined using a Realistic, Model 42-3019 sound level meter (SLM) set to "C" scale in the fast response mode. The microphone associated with the SLM was also placed 15 cm behind the outlet tube of the pneumotachograph face mask (i.e., 15 cm mouth-to-microphone distance) to monitor SPL. To maintain an utterance rate of approximately 1.5 syllables per second (SPS), an electronic metronome (Seiko, Model SQM357) providing visual (flashing light) and auditory (click) feedback was used for subject self-monitoring.

From "Laryngeal Airway Resistance of Older Men and Women as a Function of Vocal Sound Pressure Level," by L. C. Holmes, H. A. Leeper, and I. R. Nicholson, 1994, *Journal of Speech and Hearing Research, 37,* pp. 789–799. Copyright 1994 by the American Speech-Language-Hearing Association. Reprinted with permission.

With the increasing impact of rapid technological developments on the field of communication disorders, however, consumers of research will find it more and more difficult to evaluate the research in the field without some background in instrumentation. It is obviously beyond the scope of this book to attempt to teach principles of instrumentation to clinicians and students. Recent attempts have been made to make professionals aware of the need to understand instrumentation in speech and hearing. More than a decade ago, Levitt (1983) addressed this issue at the 1983 ASHA National Conference on Undergraduate, Graduate, and Continuing Education. He concisely summarized the problem when he said (Levitt 1983, p. 88):

> *In short, modern technology is transforming virtually every aspect of our profession (and of every other profession as well). It is imperative that a concerted effort be made to train professionals in our field to function effectively in this new environment.*

Levitt outlined several issues to be considered in developing guidelines for future incorporation of technological instruction in the education of communicative disorders specialists and made several suggestions to help professionals to understand and use the advancing technology in future clinical and research activities. Levitt (1983, p. 88) emphasized the importance of making technological innovations meaningful and useful to our service-oriented profession, stating:

> *It is wholly unrealistic to develop preservice and in-service training programs that will cover all aspects of modern technology. There is a need to be selective. For example, one need not understand the principles of xerography in order to use a xerox machine effectively. On the other hand, the characteristics and inherent limitations of acoustic amplifiers need to be understood in order to prescribe hearing aids properly.*

Students and clinicians must also accept some responsibility for updating their knowledge of technological innovations in the field. Many state and national conventions now offer continuing education activities that deal with the use of technical innovations, computers, and various kinds of instrumentation. Also, many recent articles have appeared in the clinical and research literature that attempt to provide knowledge about instrumentation, computer applications, and measurement techniques that are geared to clinicians. For example, Zajac and Yates (1991) discuss the accuracy of pressure-flow methods for estimating the area of the velopharyngeal orifice during connected speech; Read, Buder, and Kent (1990, 1992) detail the performance characteristics, validity, and reliability of several computer-based speech analysis systems; and Titze and Winholtz (1993) examined the effects of microphone type and placement on voice perturbation measurements. The "Research Notes" of the *Journal of Speech and Hearing Research* often presents information on instrumentation that may help clinicians update their knowledge and skills (e.g., see Orlikoff [1991]; Perlman, VanDaele, and Otterbacher [1995]).

As technological advances progress, communicative disorders specialists need to take advantage of courses and continuing education in instrumentation to keep current in their clinical work and prepare themselves to evaluate the research in the field that relies more and more on electronic instrumentation. The time has come when knowledge of instrumentation is as important a tool to communication disorders specialists as traditional tools such as knowledge of phonetic transcription, anatomy and physiology, or linguistics have been in the past.

The next excerpt (Excerpt 8.10) shows how Dalston, Warren, and Dalston use block diagrams to complement the narrative description of instruments used in a study that compared two measurement techniques (measurements of nasal resonance and measurements of nasal cross-sectional area) that can be used to assess hyponasality and/or nasal airway impairment. Calibration and specific measurement procedures are carefully explained in the prose.

EXCERPT 8.10

Instrumental Assessment of Nasal Resonance

The Model 6200 Nasometer is a microcomputer-based system manufactured by Kay Elemetrics (Figure 1). With this device, oral and nasal components of a subject's speech are sensed by microphones on either side of a sound separator that rests

Continued

EXCERPT 8.10   *Continued*

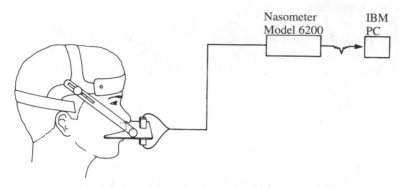

FIGURE 1   A schematic representation of the instrumentation used to obtain Nasometer measurements

on the upper lip. The signal from each of the microphones is filtered and digitized by custom electronic modules. The data are then processed by an IBM PC computer. The resultant signal is a ratio of nasal to nasal-plus-oral acoustic energy. This ratio is multiplied by 100 and expressed as a "nasalance" score.

Prior to testing, the Nasometer was calibrated and the headgear was adjusted in accordance with instructions provided by the manufacturer. Each subject was then asked to read a standard passage loaded with nasal consonants (see appendix). Those subjects who were unable to read the passage easily were asked to repeat the sentences after the examiner (Rodger Dalston).

Measurement of Nasal Cross-Sectional Area

Recent advances in respiratory monitoring technology provide the opportunity to define nasal airway impairment objectively. One approach is to measure nasal airway cross-sectional size using a technique developed by Warren for speech research (Warren & DuBois, 1964). The validity of this aerodynamic assessment technique has been substantiated in a number of laboratories (Lubker, 1969; Smith & Weinberg, 1980, 1982, 1983), and a recent study demonstrates that it can be used successfully to define airway impairment (Warren, 1984).

The method used to measure nasal cross-sectional area involves a modification of the theoretical hydraulic principle and assumes that the smallest cross-sectional area of a structure can be determined if the differential pressure across the structure is measured simultaneously with rate of airflow through it. This method, which has been used in speech research by Warren and his associates since 1961 (Warren & DuBois, 1964), was specifically modified for assessing nasal airway patency. The equation employed is

$$\text{Area} = \frac{\text{Rate of nasal airflow}}{k \left[\dfrac{2 \times (\text{oral} - \text{nasal pressure drop})}{\text{density of air}} \right]^{\frac{1}{2}}}$$

where $k = 0.65$ and the density of air = 0.001 gm/cm^2. The correction factor k was obtained from analog studies that have been reported previously (Warren, 1984; Warren & DuBois, 1964).

Figure 2 illustrates the aerodynamic assessment technique used in the current study. The oral-nasal pressure drop was measured with pressure transducers connected to two catheters. The first catheter was positioned midway in the subject's mouth, and the second catheter was placed within a nasal mask in front of the nose. Nasal airflow was measured

Continued

EXCERPT 8.10   *Continued*

with a heated pneumotachograph connected to the well-adapted nasal mask. Each subject was asked to inhale and exhale as normally as possible through the nose. The resulting pressure and airflow patterns were transmitted to the computer, analyzed, and recorded on hard copy. Although nasal areas can be measured during either inspiration or expiration, for the current study they were measured at the peak of expiratory airflow.

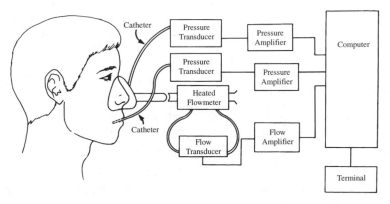

**FIGURE 2   A schematic representation of the instrumentation
used to estimate nasal cross-sectional area**

From "A Preliminary Investigation Concerning the Use of Nasometry in Identifying Patients with Hyponasality and/or Nasal Airway Impairment," by R. M. Dalston, D. G. Warren, and E. T. Dalston, 1991, *Journal of Speech and Hearing Research, 34,* pp. 11–18. Copyright 1991 by the American Speech-Language-Hearing Association. Reprinted with permission.

Calibration

Adequate calibration of instruments used in a given study is absolutely essential to the reduction of a possible threat to internal validity posed by instrumentation. Faulty calibration must lead to faulty data, either in the laboratory or in the clinic. Unfortunately, calibration procedures are sometimes given short shrift in a journal article. Thus, it is difficult to assess the adequacy of the calibration procedures used. As a result, the reader may have to rely on the integrity and honesty of the researcher in judging the adequacy of calibration.

The three major questions that the reader must ask about calibration of equipment are: (1) What was calibrated? (2) What equipment was used for calibration purposes? and (3) When was calibration performed? Excerpt 8.11 is taken from a study on a method used for fitting hearing aids. Note that in these two paragraphs the author identifies the equipment used for acoustic calibration and explains the specific reasons for the calibration procedure. The exact time that these calibration procedures were performed is not specified in these two paragraphs, but in the Speech Materials section of the article, Rankovic states that one of the calibration procedures was checked daily.

EXCERPT 8.11   Calibration and Equipment

All calibration and testing were performed in a double-walled IAC sound-treated chamber using a Telephonics TDH-49 earphone housed in a MX-41/AR cushion. Calibration measurements were made while the earphone was coupled via a NBS-9A 6-cc coupler to a sound-level meter (Bruel & Kjaer 2203) and a Hewlett-Packard 3561A dynamic signal analyzer. This configuration provided a common point of reference for speech and pure tones, allowing direct comparisons between the thresholds and speech spectrum measures.

In the amplification conditions, speech was filtered and amplified by a one-third octave band filter bank (Bruel & Kjaer 123), amplifier (Crown D-75), passive attenuator(s) (Hewlett-Packard 3500),

and/or additional high- and low-pass filter(s) (Krohn-Hite 3202). Measurements of average one-third octave band levels of a white noise calibration signal (Grason-Stadler 1724) relative to the same calibration noise measured in the 65 dB SPL speech-in-quiet equipment configuration were used to verify achievement of desired gain. Speech intelligibility testing in each condition was performed by substituting the digital-to-analog converter output for the calibration noise.

From "An Application of the Articulation Index to Hearing Aid Fitting," by C. M. Rankovic, 1991, *Journal of Speech and Hearing Research, 34,* pp. 391–402. Copyright 1991 by the American Speech-Language-Hearing Association. Reprinted with permission.

Another example (Excerpt 8.12) is taken from a study of laryngeal valving actions of normal and hearing-impaired speakers. The equipment for high-speed filming of the larynx is described briefly and reference is made to a previous study that included a more detailed description of the apparatus and procedure. The details of calibration of the filming system are described, and the authors also include a description of the expected error of measurement with the optical system. In addition, the linking of the acoustical data with the film data is described and the temporal resolution of the timing code for linking film and acoustic data is indicated. Another significant aspect of their method section is the description of the interjudge and intrajudge reliability in making the glottal area measurements from the film data.

EXCERPT 8.12

Equipment

High-speed laryngeal films (4000 frames/s) were made of each subject using the equipment and procedures described by Metz, Whitehead, and Peterson (1980). Briefly, the equipment and procedures permit making high-speed laryngeal films and obtaining noise-free high-quality acoustic recordings simultaneously. Two adjacent sound attenuating rooms isolate the subject from the camera (Redlake Hycam, 40–004) and from all noise-producing equipment. Laryngeal filming is accomplished by projecting two high-intensity light beams (Skanmart

Xenon Illuminator, XEN–300F–141) at paraxial angles to the camera lens (230mm Century Tele-Anthenar with Angenieux reflex viewfinder) through an optically flat sound attenuating window. These two light beams intersect on a specially constructed oval laryngeal mirror, which is permanently fixed in the optical path 107 cm from the focal plane of the lens. The mirror has two degrees of freedom which permit separate vertical and horizontal adjustments without changing the absolute 107-cm working distance. This optical configuration results in a 0.25 image/object ratio (lens reduction factor) if the

Continued

EXCERPT 8.12   *Continued*

plane of focus on the vocal folds is 114 cm. If the plane of focus on the vocal folds is 112 cm, the image object ratio is 0.2571. Because all film data were collected with a focus range between 112 and 114 cm, a standard image/object ratio of 0.2535 was used in all subsequent glottal area calculations. Establishing this standard was necessary because of small focusing adjustments that are required during actual filming. The resulting calibration error is negligible compared with the glottal area variations associated with phonation. For example, if the maximum glottal area was 5 mm^2, one would expect a calibration error $\pm$ .0035/5 = $\pm$ .0007 mm^2.

Acoustic data were recorded with a microphone (Electro-Voice), which was attached to the laryngeal mirror shaft 5 cm from the subject's mouth. Acoustic data were transmitted from the subject room to the equipment room via a patch panel and recorded on magnetic tape (Ampex, ATR–100). A Redlake Crystal TLG/LED Driver (13–0003) applied a timing code to the film border and a separate channel of the magnetic tape. This timing code was used to temporally synchronize the film and acoustic data with a resolution of 1 ms.

. . . .

Intra- and Interjudge Glottal Area Measurement Reliability

The research assistant remeasured 10% of the frames from each film. Intrajudge agreement coefficients (Pearson r's) ranged from .76 to 1.00 with an overall average agreement coefficient of .90 and a maximum measurement error of 1.07 mm^2($\overline{x}$ = .93 mm^2).

These same frames were remeasured by the senior author. Interjudge agreement coefficients ranged from .68 to .91 with an average agreement coefficient of .82 and a maximum measurement error of 2.33 mm^2($\overline{x}$ = 1.72 mm^2)

From "Mechanics of Vocal Fold Vibration and Laryngeal Articulatory Gestures Produced by Hearing-Impaired Speakers," by D. E. Metz, R. L. Whitehead, and B. H. Whitehead, 1984, *Journal of Speech and Hearing Research, 27,* pp. 62–69. Copyright 1984 by the American Speech-Language-Hearing Association. Reprinted with permission.

The last example in this section is taken from an article by Shipp and McGlone and is shown in Excerpt 8.13. The interesting point here is that not only was there calibration of the instruments used but a physiologic calibration procedure was also employed. The need for this latter calibration procedure is described as well.

EXCERPT 8.13

Instrumental Calibration

Calibration signals for the six physiologic data channels were recorded prior to subject preparation. To calibrate the four EMG channels, a custom-built input simulator was used that generated single pulse signals at 50, 100, 200, and 500 microvolts. The subglottal pressure channel was calibrated using a U-tube manometer, so that pressures from zero to 24 cm of water could be recorded. Calibration of the air-flow channel was conducted using a direct connection between the pneumotachograph and a Brooks flow meter attached to an air supply cylinder. Air-flow rates were recorded in 100 cc/sec steps, from zero to 1000 cc/ sec.

Physiologic Calibration

No intersubject muscle comparisons could be made from absolute EMG microvolt values, since the magnitude of the EMG signal is a function of the distance between the recording electrodes and their location within the muscle. These positions could not be replicated between subjects; therefore, a physiologic calibration measure was incorporated to normalize the data and permit intersubject

Continued

EXCERPT 8.13 *Continued*

comparisons. Immediately before the first experimental task, subjects performed the calibration maneuver of inspiring air, then phonating the vowel *a* in diatonic steps from the middle to the top of their modal registers. At different points in the performance of this calibration task, high levels of activity were picked up from each of the four muscles. From the EMG data obtained during the calibration maneuver, a metric of muscle activity was

established from 100, representing each muscle's maximum activity generated during the calibration maneuver, to zero, the average baseline noise level in that channel.

From "Laryngeal Dynamics Associated with Voice Frequency Change," by T. Shipp and R. E. McGlone, 1971, *Journal of Speech and Hearing Research, 14,* pp. 761–768. Copyright 1971 by the American Speech-Language-Hearing Association. Reprinted with permission.

Reliability and Validity of Behavioral Instruments

Under behavioral instruments, we include the enormous array of standardized and nonstandardized tests such as paper-and-pencil tests of various types, articulation tests, language tests, speech-discrimination tests, hearing tests, attitude measures, and the like. Any of these kinds of materials may be used by researchers to make measurements of independent or dependent variables. Major problems with such instruments can pose significant threats to internal or external validity. Thus, the critical reader needs to assess carefully the adequacy of behavioral instruments used in research. Most communicative disorders specialists have had a reasonable amount of exposure to behavioral instruments through academic and practicum courses and clinical work. Also, there are some sources that interested readers can consult for specific information on various behavioral instruments such as Darley (1979) or Buros (1972). In this section, we will show some examples to illustrate some of the concepts of reliability and validity of measures that were discussed in Part I.

Standardized Instruments

Many research articles in communicative disorders report the use of standardized tests for the measurement of variables in their Method section. In some cases, the researcher provides citations to the test manual that contains data on standardization or reference to previous research on the reliability and validity of the instrument used. For example, in an article comparing communication skills of late-talking young children, Paul, Looney, and Dahm interviewed the primary caregivers of each child in the study using the Vineland Adaptive Behavior Scales (VABS). Excerpt 8.14 refers to the VABS Manual for normative data and reliability and validity estimates. Additionally, secondary research is reported that attests to the VABS's criterion validity.

EXCERPT 8.14

The VABS adaptive behavior domains have been normed on 3000 individuals from birth through 18 years, 11 months, including 200 subjects in each of

15 age groups. It has undergone extensive reliability assessments and analyses of validity, both of which suggest good performance on these indices

Continued

EXCERPT 8.14   *Continued*

(VABS Manual, 1984). In addition, Rescorla and Paul (1990) found that VABS scores in Expressive Communication correlated highly ($r = .85$) with LDS scores. Comparisons of VABS Expressive Communication scores with MLUs at this age level revealed a correlation of .78 for the normal group, suggesting the VABS Expressive score is closely related to direct measures of productive language.

Excerpt 8.15 is also from the Paul et al. article. In this example the authors use previously reported research on the Language Development Survey instrument that establishes its reliability and validity. Use of the checklist format that was used in the study is justified on the basis of previous research.

EXCERPT 8.15

The Language Development Survey (*LDS*) (Rescorla, 1989) is a checklist of 300 words common to children's early vocabularies. Parent report of expressive vocabulary employing a checklist format such as that used in this study has been shown by Dale, Reznick, Bates, and Morisset (1989) and Reznick and Goldsmith (1989) to be an excellent index of expressive vocabulary size. Rescorla (1989) has reported that the Language Development Survey, using the criteria described above, is highly

reliable, valid, sensitive, and specific in identifying language delay, when compared to standardized language measures, in toddlers.

Just because a standardized test is well known or widely used does not necessarily mean that its reliability and validity are adequate. McCauley and Swisher (1984) recently reviewed the psychometric characteristics of thirty language and articulation tests intended for use with preschool children. They applied ten criteria in evaluating the thirty test manuals to assess the documentation of the reliability and validity of the tests, as well as the documentation of other factors such as size and description of the normative samples, description of test procedure, qualifications of examiners, and statistical analysis of test scores of normative sample subgroups. Their analysis found many of the tests lacking in basic documentation of factors such as reliability and validity and concluded (McCauley & Swisher, 1984, p. 41):

> *Most failures of tests to meet individual criteria occurred as a result of an absence of sought-after information rather than as a result of reported poor performance on them. The tests were not shown to be either well developed or poorly developed. This fact may falsely comfort some readers who may assume that, if collected, the data on their favorite test would be favorable. However, when given*

no information about a psychometric characteristic, the test user is realistically left to wonder whether or not a test is invalid and unreliable for his or her purposes. Stated differently, no news is bad news.

The lesson for the consumer of research is to look for evidence of reliability and validity of standardized tests used in research and not to assume that a test is reliable and valid just because it is popular.

Nonstandardized Instruments

Many studies make behavioral measurements with instruments that have not been standardized or published commercially. It is important for researchers using such behavioral instruments to indicate the reliability and validity of measurements made with such materials. Excerpt 8.16 illustrates the use of a nonstandardized behavioral instrument for measuring children's perception of vocal cues of emotional meaning. Notice how the authors describe the development of the measuring instrument and the attempts to assess its content validity. A careful rationale for the development of the instrument is presented and testing of the degree to which the items matched the intended representation is reported. Although the instrument is not a standardized test, information is reported that documents its content validity for the intended use.

EXCERPT 8.16   Development and Pretest of Instrument

The instrument used to measure the children's sensitivity to the vocal cues of emotion was developed and pretested in two stages. It is referred to subsequently as the *Measurement of Vocalic Sensitivity* (MOVS) instrument. For this initial study, only male voices were used. Even though Dimitrovsky employed both male and female voices on her stimulus tape, her findings indicated that the sex of the speaker interacted in complex ways with the emotion being presented. Because our primary interest was the exploration of differences in the interpretative skills of language-disordered and normal children, the potentially confounding influence of having both male and female speakers was not introduced.

In accordance with the recommendations of Beldoch (1964), a complete sentence containing neutral content was selected. The phrase was "Would you bring that to me." In the first stage of development, three professional actors recorded this phrase, supplying vocal cues corresponding to the emotions of happiness, anger, love, and sadness. Each actor provided numerous "takes" of each emotion, until he felt he could not improve upon his performance.

Subsequently, each take for each actor was evaluated by undergraduate students ($N = 135$). They were told the emotion each actor was portraying and were asked to rate the quality of each take. Based on these ratings, one performance of each emotion for each actor was selected as the most representative. This procedure produced a single stimulus tape containing 12 versions of the same sentence—three distinct male voices producing each of the four emotions. Both the actors' voices and the emotions were randomized on the tape to guard against order effects.

The second stage consisted of developing a method by which the children could express their recognition of these emotions. Because many of the children could not be expected to verbalize the various emotional labels, it was decided that all children would respond by pointing to the picture which matched the recorded emotional expressions. Although Dimitrovsky (1964) employed stick figures for this purpose, it was felt that pictures of actual

Continued

EXCERPT 8.16   Development and Pretest of Instrument   *Continued*

people would be more realistic and valid. Three photographs developed for training people in "recognizing emotions from facial expressions" were selected to portray the emotions of happiness, anger, and sadness (Ekman & Friesen, 1975). These photographs contained only three male faces. A fourth picture, representing loving, depicted a father hugging his child. This final picture was selected from a magazine and contained the shoulders, necks, and faces of these characters; no commercial product or trademark was visible. All photographs were enlarged to 8 × 10 inches (approx. 20 × 25 cm) in black and white and were displayed on a plain background.

To test the content validity of the MOVS instrument, a second group of undergraduate students ($N = 367$) was employed to pretest the MOVS instrument. This group was composed of adult,

native English speakers, who were judged to be normal in all aspects of speech and language production. As a group, these students successfully matched the vocal stimuli with their intended visual representations 96% of the time. Moreover, there was no indication of the tendency to select negative labels as reported by Dimitrovsky. These data, therefore, provided additional evidence that the task represented a valid indicant of the ability to interpret vocal cues of emotion.

Excerpt 8.17 is taken from an article that describes the development and administration of a test used to assess children's production and comprehension of derivational suffixes (morphemes). The production portion of the test required judgments of listeners. To establish the reliability of these judgments, Windsor calculated two different reliability estimates that are commonly used in communicative disorders literature; intrajudge and interjudge agreements.

EXCERPT 8.17   Reliability

Both intra- and interjudge reliability measures were calculated for scoring the children's responses on the production task. As scoring the comprehension task involved only circling responses, no reliability measures were obtained on this task. In order to calculate a measure of intrajudge reliability for production, 12 (20%) randomly selected response sheets were scored twice by the author. The first score was based on online judgments of the children's responses; the second was based on audiotapes of the production task. Across subjects, a mean of 99.31% agreement was obtained. To calculate interjudge reliability, the same response sheets were

scored from the audiotapes by a second, untrained judge. Across subjects, a mean of 87.84% agreement was obtained. Differences between the two judges' scores resulted mainly from like-sounding responses that were not easily differentiated from the audiotape (e.g., "BLID*ed*." versus "BLID*it*," "DAZER*ous*" versus "DAZER*ess*") and were resolved after listening again to the audiotapes.

Excerpt 8.18 shows a portion of the Method section of a study designed to investigate two different procedures for obtaining a voice range profile (VRP) or, as it is sometimes called, a phonetogram. Standard procedures for obtaining a VRP require a clinician to measure vocal sound pressure levels (SPL) throughout the speaker's fundamental frequency range using a sound level meter. Titze and his colleagues developed a fully automated, computer-based method for obtaining a VRP that used a headmounted microphone directly inputting to a computer rather than the sound level meter used for measuring SPL. Excerpt 8.18 discusses the method used to establish the validity of the computer-based SPL measurements.

EXCERPT 8.18

Two male subjects were used, RS and VV, who were able to phonate /a/ at fundamental frequencies as low as 60 Hz. They produced a series of phonations at soft and loud efforts (and for one subject, RS, a medium effort as well). Their VRPs are plotted in Figure 1 for subject RS and in Figure 2 for subject

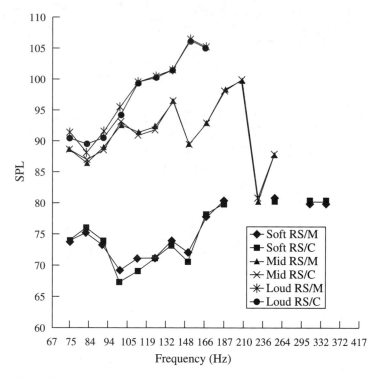

FIGURE 1 **Computer versus SPL meter low-frequency calibration, using human phonation (subject RS). /M is automated computer measurement; /C is clinician measurement using SPL meter.**

Continued

EXCERPT 8.18   *Continued*

VV. Cases where the clinician read the SPL meter are coded with a /C and cases where microphone recordings were made directly into the computer are coded with a /M.

A two-tailed *t*-test of the paired samples was calculated for each subject's effort level. There was no statistical significance at the 5% level at any effort level. Pearson correlation statistics revealed very high correlations between computer-calculated SPL levels and meter-read SPL levels ($r > 0.9$).

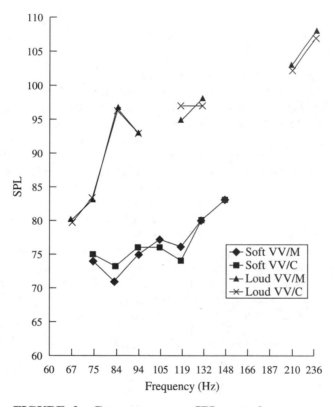

FIGURE 2   Computer versus SPL meter low-frequency calibration, using human phonation (subject VV). /M is automated computer measurement; /C is clinician measurement using SPL meter.

From "Comparison between Clinician-Assisted and Fully Automated Procedures for Obtaining a Voice Range Profile," by I.R. Titze, D. Wong, M.A. Milder, S.R. Hensley, and L.O. Ramig, 1995, *Journal of Speech and Hearing Research, 38*, pp. 526–535. Copyright 1995 by the American Speech-Language-Hearing Association. Reprinted with permission.

To summarize, the basic task in evaluating the adequacy of behavioral instruments in the Method section of a research article is to identify threats to internal validity posed by unreliable or invalid instruments. The task may be simplified if standardized tests are reported because reliability and validity information may be available for these instruments. The task may be more difficult if nonstandardized instruments are used. Here the consumer of research must evaluate the manner in which the instrument was constructed and used in order to determine its adequacy. The description of behavioral instruments used should be clear and comprehensive enough to allow the reader to determine whether the instruments can yield valid and reliable results.

Other Measurement Considerations

In addition to concern about the calibration of hardware and the reliability and validity of behavioral instruments, several other miscellaneous aspects of the measurement process should be discussed in evaluating the materials described in the Method section. These include the appropriateness of measurements made, the role of the experimenter in making the measurements, the test environment, and the test instructions.

Appropriateness of Measurements

Assuming that the instruments used provide reliable and valid measurements of the variables of interest, the reader should be concerned about the appropriateness of the measurements for fulfilling the specific purpose of the study. In other words, the Method section should be evaluated in light of the purpose and rationale spelled out in the introduction to the article. Excerpt 8.19 includes material from both the Introduction and Method sections of an article on the use of pretreatment measures to predict outcomes of stuttering therapy. The first part of the excerpt shows the author's development of a rationale for the use of measures of stuttering severity, personality, and attitudes toward stuttering as pretreatment predictors of therapy outcome in the introduction to the article. The second part of the excerpt is from the Method section and shows how the author selected instruments for measuring each of these three general variables.

EXCERPT 8.19

In all the recent studies, the only high correlation between a pretreatment measure and outcome is the finding by Gregory (1969) that pretreatment severity rating was positively correlated ($r = 0.78$) with change in severity rating from before to immediately after treatment. This result is not surprising, however, since severe stutterers enter therapy with higher levels on the severity scale and thus have a greater range to travel during treatment. Moreover, this correlation is dependent on when outcome is measured. When the nine-month posttreatment changes in severity were correlated with pretreatment severity, the correlation dropped from 0.78 to 0.48.

Changes in stuttering severity from immediately after to many months after treatment, such as shown by Gregory's subjects, are not unusual. Data are now available to support the long-standing clinical impression that many stutterers regress considerably after treatment (Ingham & Andrews, 1973; Perkins, 1973). In fact, those who improve most in treatment may show the greatest regression later (Prins, 1970). Thus, studies which measure stuttering immediately after treatment, such as those of Lanyon (1965, 1966), Prins (1968), and Gregory (1969), may not have assessed the most clinically important outcome of treatment. Long-term out-

Continued

EXCERPT 8.19 *Continued*

come is a more accurate assessment of how treatment has affected a stutterer. Of the studies cited here, only Perkins (1973) used longer term outcome in attempting to find predictors of treatment effects.

The lack of useful predictors of long-term outcome of stuttering treatment suggests a need for further investigation. Although personality measures by themselves have not been effective predictors, they might well be combined with overt measures of pretreatment stuttering for prognosis. Besides measures of personality and level of stuttering, some assessment of attitudes might also be helpful in forecasting outcome. This seems particularly possible in light of recent evidence that cognitive variables are important in determining overt behaviors (Kimble, 1973).

The present study was designed to evaluate a combination of pretreatment measures of stuttering, attitudes toward stuttering, and personality factors, as predictors of long-term outcome of treatment.

. . . .

The basic design of the study was to obtain pretreatment measures from subjects in Group 1 and then evaluate their fluency a year after treatment. Following this, multiple regression analyses were carried out to determine the degree to which pretreatment measures predicted the subjects' outcomes. Equations derived from the regressions were then used to predict the outcomes for subjects in Group 2 on the basis of their pretreatment measures. Correlations between the predicted and actual outcomes for subjects in Group 2 provided cross-validation of the findings for subjects in Group 1.

Pretreatment Measures. The pretreatment data, which included measures of personality, attitudes about stuttering, and amount of stuttering, were obtained when subjects entered the hospital.

Personality was assessed by the extroversion and neuroticism scales of the Eysenck Personality Inventory (Eysenck & Eysenck, 1963). Neuroticism and extroversion have been shown previously to be associated with success and failure on stuttering therapy programs (Brandon & Harris, 1967).

Attitudes toward stuttering were measured by the short form of the Erickson Scale of Communication Attitudes (Erickson, 1969; Andrews & Cutler, 1974) and by an abbreviated version of the

Stutterer's Self-Rating of Reactions to Speech Situations (Johnson, Darley, & Spriestersbach, 1963; Cutler, 1973). Only the avoidance and reaction responses of the Stutterer's Self-Rating form were used because these appeared to be most related to attitudes. Clinical experience suggested that those stutterers who scored high on the avoidance and reaction parts of this assessment were more likely to be emotionally affected by their stuttering, regardless of their actual level of stuttering.

In addition to the above assessments, amount of stuttering was measured when the subjects entered treatment. Stuttering was measured during conversational speech in percentage syllables stuttered (pre%SS) and syllables per minute (preSPM). These measures have been shown to correlate highly with listener judgments of severity and to be reliable (Young, 1961; Andrews & Ingham, 1971). Stuttering scores used for the multiple regression analyses were %SS and "alpha" score, a measure which combines frequency of stuttering and speech rate. The alpha score was developed because speech rate has been considered an important adjunct in the assessment of fluency (Ingham, 1972; Perkins, 1975).

Posttreatment Measures. Twelve to 18 months after the subjects completed the three-week treatment program, they were contacted by a management consultant who was unknown to them, and a meeting was arranged in his office in a different part of the city from the place of treatment. A five-minute sample of conversational speech was recorded and later scored by the experimenter. Measures of outcome were percentage of syllables stuttered (post%SS), alpha score (postalpha), and percent change in frequency of stuttering (%change). This last score, %change, was calculated by the following formula:

$$\frac{\text{pre\%SS} - \text{post\%SS}}{\text{pre\%SS}}$$

Another aspect of appropriateness is whether the researcher has selected the *most* appropriate kind of measurement from among the various options available. Different kinds of measurements are more or less appropriate for answering different kinds of questions. Many different kinds of measurements may be applied in the study of a particular problem to investigate different aspects of the problem. In the brief introduction shown in Excerpt 8.20, Kent and LaPointe justify the appropriateness of acoustic measurement.

EXCERPT 8.20

An earlier report (LaPointe & Horner, 1981) described a patient with palilalia, which is described in the literature as an acquired disorder characterized by reiteration of utterances in a context of increasing rate and decreasing loudness. The patient, J.L.B., was a 29-year-old man with palilalia of 4 years duration. The LaPointe and Horner report is apparently the first detailed description of the nature and severity of palilalic reiteration. The subject of the case study generated a large quantity of reiterative samples, as about 38% of a total speech sample of 5,489 words was reiterated.

LaPointe and Horner reported several characteristics of the pathological reiterative utterances, including reiteration types, frequency of reiteration for seven speech tasks, and consistency and adapta-tion effects. However, their report did not attempt to verify the acoustic properties that usually are mentioned as characteristic of palilalia, namely, increasing rate (accelerando) and decreasing loudness (decrescendo) over a reiteration series. The present report describes the acoustic properties of reiterated utterances and attempts to answer the general question: What is the systematic acoustic variation, if any, from item to item in a repetition series?

From "Acoustic Properties of Pathologic Reiterative Utterances: A Case Study of Palilalia," by R. D. Kent and L. L. LaPointe, 1982, *Journal Speech and Hearing Research, 25,* pp. 95–99. Copyright 1982 by the American Speech-Language-Hearing Association. Reprinted with permission.

The final concern deals with the appropriateness of the instrument for the subjects studied. A test standardized on adults may be ill suited for use with children. A test developed on children from one socioeconomic group may not be valid when administered to children from a different socioeconomic level. Arndt (1977), for instance, criticized the Northwestern Syntax Screening Test (NSST) on several grounds, one of which was that the test may have limited applicability because of the nature of the sample used for standardization, namely middle- to upper middle-class children from one geographical area. In addition, the norms do not extend beyond age six to eleven (Lee, 1977). Both the researcher *and* the clinician must recognize the limitations of the test and use the test accordingly. To reiterate, the point is simply that the critical reader of a research article must determine whether the instruments used are appropriate to the sample investigated.

Experimenter Bias in Research Measurement

Another measurement consideration is the problem of experimenter bias, or the Rosenthal effect, in the making of research measurements (Rosenthal 1966, Rosenthal & Rosnow 1969). As discussed in Part I, the Rosenthal effect can be of two types: (1) experimenter attributes that can interact with an independent variable to influence subjects' behavior or (2) experimenter expectancies that bias an observer's measurement of the behavior of subjects.

The first type actually changes subjects' behavior, whereas the second type does not change the subjects' behavior but changes the way it is measured. It is important to note that expectancy effects have been identified in a wide variety of areas, including learning studies, reaction-time studies, psychophysical studies, and animal research (Christensen, 1988).[1]

There are several different methods that an experimenter can use to reduce or control experimenter bias. The critical reader of research should be alert to these methods and attempt to identify them *somewhere* in the Method section. One way of controlling experimenter expectancy is to use a blind technique whereby the experimenter knows the hypothesis but does not know in which treatment condition the subject is. Barber (1976) makes a distinction between an investigator (designs, supervises, analyzes, and reports the study) and an experimenter (tests subjects and collects data) and urges, as another way of controlling experimenter bias, that the investigator and experimenter *not* be the same person. Still another method is to automate procedures and, where possible, to record and analyze responses by mechanical or electrical devices. Experimenter bias can also be reduced, according to Barber (1976), by the use of strict experimental protocols and by frequent checks to determine if the protocol, designed by the investigator, is being followed by the experimenter. To control for experimenter attributes, different experimenters, with different attributes, could be used in a given study. Or a study could be replicated using a different experimenter, especially if experimenter attributes were believed to have confounded the data of the first study.

Surprisingly little attention has been paid to the problem of experimenter bias in communicative disorders research. One study (Hipskind & Rintelmann, 1969) did investigate the effect of experimenter bias on pure-tone and speech audiometry and found no influence of attempts to bias experienced or inexperienced testers with true or false information about prior audiometric results. No systematic research has been published to identify areas of speech and hearing research that are more or less susceptible to experimenter bias, however. A few studies may be found in the communicative disorders literature that have introduced some control procedures to attempt to reduce or eliminate problems of experimenter bias.

The examples shown in the next three excerpts may help readers to identify how researchers have tried to reduce experimenter bias threats to internal validity. Excerpt 8.21 shows two portions of the Method section taken from a multidiscipline study of functional hearing loss, an area where tester or investigator bias has long intruded. The last sentence of the first part of the excerpt is the key one and indicates that of the several investigators involved in the evaluation of subjects (including a psychologist and a psychiatrist), only the audiologists knew what subjects were in the control (nonfunctional) group or in the experimental (functional) group. The other experimenters did "blind" evaluations. How did the audiologists control for their bias? Because they knew which subjects were in which group, experimenter expectancy could not be totally controlled. However, expectancies with regard to certain aspects of the data were controlled, in part, as shown in Excerpt 8.21. Test-retest measurements constituted an important part of the audiologic evaluation and the RVA controlled, to some extent, experimenter bias from influencing the test-retest measurements. In addition, a rigid test protocol was followed by the entire research staff.

---

1. There is some controversy over the existence and magnitude of experimenter-expectancy effects. For a detailed discussion of this issue, the reader is urged to see Barber and Silver (1968) and Barber (1976).

EXCERPT 8.21   Subject Selection

Methodological and procedural inadequacies of subject selection in previous studies have been fully discussed (Chaiklin & Ventry, 1963). In this study an effort was made to develop precise sampling procedures, objective general and medical eligibility criteria, and specific audiometric criteria.

A monthly schedule of appointments (covering a 25-mo period) was established specifying the random order in which subjects for the two major groups would be hospitalized for evaluation. The appointment designations referred not to individual subjects but only to the order in which subjects for the two groups would be evaluated. Twice as many functional as nonfunctional subjects were included in the schedule. The order in which subjects were scheduled was known only to the project audiologists. Thus all research evaluations, except the audiological evaluation, were performed without examiners knowing to which group a subject was assigned.

. . . .

All inpatient examinations for both groups were conducted in the suite containing the I.A.C. 1201

booth. In addition, this suite contained a Grason-Stadler Békésy audiometer Model E 800, and an accessory Random Variable Attenuator (RVA) that allowed six different values of attenuation (0 to 25 dB in 5-dB steps) to be introduced into the earphone line before each repeat measurement.

The face of the RVA is blank but there is provision for quick read-out of the amount of attenuation introduced into the line. The six attenuation values are arranged randomly on the RVA's selector switch. Before a repeat measurement the experimenter rotated the dial to introduce one of the attenuation values. After the repeat measurement the RVA value was determined and then subtracted from the hearing level dial reading to produce the correct measurement figure. The use of the RVA made test–retest measurements relatively free from tester bias. The RVA was designed and constructed by Mr. L. G. Pew, Electro-Acoustic Co., San Carlos, California.

From "Introduction and Research Plan," by J. B. Chaiklin and I. M. Ventry, 1965, *Journal of Auditory Research, 5,* pp. 179–190. Reprinted by permission of the authors.

The next example, shown in Excerpt 8.22, is from a study of stuttering in monozygotic and dizygotic twins. Note that two diagnoses had to be made: one for zygosity and one for stuttering. In both instances "blind" judges were used who had no knowledge of the other diagnosis while making the diagnosis for which they were responsible. Also note the use of two judges for zygosity, one of whom had contact with the twins and one of whom did not, in order to have no information available to that judge about stuttering concordance.

EXCERPT 8.22

Diagnosis of Zygosity

Twin pairs were classified as either monozygotic (MZ) or dizygotic (DZ), based on the following four criteria: (a) blood grouping for nine systems: ABO, Rhesus, MNSs, P, Lutheran, Kell, Lewis, Duffy, Kidd (Race & Sanger, 1968). Permission for blood tests was granted by 22 pairs, six of whose HLA tissue typing was also available; (b) total ridge counts and maximal palmar ATD angle (Holt, 1968); (c) cephalic index (Weiner & Lourie, 1969); and (d) height.

In seven pairs, DZ classification was certain because of the presence of at least one blood type difference. For each remaining pair, the probability of dizygosity was calculated, given the observed intrapair differences and similarities on the four criteria (Maynard-Smith & Penrose, 1955; Race & Sanger, 1968). The calculated probability of dizygosity was less than .05 in all but three of the pairs classified as MZ and greater than .95 in all but four of the pairs classified as DZ. Final classification

Continued

EXCERPT 8.22   *Continued*

was based on the probabilities examined in conjunction with intrapair differences in iris color, hair color and form, earlobe attachment, and finger ridge patterns. Zygosity was assessed by two judges, one of whom had direct contact with the twins, while the other made the diagnosis on the basis of profile and full-face photographs and all the relevant data. Thus, the second judge had no information about stuttering concordance. The zygosity classifications of the two judges agreed in every case.

Speech Samples and Diagnosis of Stuttering

For each subject, two 500-word speech samples were recorded: a monologue with standard instruc-

tions ("Tell the story of a book or film"); and a conversation with the experimenter on standardized topics. The recordings of the 60 subjects were arranged on audiotape in random order, and stuttering was diagnosed by a speech pathologist who had never met the twins and had no knowledge of twin pair membership or zygosity, thus ensuring independence of stuttering diagnosis and zygosity classification.

The third example illustrates the importance of eliminating experimenter bias during acoustic measurement procedures. Excerpt 8.23 is from a study that examined the effect of familiarity on word durations in children's speech over a four-week period. Novel words were introduced to the children in the "early" sessions of the experiment, and the durations of their productions were compared to the durations of the same words that were produced during the "late" sessions of the experiment. An acoustic analysis was used to obtain the word durations. In an effort to eliminate potential experimenter bias, the person conducting the acoustic measurements did not know whether the words came from the early or late experimental sessions.

EXCERPT 8.23

Word and vowel duration were measured using a Kay 5500 sonograph with a wideband setting (300 Hz). Measurements were made from a master tape constructed by dubbing from a mixed order of session tapes. The primary judge was not aware of the designation of tokens as early or late. Both the amplitude and the spectrographic display were used in determining the beginning and endpoints of measurement. Word onsets were measured from the first visible increase of amplitude from zero and the cor-

responding onset of voicing or the burst on the spectrographic display or from the onset of visible noise in the case of fricatives. Word offsets were measured at the end of closure or the release of final stops.

The problem of experimenter bias is basically a problem in determining the *validity* of the measures made by an experimenter. The more free of bias an experimenter is, the more valid are the measurements made by that experimenter. An issue that is closely related to experimenter bias, then, is the *reliability* of the experimenter in making these measurements. Researchers can check an experimenter's reliability in one of two ways.

Inter-experimenter reliability is the consistency among two or more experimenters in making a measurement. *Intra-experimenter* reliability is the consistency of one experimenter in remaking a particular measurement. Excerpt 8.24 shows information on experimenter reliability taken from the method section of an article on laryngeal behavior during the production of voiced and voiceless consonants. Both intrajudge and interjudge reliability are assessed for both the laryngeal behavior judgments and the phonetic transcriptions of the voiced and voiceless consonants.

EXCERPT 8.24   Intra- and Interjudge Reliability

To assess the intrajudge and interjudge reliability of the laryngeal behavior judgments, 52 randomly selected consonantal utterances (9% of the total) were selected for remeasurement. From four to eight productions were selected from each of the eight speakers, so that the sample consisted of 28 plosives (15 voiced and 13 voiceless) and 24 fricatives (13 voiced and 11 voiceless).

The first author rejudged the vocal fold behavior associated with the 52 consonantal productions while the second author separately analyzed the same subset of samples. Analysis of intrajudge agreement of laryngeal behavior determined for the 52 samples (agreement/disagreement + agreement, after Sander, 1961) revealed considerable agreement (.98), ranging from .84 to 1.00 for individual subjects. Interjudge agreement was .87 for all subjects combined (range = .66–1.00 for individual subjects' productions).

To assess the intratranscriber reliability of phonetic transcription, a subset of 64 randomly selected samples (8 productions from each speaker for 13%

of the total) were retranscribed by the first author. Of the 64 test words, 35 were word-initial plosives (19 voiced and 16 voiceless) and 29 were word-initial fricatives (18 voiced and 11 voiceless). Comparison of the first author's original and second transcription revealed intratranscriber agreement of .97 (range = .87–1.00).

Intertranscriber reliability of phonetic transcription was assessed by having two judges (R1 and R2) transcribe each speaker's second production of the entire stimulus set. Interjudge agreement (Sander, 1961) between the first author and R1 was .91 (range = .70–1.00 for transcriptions of individual speakers), whereas intertranscriber agreement between the first author and R2 was .93 (range = .83–1.00).

From "Deaf Speakers' Laryngeal Behavior," by J. J. Mahshie and E. G. Conture, 1983, *Journal of Speech and Hearing Research, 26,* pp. 550–559. Copyright 1983 by the American Speech-Language-Hearing Association. Reprinted with permission.

One final example should suffice. Caruso and his colleagues investigated the effects of three different levels of cognitive stress on the articulatory coordination abilities of stutterers and nonstutterers. Articulation coordination abilities were assessed using a variety of acoustic measurements. Excerpt 8.25 shows that both intrajudge and interjudge acoustic measurement reliabilities were assessed. Reliability coefficients are not reported. Rather, the actual measurement-remeasurement differences are reported. As such, the consumer of research knows the exact magnitude of both the intrajudge and interjudge measurement differences and can thus interpret directly the measurement reliability. Conversely, intrajudge and interjudge reliability of the identification of disfluencies is reported using a well-established agreement index.

EXCERPT 8.25   Reliability

A random subset of approximately 10% of the speech samples from stutterers and nonstutterers under all three conditions were re-analyzed by the examiner and also analyzed by a second judge to assess reliability. The mean intrajudge measurement difference and range (shown in parentheses) for each acoustic measure were as follows: word duration—1.41 msec (0–29 msec); vowel duration—4.59 msec (0–26 msec); consonant-vowel transition extent—15.00 Hz (0–62 Hz); consonant-vowel transition duration—4.00 msec (0–22 msec); first formant center frequency—12.26 Hz (0–62 Hz); second formant center frequency—14.83 Hz (0–93 Hz). The mean interjudge measurement difference for each acoustic measure was as follows: word duration—1.88 msec (0–33 msec); vowel

duration—3.11 msec (0–39 msec); consonant-vowel transition extent—13.74 Hz (0–93 Hz); consonant-vowel transition duration—4.67 msec (0–30 msec); first formant center frequency—4.63 Hz (0–62 Hz); second formant center frequency—18.59 Hz (0–93 Hz). Measures of agreement (Sander, 1961) were computed for the identification of dysfluencies (agreement/disagreement + agreement). Intrajudge agreement was 90% and interjudge agreement was 92% for judgments of dysfluency.

From "Adults Who Stutter: Responses to Cognitive Stress," by A. J. Caruso, W. J. Chodzko-Zajko, D. A. Bidinger, and R. K. Sommers, 1994, *Journal of Speech and Hearing Research, 37*, pp. 746–754. Copyright 1994 by the American Speech-Language-Hearing Association. Reprinted with permission.

Test Environment

The environment within which research measurements are made may be an important aspect of measurement in many studies. Test environment may affect both internal and external validity. With regard to internal validity, test environment should be specified if measurements could vary from one environment to another. Also, the constancy of environments across all measures should be ascertained if measurements need to be made in different environments. If environmental variables need to be controlled, sufficient detail should be provided to allow the environment to be replicated in future research. Excerpt 8.26 is from an article regarding sound localization and sound tracking abilities of children. Sound localization and sound tracking experiments require the control of environmental echoes. Excerpt 8.26 explicitly details the nature and characteristics of the test environment.

EXCERPT 8.26

Subjects were tested inside a double-walled IAC test booth that had all internal surfaces lined with special 4-inch-thick absorbent foam (Peabody Noise Control Co.) to minimize sound reflections or echoes. The mean RT_{60} reverberation times of the booth at 0.5, 1, 2, and 4 kHz measured less than 0.10 sec. Subjects were seated with the head positioned against a headrest designed to minimize head movement during testing. Three acoustically matched

5-inch loudspeakers were positioned forward of the subject, one directly in front, and one each situated 45 degrees to the left and right of midline. Each loudspeaker was 150 cm from the subject's head.

From "Tracking of 'Moving' Fused Auditory Images by Children," by J. L. Cranford, M. Morgan, R. Scudder, and C. Moore, 1993, *Journal of Speech and Hearing Research, 36*, pp. 424–430. Copyright 1993 by the American Speech-Language-Hearing Association. Reprinted with permission.

Research studies in communicative disorders report the kind of test room used and the background noise levels because of the importance of maintaining an adequately low background noise level to eliminate masking in audiology studies and to yield noise-free recordings for speech analysis. Studies of lipreading often report the illumination characteristics of the room because of the importance of lighting for lipreading. Any time environmental variables can affect measurements taken in a given research study, they should be specified.

With respect to external validity, the environment may serve as a "reactive arrangement" so that generalizations may be limited to individuals functioning only in that particular environment. The question facing the critical reader is whether the test environment is so different from environments to which the reader wishes to generalize as to preclude such generalization. An adequate description of the environment in which testing or treatment took place can help the reader judge the possible reactivity of the environment. It would be even better for the researcher to discuss the possible threat to external validity of reactive arrangements or to test the generality of results to other environments with a systematic replication.

Excerpt 8.27 is from a study by Andrews and Ingham that addresses the issue of generalization of the results of stuttering therapy to other environments. The first part of Excerpt 8.27 is from their Introduction section, and the second part is from their Results section. We have italicized a portion of the excerpt to highlight the authors' concern about external validity of stuttering-treatment effects. Note the authors' expression of concern regarding the lack of information about generalization in the reporting of results of many treatments and the unique feature of a generalization probe to test the degree to which their results were "laboratory-bound."

EXCERPT 8.27

This paper is addressed to the problem of evaluating the effects, or outcome, resulting from the treatment of stuttering. It will be argued that a satisfactory procedure for evaluating the outcome of treatment must establish a method of measuring stuttering behavior, *must show that changes occurring in the treatment situation carry over into the outside world,* and must be capable of estimating the degree to which the results achieved prove stable over time. The stuttering therapy literature is generally bereft of reports which fulfill these suggested criteria. Genuine therapeutic success in individual cases is probably not uncommon and apparently occurs with many of the currently used therapies. But lack of preparedness to systematically measure progress and assess out-

come of treatment may have led to the present crisis in confidence over the efficacy of treatments for stuttering (Van Riper, 1970; Wingate, 1971).

. . . .

One strangely neglected feature of many treatments is the absence of a design which ensures that improvements attained within the laboratory generalize to the outside world, or are not "laboratory-bound." In the present program, generalization of treatment gains was assessed by the use of a "probe" measure of speech performance during treatment. Each evening the subjects were assessed in conditions which were independent of most stimuli associated with the laboratory. From this measure it was found, for example, that subjects who

Continued

EXCERPT 8.27 *Continued*

were treated by a regular contingent token-system schedule displayed improved performance in both the probe and laboratory situations. However, when subjects were treated with a mixed noncontingent and contingent token system schedule, they did not show significant improvement in the probe measure, despite concurrent laboratory improvement. Thus the contingent token-system schedule, as used in this therapy program, was demonstrated to produce treatment and token control effects over stuttering (Ingham, 1972).

From "An Approach to the Evaluation of Stuttering Therapy," by G. Andrews and R. J. Ingham, 1972, *Journal of Speech and Hearing Research, 15,* pp. 296–302. Copyright 1972 by the American Speech-Language-Hearing Association. Reprinted with permission.

In summary, the test environment is an important part of the Materials section of an article for two reasons. First, the environment may be important in determining the internal validity of the study by assessing the degree to which the environment affects the measurements made. Second, the nature of the research environment is important in determining the external validity of the results with regard to generalizing to other settings.

Instructions

The final consideration in this section has to do with instructions. Instructions to subjects can be thought of as part of instrumentation because instructions are the tools by which the researcher attempts to elicit the desired response or behavior and to maintain a consistent response set across subjects. Inadequate, inappropriate, poorly worded instructions thus pose an instrumentation threat to internal validity. In many circumstances, instructions are rather straightforward and, in fact, are specified in the administration of standardized test instruments. In other instances, the researcher may have to develop a set of instructions. The intent of the instructions, the thrust of the instructions, if not the instructions themselves, need to be specified by the researcher. The critical evaluator needs to ask two questions: (1) Are the instructions appropriate to the task at hand? and (2) Is sufficient detail provided to allow for replication or for clinical application?

Excerpt 8.28 is a fairly lengthy section that details the instructions given to two different groups of raters in a study that investigated the construct validity of interval rating procedures for judging nonstutterers' and stutterers' speech naturalness from audiovisual recordings. The equal-appearing interval (EAI) rating procedure that was used replicated an earlier study by Martin and Haroldson. As such, the instructions given to the EAI raters were taken verbatim from Martin and Haroldson's study. The instructions given to the raters using the direct magnitude estimation (DME) procedures were similar to those used in a study by Metz, Schiavetti, and Sacco that evaluated the construct validity of interval scaling procedures for judging stutterers' speech naturalness from audio recordings.

EXCERPT 8.28

Equal-Appearing Interval (EAI) Rating

Twenty raters were assigned randomly to use the EAI rating procedure. No more than five raters participated in a given session. In general, the rating procedures and instructions were the same as those employed in the Martin et al. (1984) and the Martin and Haroldson (1992) studies. Raters were seated in front of a video monitor and given a packet of 20 numbered 9-point naturalness scales on which 1 was labeled "highly natural" and 9 was labeled "highly unnatural." Raters were asked to read the following instructions:

> We are studying what makes speech sound natural or unnatural. You will see and hear a number of short speech samples. The samples will be separated by a few seconds of silence. Each sample will be introduced by the sample number. Your task is to rate the naturalness of each speech sample.
>
> If the speech sample sounds highly natural to you, circle the 1 on the scale. If the speech sample sounds highly unnatural, circle the 9 on the scale. If the sample sounds somewhere between highly natural and highly unnatural, circle the appropriate number on the scale. Do not hesitate to use the ends of the scale (1 or 9) when appropriate.
>
> "Naturalness" will not be defined for you. Make your ratings based on how natural or unnatural the speech sounds to you.

Direct Magnitude Estimation (DME)

The other 20 raters participated in the DME rating procedure. Again, no more than five raters participated in a session. The DME rating procedures and instructions were similar to those used with DME raters in the Metz et al. (1990) experiment. Raters were seated in front of a video monitor and given a protocol sheet on which were listed samples 1 through 20 with a blank space beside each number. Raters were asked to read the following instructions:

> We are studying what makes speech sound natural or unnatural. You will see and hear a number of short speech samples. The samples will be separated by a few seconds of silence. Each sample will be introduced by the sample number. Your task is to rate the naturalness of each speech sample.
>
> When you have seen and heard the first sample, give its naturalness a number—any number you think is appropriate. You will then be presented the second sample to rate. If the second sample sounds more natural than the first sample, give it a lower number. If the second sample sounds more unnatural than the first sample, give it a higher number. Try to make the ratio between the two numbers correspond to the ratio of the naturalness between the two samples. The higher the number, the more unnatural the second sample sounds relative to the first sample; the lower the number, the more natural the second sample sounds relative to the first sample. If you assigned the first sample the number "10," and the second sample sounds twice as natural, give the second sample a rating of "5." If the third sample sounds twice as unnatural as the first sample, give the third sample a rating of "20."
>
> "Naturalness" will not be defined for you. Make your ratings based on how natural or unnatural the speech sounds to you.

We followed the suggestions of Engen (1971) for the use of DME with no standard/modulus so that raters were free to rate the first speaker with any number they chose and to scale the speech naturalness of all subsequent speakers with numbers proportional to the perceived naturalness or unnaturalness of each speaker. Further details on the use of direct magnitude estimation with and without standard/modulus can be found in Engen (1971); Lane,

Continued

EXCERPT 8.28   *Continued*

Catania, and Stevens (1961); and Schiavetti, Sacco, Metz, and Sitler (1983). In a manner similar to that described by Metz et al. (1990), both the DME and EAI raters practiced their respective rating procedures by scaling the relative lengths of a number of horizontal lines.

From "Psychophysical Analysis of Audiovisual Judgments of Speech Naturalness of Nonstutterers and Stutterers," by N. Schiavetti, R. R. Martin, S. K. Haroldson, and D. E. Metz, 1994, *Journal of Speech and Hearing Research, 37,* pp. 46–52. Copyright 1994 by the American Speech-Language-Hearing Association. Reprinted with permission.

The example shown in Excerpt 8.29 is from a study of vocal characteristics of stutterers and normal speakers during choral reading. The authors not only describe their instructions to the subjects but also provide a detailed rationale for the specific instructions used relative to the purpose of the study. The instructions are presented in sufficient detail for another investigator to replicate the procedure.

EXCERPT 8.29

Subjects were tested individually in a sound-treated room. The conditions were presented in a counterbalanced order with at least a 20-minute rest period between them to minimize adaptation (Jamison, 1955).

Each condition began with a subject receiving a standard set of instructions. In the experimental condition, these directions included the statement, "If you experience a disfluency, stumble over or misread a word as you are reading in unison, don't try to rush to catch up. Just skip ahead in the reading to the word you hear the model speaker producing." These instructions were given for the following reasons: It was assumed that a subject who experienced any of the speech production lapses mentioned above, would as a result, fall behind and out of unison with the model speaker. Consequently, the subject might be tempted to shorten his subsequent vowel durations in an effort to speed up, catch the model and get back in unison with him. We wanted to discourage such a

reaction. Had we failed to do this, the subject could have modified his vowel durations for reasons that had nothing to do with any effect that the independent variable might have had on them. When signalled to begin, the subject read aloud into a microphone (Sony ECM 50) that was positioned and maintained a set distance from his mouth. During the experimental condition only, the subject wore earphones in order to hear the tape of the speaker with whom he was instructed to read in unison. This taped signal was presented to subjects at a comfortable loudness level with the playback volume setting fixed. Subjects' oral readings were audio-taped (Ampex AG 350).

From "Vocal Characteristics of Normal Speakers and Stutterers during Choral Reading," by M. R. Adams and P. Ramig, 1980, *Journal of Speech and Hearing Research, 23,* pp. 457–469. Copyright 1980 by the American Speech-Language-Hearing Association. Reprinted with permission.

In conclusion, the major emphasis of this section on materials has been to identify instrumentation threats to internal validity. Inadequate instrumentation and inadequate materials can vitiate the value of an elegant design, but, to reiterate, a poor problem cannot be salvaged with even the most sophisticated instrumental array. Thus, the need for the enlightened consumer of research to put the Materials section of the research article into proper perspective. The Materials section is important but constitutes only one portion of the research article.

Procedures

The Procedure section of the research article usually concludes the Method section. It is here that the researcher describes what is done to the subjects with the materials. It must be recognized that for convenience and simplicity, we have divided the present chapter into the three *typical* parts of a Method section. Reading just a few issues of selected journals will quickly reveal that there may be considerable overlap among parts; some procedures may be described in the Materials section, subject-selection procedures might be handled in the Procedures section, and so on. Despite the variety of formats used, the critical reader's responsibility is to identify how the researcher has dealt with the threats to internal and external validity detailed in Part I. Because the preceding sections of this chapter have dealt primarily with the threats to validity posed by subject-selection procedures and instrumentation (materials), this section will deal with the remaining threats to validity.

It should be apparent by now that principal ways to reduce threats to validity are through the use of an appropriate experimental design or through the use of special precautions when employing a descriptive design. For example, the one-group pretest–posttest design is far weaker than the randomized pretest–posttest control-group design. A between-subjects design with faulty subject-selection criteria is far less adequate than a within-subjects design where appropriate attention has been given to counterbalancing or randomizing test conditions. However, a within-subjects design can be faulted if, for example, randomization or counterbalancing has not been used. The point, then, is for the critical evaluator to identify the type of design employed by the researcher and to assess the adequacy of the design, keeping in mind the advantages and disadvantages of the various designs described in Part I. To help develop this critical skill, the remainder of the chapter includes some rather lengthy excerpts from the research literature. Our accompanying narrative shows how the reader can identify the type of research design used and how the researcher has dealt with threats to validity.

Within-Subjects Experimental Designs

Excerpt 8.30 is taken from the Method section of a study by Conture on the effects of loudness and frequency spectrum (two independent variables) on stuttering frequency, reading rate, and vocal level (three dependent variables). The design is within-subjects because all the stutterers were exposed to all levels of the independent variables and there was only one group of subjects. Each subject participated in all four sessions in this experiment, and several important design strategies were used to reduce threats to internal validity. Note, first, that a measure of TTS was used each day to ensure that no threshold shifts would contaminate the data with a carry-over effect from the previous day's noise exposure. Also note that rest periods were used to reduce short-term maturation (fatigue), and an adjustment period was used before the preexposure period to stabilize subjects' speaking behavior. The sequences of conditions and passages read during each condition were both randomized to control for sequencing effects. This within-subjects experimental design, then, shows several concerted attempts to minimize threats to internal validity.

EXCERPT 8.30

Subjects

The subjects were nine adult male stutterers who were receiving speech therapy at the Wendell Johnson Speech and Hearing Center at the University of Iowa. All nine subjects had hearing threshold levels of better than 15 dB (re ANSI, 1969) at 500, 1000, and 2000 Hz.

Stimulus Material

The stimulus material consisted of five prose readings taken from the same level of the *Reader's Digest Reading Skill Builder* series (ninth-grade level, Part 3). A random sample of 100 words was taken from each of the five readings and rated according to Brown's (1945) "word weights." The similarity of the average word weight among the five readings indicated that the five passages were suitably equated with regard to Brown's four linguistic factors (Conture, 1972).

Experimental Conditions

Each subject read during four sessions separated by at least 24 hours. There were two conditions in three sessions and one condition in the fourth. At the beginning of the first session, and at the start of every subsequent session, each subject performed a fixed frequency (4000 Hz) Bekesy tracing for two minutes in each ear. The middle one-minute segment from each ear was used to determine

whether a subject's exposure to noise from the previous session might have produced a temporary threshold shift (TTS). If a shift of 5 dB or greater was noted on this task at the beginning of any session, then the subject was asked to leave and to come back another day.

After the TTS check, the subject began to read aloud continuously from the prepared readings while two conditions were presented. The sequence of presentation of the six experimental conditions and one control condition was as follows: the subject read for five minutes (adjustment period), then for another five minutes (preexposure period), followed by a 10-minute rest period. The same sequence was presented after the rest period, except that a different condition was presented during the exposure period. Sessions 2, 3, and 4 were identical to Session 1 except for the type of experimental or control conditions presented during the exposure period. The sequence of conditions and the particular passage that was read during a condition were all determined by chance through the use of a table of random numbers.

From "Some Effects of Noise on Speaking Behavior of Stutterers," by E. G. Conture, 1974, *Journal of Speech and Hearing Research, 17,* pp. 714–723. Copyright 1974 by the American Speech-Language-Hearing Association. Reprinted with permission.

Between-Subjects Experimental Designs

Excerpt 8.31, taken from a study of the effect of treatment on language recovery in aphasia, quickly identifies the research as a between-subjects experimental study. In this study, thirty-one severely impaired aphasic subjects were assigned to three groups; one group received programmed instruction, one group received nonprogrammed speech treatment, and one group received no intervention. Note the authors' implicit recognition of the value of random assignment to treatment groups, as well as the reason why this was not possible. At first glance, this design could be diagrammed as follows, maintaining the notation system described in Part I:

$$
\begin{array}{ccc}
O_1 & X_{PI} & O_2 \\
\hline
O_3 & X_{NPI} & O_4 \\
\hline
O_5 & & O_6
\end{array}
$$

Here X_{PI} represents programmed instruction, X_{NPI} represents nonprogrammed instruction, and the third group received no treatment. The reader should recognize this as the non-equivalent control-group design. Recall that a major shortcoming of this design is the subject-selection factor. That is, because subjects are not selected randomly or randomly assigned to the control or experimental group, subjects may, in fact, be quite different on certain extraneous variables that may interact with the independent variable. Sarno and her associates recognized this problem and determined that the subjects in the three groups were not different on six extraneous variables: age, symptom duration, Functional Communication Profile (FCP), previous treatment, time in treatment, and number of treatment sessions. In a sense, the groups were matched on those dimensions that might interact with the treatment.

EXCERPT 8.31   Subjects

Patients were at least 18 years old, had suffered a CVA with right hemiplegia, were premorbidly right-handed, and spoke fluent American English. There was no upper age limit. All patients exhibited severe aphasic symptomatology of at least three months duration. This cutoff point was chosen to avoid biasing the results with the possible effects of spontaneous recovery (Eisenson, 1964; Lenneberg, 1967). There was no upper limit on duration of symptoms. Severe aphasia was operationally defined as an Overall Functional Communication Profile (see Materials section) score of below 31%. For the most part patients in this category had no speech function and little understanding of speech. At best, some were able to say a few words and understand some simple commands. Despite the severity of their language impairment, the majority of the patients were alert.

Those who did not have adequate motor and sensory function in at least one hand, and vision and hearing adequate for the task requirements were excluded, as were those who were heavily medicated or had a premorbid language impairment. The presence of a right homonymous hemianopsia was not considered sufficiently incapacitating to preclude participation in the study. All study candidates were examined by a neurologist to exclude patients who showed signs of bilateral brain damage.

Patients with aphasia secondary to brain trauma or tumor were excluded since their recovery process is known to be different from that of the post-CVA patient.

A total of 31 patients were assigned to three groups: programmed instruction, nonprogrammed speech therapy, and an untreated control group. It was virtually impossible to balance the treatment groups by random assignment due to the varied location of patients, limitations in the availability of a programmed-instruction clinician and/or a

Continued

EXCERPT 8.31   Subjects   *Continued*

nonprogrammed clinician. However, all groups were found to be equivalent with regard to age, symptom duration, Functional Communication Profile (FCP) scores, previous speech therapy, total time on program, and number of treatment sessions. (See Tables 1 and 2.)

TABLE 1   Range, median, and means for age, overall FCP scores, duration of symptoms for all treatment groups

Treatment Group	Age			Duration of Symptoms			FCP Overall Scores		
	Range	Mean	Median	Range	Mean	Median	Range	Mean	Median
Programmed instruction	46–80 $n = 16$	63.81 $n = 16$	63.50 $n = 16$	3–144 months $n = 16$	33.69 $n = 16$	19.50 $n = 16$	15–31 $n = 16$	17.06 $n = 16$	18.00 $n = 16$
Nonprogrammed	54–83 $n = 7$	66.86 $n = 7$	64.00 $n = 7$	3–72 months $n = 7$	27.00 $n = 7$	18.00 $n = 7$	11–27 $n = 7$	16.29 $n = 7$	14.00 $n = 7$
Control	54–70 $n = 7$	63.71 $n = 8$	65.00 $n = 8$	18–72 months $n = 7$	41.14 $n = 8$	45.00 $n = 8$	5–29 $n = 8$	17.75 $n = 8$	20.00 $n = 8$

TABLE 2   Comparisons between subjects assigned to programmed instruction, nonprogrammed instruction, and control groups

Groups	Age		Symptom Duration		FCP		Previous Speech Therapy		Time in Therapy (Weeks)		Therapy Sessions	
	t	df	t	df	t	df	t	df	t	df	t	df
PI-NPI	0.70	21	0.41	21	0.23	20	0.75	19	0.53	20	0.91	19
PI-C	0.03	21	0.47	21	0.19	21	0.90	20	—	—	—	—
NPI-C	0.66	12	1.13	12	0.36	13	0.26	13	—	—	—	—

Note: None of the *t*-values were significant at the 0.05 level.

It should be apparent to the reader that this type of treatment study is exceedingly difficult to design so that all threats to internal and external validity are circumvented. Even with the care taken by Sarno, Silverman, and Sands, history and the reactivity of the measures employed could affect internal validity, and pretesting and reactive arrangements could affect external validity. It is interesting to note that the results of this study led the authors (p. 621) to conclude that "severe aphasic stroke patients do not benefit from speech therapy." Recognizing that only two types of therapy were employed for a relatively small group of subjects, they recommend "further studies using other methods of treatment and a larger group of patients."

Sarno, Silverman, and Sands could not randomly assign subjects to treatment groups; instead, they had to employ an overall matching procedure. Wilson, on the other hand, used a stronger procedure in his 1966 study of speech treatment with educable mentally retarded children (Excerpt 8.32). In this large-scale study, Wilson first drew a sample of one-thousand children. Although we do not know if this is a random sample, we do know that it is a large sample and, in fact, may include *all* of the educable mentally retarded children enrolled in the Special District program. The sample size was then reduced to 777 when the three exclusion criteria identified in the first paragraph were applied. Subjects were then divided into two groups, those with speech deviations and those without. The third paragraph of the excerpt is the key in identifying this study as a between-subjects experimental study. Three groups were formed and most important, the speech-deviant subjects were *randomly assigned* to one of the three groups. As we have emphasized previously, random assignment to treatment and control groups is the best way to minimize such threats to internal validity as history, subject selection, and maturation. Although the Wilson study is superior in this respect to the Sarno, Silverman, and Sands study (random assignment vs. overall matching), Wilson's research suffered a mortality problem that did not exist in the Sarno research. Because Wilson's study was three years in duration, subjects dropped out and, although random assignment should, in theory, produce a comparable mortality rate across treatment groups, it is apparent that this was not the case here. The mortality rate was 18 percent for the experimental group, 26 percent for the control group but *50 percent* for the placebo group. Interestingly enough, Wilson's results did not demonstrate significant group differences in phoneme errors over the three-year duration of the study. Further investigation would be necessary to assess the influence of the differential mortality rates on the results of the study.

EXCERPT 8.32   Method

Subjects

A sample of 777 children between the ages of six and 16 years was drawn from the 90 classes of educable mentally retarded children[1] of the Special District for the Education and Training of Handicapped Children of St. Louis County, Missouri.

[1]The IQ range of children in classes for educable mentally retarded children in the state of Missouri is 48–78.

This sample of 777 children was derived from a larger group of 1000 by eliminating children with hearing disabilities, severe organic problems, and no current intellectual assessments.

The initial classification of children established two basic groups: (1) a group with normal speech, and (2) a speech-deviant group. The classifications were based on the results of the Hejna Articulation Test administered by three speech clinicians. A scale of articulatory severity that had been used by

Continued

EXCERPT 8.32   Method   *Continued*

Special District speech clinicians for five years was applied to the speech-deviant group. From the criteria on the scale, a rating from least to most severe was made. The severity scale rating for the speech-deviant group was made by one clinician. Of the 777 children tested, 415 children (53.4%) had speech deviations. The remaining 362 children (46.6%) had normal speech. The median chronological age (CA) of the deviant group was 10.6 years, and the median CA of the nondeviant group was 12.5 years. The median mental age (MA) of the speech-deviant group was 6.8 years and the median MA of the nondeviant group was 8.5 years. These scores were based on current psychological evaluations using an individual intelligence test. Based on the intelligence test, the median IQ for the speech-deviant group was 63 and for the nondeviant group 68. There were 461 males, with 251 speech-deviants and 210 normals. There were 316 females, with 164 speech-deviants and 152 normals.

The 415 speech-deviant children were randomly divided into three groups labeled Experimental ($N =$ 140), Placebo ($N = 130$), and Control ($N = 145$). The number of children remaining in each category after a three-year program was 115, 65, and 107, respectively. The decrease in number was due primarily to the transient nature of the population.

In this particular project, speech therapy was limited to specific articulation therapy. The program of treatment for each of the three groups was as follows:

Experimental.   Children in this group received two half-hour sessions of direct speech therapy per week, as previously defined. Each child had some individual and some group therapy. At no time did group size exceed four. The three clinicians who performed the initial evaluation were assigned to provide therapy. They were not given specific, detailed instructions or therapy lesson plans, but were directed to plan a corrective speech program for each child within the framework suggested by Van Riper (1956).

Placebo.   Children in this group received two half-hour sessions of nonphoneme-oriented speech and language stimulation per week. They did not receive specific guidance in correcting individual sound errors. The purpose of the placebo segment of the sample was to offset the possibility that alterations in the speech of the experimental group, either positive or negative, might have resulted primarily from the special attention derived from the therapy situation.

Control.   Children in this group were given articulation tests at the same intervals as those in the other groups. No therapy was administered, and the testing situation was their only contact with the speech clinician.

From "Efficacy of Speech Therapy with Educable Mentally Retarded Children," by F. B. Wilson, 1966, *Journal of Speech and Hearing Research, 9,* pp. 423–433. Copyright 1966 by the American Speech-Language-Hearing Association. Reprinted with permission.

The two previous examples of between-subjects designs (Excerpts 8.31 and 8.32) are from experimental studies of the effects of treatment that involve rather long-term studies of the subjects. Most short-term experiments, like the one by Conture of the effects of noise on stuttering shown in Excerpt 8.30, use within-subjects designs because allowing subjects to act as their own controls by participating in all experimental conditions eliminates problems of differential subject selection. The example shown in Excerpt 8.33 illustrates a short-term experiment on the effects of practice and instructions on lingual vibro-tactile thresholds using a between-subjects design. A between-subjects design was used because of the probability that a permanent carry-over effect could not be eliminated with counterbalancing or randomization of the conditions presented to the subjects. Note the authors' rationale for using the between-subjects design instead of counterbalancing conditions because subjects could not become naive again after having been exposed to the instructions. Thus, a within-subjects design would be exposed to the danger of carryover of the effect of one instruction set onto another subsequent instruction set in later conditions. Note also that the authors dealt with the problem of differential subject selection by randomly assigning subjects to one of the three conditions.

EXCERPT 8.33   Procedure

The 30 subjects were divided randomly into three groups of 10 each. Each group was assigned to a condition involving a different instructional set for obtaining their lingual vibrotactile thresholds. A counterbalancing design, although desirable, could not be employed since naiveté was a prerequisite for each subject to be used in the study. Once a subject received an instructional set, that subject would no longer be naive; therefore, it would be difficult to determine whether the instructions previously given interacted with a new instructional set. The instructional sets were as follows:

Condition 1—Strict instructions.   Subjects were given simple but relatively strict instructions to raise their hands as soon as they felt the stimulus on their tongue.

Condition 2—Comprehensive instructions.   Subjects were given more comprehensive instructions in which the idea of threshold was stressed. This set of instructions told the subjects to raise their hands as soon as they felt the stimulus, no matter how faint it appeared to be. They were encouraged to respond even if they only thought the stimulus was present.

Condition 3—Comprehensive instructions with examiner reinforcement.   Subjects were given the same instructions as in the second condition, but appropriate examiner feedback was supplied regarding the accuracy of their responses. If their responses did not conform to what we have experi-

enced as fitting within the range of previously generated normative threshold data, appropriate feedback was provided. The following subject responses and examiner feedback occurred during this experimental condition:

Subject Responses

1. False alarm.
2. Should be responding earlier.
3. Appropriate response.

Examiner Feedback

1. Make sure you are feeling the tickling before you raise your hand.
2. You probably feel the stimulus before you raise your hand.
3. You are responding right about where I would expect you to.

Examiner feedback used in Condition 3 was based on normative lingual vibrotactile threshold data obtained from 110 normal young adults (Telage, Fucci, & Arnst, 1972).

Mixed (Between-Subjects and Within-Subjects) Designs

The example shown in Excerpt 8.34 illustrates a mixed design in which one independent variable is studied with a between-subjects design and another independent variable is studied with a within-subjects design. This study is also an example of combined experimental–descriptive research because one independent variable is manipulable and the other independent variable is subject classification. The between-subjects independent variable is the subject classification (normal vs. defective articulation), or the nonmanipulable, descriptive independent variable. The within-subjects independent variable is the manipulable, experimental independent variable (type of recall stimuli). The dependent variable is performance on the recall task.

The between-subjects component of the study is identified in the Subjects section of Excerpt 8.34. This section describes the subject-classification independent variable and reveals the comparative (descriptive) aspect of the study. Note the care taken to ensure that the two groups of subjects are comparable on important extraneous variables (e.g., chronological age, gender, race). The exclusion criteria described in the last paragraph of this section (no subjects with hearing loss, stuttering, bilingual background, and so forth) also helped to reduce the threat to internal validity posed by differential selection of subjects. It is clear, then, that the subject-selection procedure employed by Saxman and Miller produced two groups of comparable subjects that differed primarily (if not solely) in articulation skills.

EXCERPT 8.34

Subjects

The subjects used in this study were 28 public school kindergarten children with defective articulation and 28 subjects with normal articulation. The group with defective articulation, 17 boys and 11 girls, performed one standard deviation or more below the norms for their age and sex on the Templin-Darley 176-item diagnostic test of articulation. They ranged in age from five years six months to six years seven months, with a mean age of six years.

The group with normal articulation, none of whom had more than one articulation error, were selected and matched with the subjects who had defective articulation. Subjects were matched on the basis of chronological age, sex, race, and father's occupation and level of education.

All subjects were screened for normal hearing (25 dB ISO; 0.25 to 8 kHz) and had no obvious motor disabilities or apparent organic deviation determined by an oral peripheral examination. In addition, no subject was from a bilingual home, was a twin or a stutterer, or was considered by his classroom teacher to have a significant intellectual deficit.

Materials

The materials for the immediate recall tasks consisted of three lists: strings of randomized digits, random-word strings, and active-declarative sentences. The digit strings were constructed by drawing digits from a table of random numbers with replacement resulting in strings from two to nine digits in length. There were two strings at each length level for a total of 16 strings. Fourteen active-declarative sentences were constructed using the controlled vocabulary of Rinsland (1945). The sentences ranged from four to 10 words in length with two sentences at each length. The random-word strings were constructed by numbering consecutively each word in the sentence list. A table of random numbers was used to make word strings of two to nine words in length. There were two word strings at each length for a total of 16 random-word strings. This procedure insured the same vocabulary for both the sentences and random-word strings.

Procedure

Each subject was seen individually for the immediate recall tasks. The subject was instructed to repeat the materials read by the examiner. For example, the examiner would read, "I want you to say exactly what I say. If I say 6–2–3, what do you say?" The child would respond, "6–2–3." Several examples of each of the three types of materials were given as practice items to insure that the subject understood the task. The materials were read

Continued

EXCERPT 8.34 *Continued*

by the examiner at a practiced constant rate of approximately one word per 0.75 seconds and with a flat intonational contour.

In presenting each of the three lists, the items were read in the order of shortest to longest items. When the child missed three consecutive items on a list, testing was stopped for that list. The lists were presented in random order. All responses were

recorded on a Nagra IV tape recorder for later transcription and analysis.

From "Short-Term Memory and Language Skills in Articulation-Deficient Children," by J. H. Saxman and J. F. Miller, 1973, *Journal of Speech and Hearing Research, 16,* pp. 721–730. Copyright 1973 by the American Speech-Language-Hearing Association. Reprinted with permission.

The within-subjects component of the study is described in the Materials and Procedures sections. Three kinds of recall stimuli were presented to the subjects: randomized digits, random-word strings, and active-declarative sentences. The Procedures section reveals two important aspects of the within-subjects design: (1) all subjects received all levels of the experimental independent variable (stimuli) and (2) the three stimuli were presented in random order.

The Saxman and Miller study, then, illustrates both the use of a mixed (between-subjects and within-subjects) design and the use of combined experimental–descriptive research. The study examines the effect of the experimental independent variable on subjects in two different classifications. Careful attention should be given to this type of research design because it is so commonly encountered in the literature.

Within-Subjects Time-Series Experiments

The next example is the Procedure section taken from a within-subjects time-series study by Williams on the relationship between productive phonological knowledge and generalization of learning patterns in nine phonologically disordered children. Excerpt 8.35 describes a multiple-baseline design to evaluate the effects of consonant cluster training on the production of that cluster, as well as potential production generalization to a different consonant cluster. A basic AB design is used. During the baseline segment *(A),* both consonant clusters were measured to provide an index of each subject's pretreatment production performance. During the treatment segment *(B),* test probes were administered for both consonant clusters at the end of every third training session. Training was initiated on one of the consonant clusters at the start of the *B* segment and continued until the child achieved 70 percent production accuracy or had completed twenty-one training sessions. When the child had completed training on the first cluster, training on the second cluster began. Excerpt 8.35 also shows the test probe results for three of the nine subjects in the Williams study. Observe the relatively stable baselines during the *A* segment and the influence of training a particular consonant cluster in the *B* segment.

EXCERPT 8.35

Experimental Design

A multiple-baseline design across behaviors was used with a counterbalanced training order. The two cluster classes, [st] and [tr], were the two behaviors forming the dependent variable. The independent variable, treatment, was applied to the first behavior while the second behavior continued to be measured in baseline. Training was shifted to the second behavior when training was completed for the first behavior.

In this design, both behaviors were measured initially during a baseline period, then treatment was applied to the first behavior while the second behavior remained in baseline. When treatment on the first behavior was completed, the second behavior was treated. Thus, there were two points of evidence in the multiple baseline across behaviors design that demonstrated experimental control: (a) the point that occurred at the end of baseline and the beginning of treatment for the first behavior and (b) the point that occurred at the end of baseline for the second behavior and the beginning of treatment for that behavior (McReynolds & Kearns, 1983).

Procedures

Prior to training, each child's phonological knowledge was assessed using the procedures of standard generative phonology as described in Dinnsen (1984), Elbert and Gierut (1986), and Kenstowicz and Kisseberth (1979). The analyses were based on data from a 20-min conversational sample and a 306-item analysis probe (adapted from Gierut, 1985). The items were elicited by utilizing a cueing hierarchy that began by requesting spontaneous production of the target item. If needed, additional cues (i.e., sentence completion, delayed imitation, direct imitation) were systematically provided to elicit the form. The analysis probe sampled each English phoneme a minimum of five times in all permissible word positions, included potential minimal or near-minimal pairs and morphophonetic alternations, and included word-initial and word-final consonant clusters. Each child's phonological system was described in terms of phonetic and phonemic inventories, phonological rules, phonotactic constraints, and underlying representations.

Following the description of each child's unique phonological system, a hierarchy of knowledge was constructed that compared the child's system to the target phonological system. From this analysis, it was determined that all subjects exhibited nonambient knowledge, or incorrect underlying representations, of the sounds [s] and [r]. According to the classification system discussed by Dinnsen et al. (1987), Elbert and Gierut (1986), and Gierut et al. (1987), these sounds were characterized by inventory constraints. Hierarchies constructed for each child prior to treatment are presented in Table 3 and discussed in the Results section.

A generalization probe was constructed to measure each subject's baseline and generalization performance on /s/ and /r/ clusters. The probe consisted of 40 items each of /s/ and /r/ word-initial clusters. Included were the five /st/ and five /tr/ training words plus five untrained /st/ and /tr/ word-initial clusters. Five additional /s/ and /r/ clusters of the following were included: /sl/, /sp/, /sk/, /sm/, /sn/, /sw/, /pr/, /dr/, /gr/, /kr/, /θr/, and /fr/. The generalization probe is shown in the Appendix.

The generalization probe was administered on three separate occasions prior to treatment, which constituted the baseline period. After the initiation of training, the probe was administered at the end of every third training session. A delayed imitation elicitation procedure was utilized. For example, "Do you climb a tree or a banana?"

The training items consisted of five initial /st/ words and five initial /tr/ words, as shown in the Appendix. Training continued for each cluster until the child achieved 70% accuracy for the target

Continued

EXCERPT 8.35 *Continued*

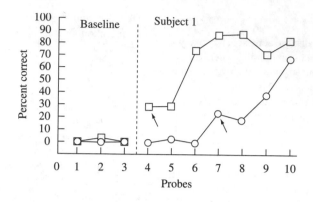

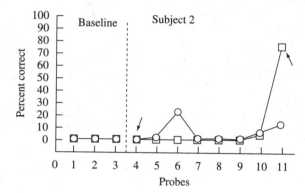

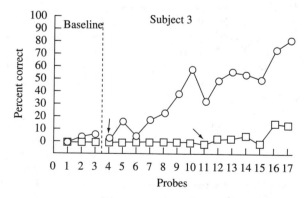

FIGURE 1a **Generalization learning curves for all subjects for target /s/ and /r/ clusters. Squares represent target /s/ clusters and circles represent target /r/ clusters. The arrows indicate initiation of treatment.**

Continued

EXCERPT 8.35 *Continued*

cluster on the generalization probe or until a total of 21 sessions were completed.

Training consisted of three phases. In Phase 1, children imitatively produced the pictorially represented training items following the clinician's model. A continuous reinforcement schedule was utilized. Phase 2 was identical to Phase 1 except the reinforcement schedule was shifted to a variable reinforcement schedule in which approximately every third correct response was reinforced. During Phase 3, the children spontaneously produced the training items when the experimenter presented the

pictures without a verbal model. The variable schedule of reinforcement was continued in this phase. Criterion to move from each phase was 90% accuracy of production across three training sets. A training set consisted of 20 responses, and each training session involved five training sets, or 100 trials.

From "Generalization Patterns Associated with Training Least Phonological Knowledge," by A. L. Williams, 1991, *Journal of Speech and Hearing Research, 34,* pp. 722–733. Copyright 1991 by the American Speech-Language-Hearing Association. Reprinted with permission.

Excerpt 8.36 shows portions of the Method and Results sections of an article by Costello and Hurst that used a time-series design in an experiment with three subjects over a longer period of time. The subject for whom the data are shown participated in twenty-seven sessions over a period of about nine weeks. This particular example illustrates several other points about time-series designs. First, the speaker participated over a longer term for more extended analysis of their behavior. The Experimental Design section explains how the ABABAC time-series design was executed. Second, the design used two reversals of baseline *(A)* and experimental segment *(B),* with several sessions included in each segment. Note the first paragraph of the Experimental Design section where the authors discuss the reasons for using this repeated reversals design. Third, the authors studied the effects of the experimental manipulations on different dependent variables (two stuttering behaviors for Subject 1 and three behaviors each for Subjects 2 and 3). This allowed them to check the effect of manipulations on "target" behavior, as well as generalization to other behaviors. After the second baseline, the manipulation was changed to the nontarget behavior to evaluate the effect on both behaviors.

Figure 1 in Excerpt 8.36 illustrates the data for the first subject. The two dependent variables (stuttering behaviors) are indicated by the two lines with open and filled circles. Note reasonable stability of both behaviors in the first *A* segment, a decrease in both behaviors in the first *B* segment, an increase back toward the first baseline levels in the second *A* segment, and another decrease in both behaviors in the second *B* segment. Both behaviors increased again in the third *A* segment and decreased in the *C* segment, although tremor disfluencies (which became the *non*target behavior in the *C* segment) began to increase again when they were no longer punished. Excerpt 8.36 illustrates the many possibilities for variation with multiple treatments, and multiple dependent variables with time-series designs. One caution that must be entertained in discussing these variations is that multiple-treatment interference is a threat to external validity that can best be dealt with through multiple replications to ferret out individual treatment effects and interactions among treatments.

EXCERPT 8.36

Experimental sessions were approximately 40 minutes in length. Subjects 1 and 3 attended sessions three days per week, while Subject 2 came for sessions four days per week. Subject 1 participated in 27 sessions, Subject 2 in 51, and Subject 3 attended 39 sessions.

Experimental Design

The stuttering behavior of each subject was studied through a within-subject repeated reversals experimental design. For each subject, two or three selected types of stuttering behavior were separately and concurrently measured and one of them was directly manipulated by a punishment procedure. Experimental and baseline/reversal conditions were systematically alternated over several sessions yielding a repeated reversals design, often referred to as an ABAB design (Hersen & Barlow, 1976, p. 185). This design allows repeated observations of the effects of the independent variable on the form of stuttering behavior being manipulated (the target disfluency), as well as on the unmanipulated disfluency types being measured concurrently.

Baseline condition. During baseline (Condition A) the clinician instructed the subject to speak in monologue or to read for the entire 40 minutes. Noncontingent (never following a moment of stuttering) social reinforcers in the form of smiles and nods from the clinician were provided on the average of every 60 seconds while the subject was speaking. Further, the clinician maintained continuous attention to the subject's speaking throughout each session by maintaining eye contact. During the baseline sessions the experimenter differentially counted the frequency of occurrence of each selected stuttering topography. Baseline sessions were continued until stuttering was stable or was not systematically decreasing. Stability was said to have been achieved when the within-session average disfluency rate of each disfluency type showed variation no greater than plus or minus one disfluency per minute in three consecutive sessions. When the baseline data indicated stability, the experimental condition was introduced. All changes in conditions were introduced within sessions.

Experimental condition. As in the baseline sessions, subjects continued speaking in monologue or reading during experimental (Condition B) sessions, and the clinician provided continuous social reinforcement in the form of attention as long as the subject was speaking fluently. However, during experimental sessions every occurrence of the target disfluency was consequated by one of two punishment procedures. In one, referred to as time-out from positive reinforcement (Costello, 1975), each occurrence of the target disfluency was immediately followed by the clinician saying, "Stop," and looking away from the subject for ten seconds. The subject was required to stop speaking immediately. After the time interval had elapsed the clinician looked up, smiled, and said, "Begin." In the other punishment procedure each occurrence of the target disfluency was followed by the immediate presentation of a one-second burst of a 50-dB, 4000-Hz tone through headphones, a procedure similar to that described by Flanagan, Goldiamond, and Azrin (1958).

During the experimental condition the experimenter continued counting the frequency of occurrence of all of the selected stuttering behaviors for each subject. The experimental condition was continued until the data were stable or until the direction and nature of change were clear. At this time Condition A was reintroduced in order to assess whether changes produced by the introduction of the independent variable could be reversed by its withdrawal. Following this the experimental condition was reintroduced in order to demonstrate further the control of the independent variable over the dependent variables by replication of the original effect.

Subsequent manipulations. Following the last reversal session (Condition A) for Subject 1, the target disfluency was changed to the previously nonmanipulated disfluency form. This was continued for three sessions. For Subject 2, during the final experimental condition, all disfluencies regardless of topography became the targets for punishment by time-out. This condition continued until the end of the study.

. . . .

Continued

EXCERPT 8.36   *Continued*

Experimental Findings

The data from each of the three subjects indicate that stuttering behaviors tended to covary directly with one another. When a punishing stimulus was applied to one topography of disfluency, other topographies were seen to decrease in frequency of occurrence, even though they were never directly manipulated.

Subject 1. Figure 1 shows the session-by-session data collected for Subject 1 across all experimental conditions. The speaking modality for this subject was reading and the two topographies of disfluency selected for measurement were: (1) jaw tremors; and (2) unitary repetitions of phonemes, syllables, and monosyllabic words. Jaw tremors were chosen as the

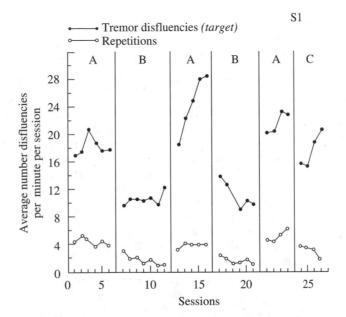

FIGURE 1   **Disfluency data for Subject 1. The ordinate indicates the number of disfluencies per minute averaged across each session; the abscissa represents individual sessions, except where changes in condition occurred. The last data point in each condition is from the same session as the first data point in the subsequent session. Experimental conditions are indicated at the top of the graph and are separated by dark vertical lines. The selected stuttering topographies measured for Subject 1 are defined in the legend at the top of the graph, and the one which served as the target disfluency is also indicated.**

Continued

EXCERPT 8.36   *Continued*

target disfluency for the application of punishment contingencies during experimental conditions.

Condition A (baseline) was conducted for five complete sessions. Jaw tremors averaged 18.20/min while repetitions averaged 4.45/min. After the first ten minutes of Condition A in session 6, Condition B was initiated. A time-out interval of ten seconds was presented contingent upon every instance of tremors. The experimental condition was in effect for seven sessions wherein a decrease in the frequency of occurrence of tremors was noted, as well as a progressive decrease in the frequency of occurrence of untreated repetitions. Condition A was reinstated for five sessions after the first ten minutes of session 12. An immediate increase in the frequency of tremors and of repetitions demonstrated the functionality of the punishing stimulus and the reliability of the direct covariation phenomenon. During session 16 the experimental condition was reinstated for six sessions. Time-out contingencies applied to all tremors once again produced a decrease in the frequency of occurrence of these behaviors and direct covariation of untreated repetitions, thus replicating the effects of the first experimental condition and further verifying the response class relationship between tremor and repetition disfluencies for this subject. During the third session of this condition (session 18), the time-out interval was decreased

from ten to five seconds, with no apparent influence on the data. Reversal Condition A was once again instated during session 21 for four sessions, resulting in an immediate increase in the frequency of occurrence of tremors and repetitions to their original baseline levels. It is unlikely that changes in speaking rate (word output) systematically varying across conditions would have accounted for these ABABA results because speaking rate has been shown to remain independent of disfluency rates in studies using procedures similar to those of this study (e.g., Costello, 1975; Martin, 1968).

In Condition C, introduced during session 24 for four sessions, time-out was no longer presented contingent upon tremors, but rather contingent upon repetitions, heretofore untreated. The frequency of occurrence of repetitions was observed to decrease. A corresponding initial decrease in the rate of now untreated tremors was noted, but this was followed by a gradual increase toward the baseline level. Thus the direct covariation observed to occur reliably across behaviors when tremors were treated was not replicated clearly when the treatment target was changed.

From "An Analysis of the Relationship among Stuttering Behaviors," by J. M. Costello and M. R. Hurst, 1981, *Journal of Speech and Hearing Research, 24,* pp. 247–256. Copyright 1981 by the American Speech-Language-Hearing Association. Reprinted with permission.

Between-Subjects Comparative Design

The basic structure of a descriptive study using a comparative design has already been illustrated in the subject-selection section of this chapter (see Excerpts 8.5 and 8.6). Because of the frequency with which this type of design has been employed, another brief example is appropriate with respect to procedural considerations.

Excerpt 8.37 is from a comparative study that examined the effect of emotional content on verbal pragmatic aspects of discourse production in right-brain-damaged, left-brain-damaged, and normal adults. The research question describes the groups of adults to be studied and the dependent variables to be compared. The Subjects part of the Method section describes the three groups of adults, indicates how they were selected, and displays data regarding relevant subject characteristics in Table 1. Additionally, the brain-damaged adults were screened extensively before being included in the study to ensure that they could adequately participate in the study. The results of the screening tests and group matching procedures (demographic information) are also presented in Table 1. The Procedures section of the Method section details the manner in which discourse was elicited and how emotional content was varied.

EXCERPT 8.37

In this study, we attempted to clarify whether there is a breakdown in the verbal pragmatic aspects of narrative discourse in right-brain-damaged patients and in left-brain-damaged aphasics. Further, we attempted to determine the extent to which emotional versus nonemotional (i.e., visuospatial and procedural) content contributes to pragmatic discourse deficits when they occur.

To characterize the pragmatic rules used to produce discourse, seven verbal pragmatic features were evaluated: topic maintenance, conciseness, specificity, lexical selection, revision strategy, quantity, and relevancy. The pragmatic features used in this analysis have been described by Grice (1975), who proposed that people adapt to certain cooperative principles when they communicate. Accordingly, raters in this analysis evaluated a speaker's adherence to the rules that enable an efficient exchange of information between communication partners. A variation of this pragmatic analysis has been used previously by Prutting and Kirchner (1987) for describing populations with communication disorders.

In the current study, a picture-story task (Bloom et al., 1992) was used to elicit narratives from all subjects in emotional and nonemotional conditions. The nonemotional conditions included a visuospatial one and a procedural/neutral one for baseline comparison.

Method

Subjects

Brain-damaged subjects were 21 right-handed adults, 9 with unilateral right hemisphere pathology (RBDs) and 12 with unilateral left hemisphere pathology (LBDs). Twelve neurologically healthy adults served as normal controls (NCs). All subjects were recruited from hospitals and rehabilitation agencies within the greater New York City area.

In order to be included in the study, patients had to meet the following criteria: (a) unilateral left or right hemisphere damage resulting from a single thrombotic or embolic cerebrovascular accident (CVA) confirmed by CT scan; (b) at least 6 months post CVA onset; (c) righthanded by self-report and confirmed by a score of +80 or higher on the Modified Edinburgh Handedness Inventory (Oldfield, 1971); (d) monolingual English speaker; (e) at least 11 years of education; (f) no history of psychiatric or prior neurological disorder, dementia, or substance abuse; and (g) no uncorrected peripheral visual or auditory impairment. Nominal controls also met the above criteria with the exception of (a) and (b).

The LBDs were referred by speech-language pathologists on the basis that the patients demonstrated a mild to moderate aphasia as measured by standard aphasia batteries (i.e., Goodglass & Kaplan, 1983; Schuell, 1965). Global or severe aphasic patients were not included because subjects needed to produce sufficient discourse for analysis. The RBDs were recruited through medical chart review and were referred through speech-language pathologists. None of the RBDs demonstrated any clinical signs of aphasia or specific deficits on the four subtests of the auditory comprehension section of the Boston Diagnostic Aphasia Examination (Goodglass & Kaplan, 1983).

In order to be included in the study, subjects were tested to ensure that they had adequate cognitive, perceptual, temporal-sequencing, and auditory comprehension abilities. For cognitive screening, subtests of the Wechsler Adult Intelligence Scale-Revised (WAIS-R) (Wechsler, 1981) were selected to tap into the presumably intact functions of the nonlesioned hemisphere—a WAIS-R Verbal subtest for the RBDs and a WAIS-R Performance subtest for the LBDs. The Information subtest was administered to the RBDs, the Block Design was administered to LBDs, and both subtests were administered to the NCs. These two particular subtests were selected because of their high correlation with the overall WAIS-R IQ scores. An age-corrected scaled score of 8 or better on each subtest was required to participate in the study. For visual perceptual

Continued

EXCERPT 8.37   *Continued*

TABLE 1   **Screening, demographic, and lesion site variables for each subject group**

Category	Variable	Measure	RBDs M	RBDs SD	LBDs M	LBDs SD	NCs M	NCs SD
Screening	Intelligence	WAIS-R age-corrected scaled score (≥8)[a]	10.3	1.9	10.3	1.6	11.8	1.4
	Visual perception	BVFDT (≥26)	28.1	2.9	29.5	1.8	29.4	1.8
	Handedness	MEHI (≥80)	97.2	6.7	97.5	4.5	94.6	8.4
	Auditory comprehension	BDAE (≥60 for LBDs, ≥80 for RBDs)	90.2	6.6	79.9	10.8		
Demographic	Gender	males/females	6/3		9/3		8/4	
	Age	years	64.2	7.5	63.3	10.4	62.8	8.0
	Education	years	12.8	1.6	12.8	2.2	13.2	2.0
	Occupation	9-point scale[b]	5.1	1.5	4.7	1.6	5.1	2.2
Lesion site	Frontal	number of subjects	2		3		—	
	Parietal		3		3		—	
	Temporal		1		2		—	
	Parietal/frontal		2		1		—	
	Parietal/temporal		1		3		—	

Note. [a]WAIS-R Information subtest for RBDs, Block Design subtest for LBDs, and Information and Block Design subtests for NCs. [b]Hollingshead Scale (1977), where 1 = unskilled worker, 5 = clerical or sales worker, and 9 = major professional. WAIS-R = Wechsler Adult Intelligence Scale-Revised. BVFDT = Benton Visual Form Discrimination Test. MEHI = Modified Edinburgh Handedness Inventory. BDAE = The mean percentile score for the four subtests from the auditory comprehension section of the Boston Diagnostic Aphasia Examination.

screening, the Visual Form Discrimination Test (Benton, Hamsher, Varney, & Spreen, 1983) was administered. In order to participate, a score of 26 or better (of 32 possible points) was required. Screening data are displayed in Table 1.

A picture sequence task was designed as a screening device to ensure that a subject could adequately process temporal information. The content of the picture sequences was equivalent in length and complexity to the pictures used in the study to elicit discourse. Three sets of three-picture sequences were presented. In order to participate in the study, a subject was required to demonstrate appropriate left-to-right placement of the cards for at least two of the three sets.

Additional language screening was conducted on the LBDs (aphasics) to control for complicating linguistic factors. On the Auditory Comprehension Subtests of the Boston Diagnostic Aphasia Examination (Goodglass & Kaplan, 1983), a mean percentile score of 60 or better was required to be included in the study (see Table 1). To ensure that the LBDs had sufficient quantity of verbal output, the Picture Description Subtest of the Minnesota

Continued

EXCERPT 8.37   *Continued*

Test for the Differential Diagnosis of Aphasia (Schuell, 1965) was administered. A minimum score of 2 ("uses phrases and sentences and names at least 10 objects correctly") was required on this measure.

The three subject groups were matched for gender, age, education, and occupational status (see Table 1). No significant group differences were found when one-way analyses of variance (ANOVAs) or chi square tests were conducted on the four demographic variables. RBDs ($M = 39.2 \pm 31.9$) and LBDs ($M = 44.7 \pm 51.9$) did not differ significantly on months post CVA onset at the time of testing. The number of patients with lesions in a particular site is specified in Table 1. Sites include the frontal lobe, parietal lobe, temporal lobe, parietal and frontal lobes, and parietal and temporal lobes. Site of lesion information was taken directly from the neuroradiological report of the CT scan results in the medical chart of each person. Fisher exact tests revealed that the distributions of patients with and without lesions in each of these sites were not significantly different from each other.

Procedures

Picture story test.   Discourse was elicited in response to three sets of sequential pictures presented with the examiner seated directly across from the subject. Each stimulus set contained three 5×5-inch line drawings mounted horizontally on cardboard (Bloom et al., 1992). The stimulus sets were designed to elicit emotional content (a story about a girl whose dog is hit by a car), visuospatial content (about moving a box by climbing on books piled on a chair), or procedural/neutral content

(about how to fry an egg). Each stimulus set was designed to contain seven predictable content elements. The stimulus sets were piloted on three naive normal subjects to ensure that the seven content elements, and not others, were reliably produced.

To orient the subjects to the storytelling task, the examiner first displayed a practice set of pictures and modeled a narrative (Bloom et al., 1992). Using the procedures described above, the practice stimulus set and modeled narrative were designed to contain approximately equal amounts of emotional, visuospatial, and procedural content elements. After the examiner modeled the sample narrative, subjects were then instructed to tell a story about each of the three stimulus sets. Stimulus set presentation order was randomized within subject and across groups. The development and rationale of the picture story test are further described in Bloom et al. (1992).

The stories were audiotaped and transcribed verbatim for analysis. The audiotapes were reviewed independently by two trained professionals. Percentages of agreement were calculated for each transcript (Sackett, 1978) and revealed a 96.7% mean level of interrater reliability. Written transcripts were used to eliminate the effects of prosody.

From "Suppression and Facilitation of Pragmatic Performance: Effects of Emotional Content on Discourse Following Right and Left Brain Damage," by R. L. Bloom, J. C. Borod, L. K. Obler, and L. J. Gerstman, 1993, *Journal of Speech and Hearing Research, 36,* pp. 1227–1235. Copyright 1993 by the American Speech-Language-Hearing Association. Reprinted with permission.

Developmental Research Designs

The characteristics of developmental research were discussed in Part I. Three basic designs for developmental research were discussed: cross-sectional (between-subjects design), longitudinal (within-subjects design), and semilongitudinal (mixed design). In this section, we will present excerpts from each of these three different types of developmental studies to illustrate the way subjects were selected and procedures were outlined for studying the development of their behavior. Note that two of the studies are concerned with the development of young children and one of them concerns the geriatric population. As mentioned earlier, these are the two age ranges of greatest concern in developmental research because the greatest maturation occurs in the younger and older years.

Excerpt 8.38 is taken from a developmental study of voice onset time in a normal-aged population. As stated in the purpose shown in the excerpt, the authors wished to extend the developmental model of speech timing to older subjects. The study was cross-sectional, in that it used a between-subjects design to compare the behavior of a group of 25- to 39-year-old adults, a group of 65- to 74-year-old adults, and a group of adults over 75. In other words, three *different* groups of subjects representing three different levels of maturation were compared with each other to examine developmental trends. The excerpted material shows a brief statement of the specific purpose of the study followed by a portion of the Method section that describes the three groups of subjects who were compared in this cross-sectional developmental study. Note the selection criteria that were used to ensure that adults were selected who were normal with respect to various health measures and the use of a physician to examine the older subjects. The subjects' ages are shown in the excerpted table (along with their gender and vital-capacity data). Inspection of the table shows that the groups represent three well-separated age groups with no overlapping among the ages of the three groups and that males and females are equally represented in all three groups.

EXCERPT 8.38

The purpose of this descriptive study, therefore, was to obtain measures of VOT and vowel duration in healthy older subjects as a necessary first step in the extension of a developmental model of speech timing control to the later years. Results relating to voice onset time are reported in this paper.

Method

Subjects

Three groups of 10 subjects were used. The control group, Group 1, was composed of subjects between 25 and 39 years of age. Groups 2 and 3 subjects were 65–74 years and over 75, respectively. Subject characteristics are summarized in Table 1.

All subjects were living independently, were considered to be embedded in the social structure of the community, were free of any chronic or debilitating disease, had measured vital capacities within the normal range, and presented negative histories for hearing problems, cardiovascular, respiratory, neurological and laryngeal disorders. All were native speakers of English and had been raised in homes in which only English had been spoken. Within 15 days of testing, each of the Groups 2 and 3 subjects was seen by a physician who was aware of the subject criteria of the study and who certified that the heart and lungs were normal on auscultation and percussion, that blood pressure was within normal limits, and that there was no apparent neuropathology.

Continued

EXCERPT 8.38 *Continued*

TABLE 1 Characteristics of the 30 subjects

Subjects by Group	Age	Sex	Vital Capacity (liters)
Group 1			
Age 25–40			
1-1	39	M	4.5
1-2	38	F	3.1
1-3	29	F	2.8
1-4	38	F	2.9
1-5	30	M	4.7
1-6	32	F	3.1
1-7	28	M	6.4
1-8	30	F	2.5
1-9	30	M	4.6
1-10	36	M	4.4
Mean age	33		
Group 2			
Age 65–74			
2-1	71	M	3.0
2-2	71	M	2.8
2-3	73	M	3.3
2-4	66	F	2.0
2-5	66	M	4.4
2-6	69	F	1.9
2-7	69	F	1.8
2-8	66	F	3.0
2-9	67	F	2.2
2-10	68	M	3.7
Mean age	68.6		
Group 3			
Age 75 and over			
3-1	88	M	1.9
3-2	77	M	3.1
3-3	75	F	2.1
3-4	77	F	2.3
3-5	81	F	2.0
3-6	76	F	2.5
3-7	91	M	1.9
3-8	87	F	1.9
3-9	79	M	3.2
3-10	82	M	1.8
Mean age	81.3		

From "Voice Onset Time in a Normal-Aged Population," by P. M. Sweeting and R. J. Baken, 1982, *Journal of Speech and Hearing Research, 25,* pp. 129–134. Copyright 1982 by the American Speech-Language-Hearing Association. Reprinted with permission.

Portions of a longitudinal developmental study are shown in Excerpt 8.39. This study examined the concept of agent in the emerging language of three children as they developed from about age eleven months to age two years. The first part of the excerpt shows the research questions posed. This is followed by a description of the three subjects who were studied and the method of observing them. Note that the children were observed ten times over a twelve-month period of development. The observation sessions and the children's ages at each session are detailed in Table 2 shown in Excerpt 8.39. Whereas the cross-sectional study shown in Excerpt 8.39 used a between-subjects design, this longitudinal study used a within-subjects design to observe the children repeatedly over the developmental span and to watch their behavior change directly. Note that a larger number of subjects was employed in the cross-sectional study ($N = 30$) and a smaller number of subjects was used in the longitudinal study ($N = 3$), as is usually the case.

EXCERPT 8.39

The research that follows examines the emergence of the cognitive concept of agent as hypothesized in Table 1. This was done by observing those overt, nonverbal behaviors (i.e., gestures) assumed to be indicative of the cognitive notion of agent, and subsequently describing the evolution of these behaviors over time in three children. Specifically the following questions were addressed: What gestural behavioral sequences indicate the child's nonverbal concept of agent? To what extent does actual development of the cognitive notion of agent match the hypothesized 5-level developmental sequence proposed in Table 1?

Method

To discover behavioral changes which emerge over the course of a child's early development, a descriptive, longitudinal study was conducted. The methodology used a modification of the traditional observation approach (Bloom, 1970, 1973; Bloom, Lightbown, & Hood, 1975; Bowerman, 1973; Brown, 1973; Carter, 1974; Greenfield & Smith, 1976). Rather than using only diary-like observations of free unstructured sessions in which no specific activities are scheduled for administration and observation, this study included several activities having a high probability of eliciting the behaviors hypothesized in Table 1, depending on the child's current concept of agent (Edwards, 1974; Ingram, 1971; Lock, 1976; Piaget, 1952, 1954; Snyder, 1975; Sugarman, 1973).

Subjects

The three subjects were selected on the basis of a normal prenatal and perinatal history, meeting developmental milestones as determined by the *Bayley Scales of Infant Development* (Bayley, 1969) and the Uzgiris and Hunt scales (Uzgiris & Hunt 1975), and by a normal medical history. At the beginning of the study, all three children were 11 months old, and according to the author's interpretation of the Uzgiris and Hunt scales their performance was most characteristic of Piaget's sensorimotor Stage IV (see Appendix A). The subjects, two boys and one girl, were from upper-middle-class families; the mothers of all three children either worked or attended school, resulting in the children spending at least part of the day with babysitters. One boy had an older sibling, whereas the other two subjects had none. At the beginning of the study, all three subjects were producing prelinguistic vocalizations (i.e., consonant-vowel combinations, fussing, whining); according to the parents, none of the children had used any consistent phonetic forms to label people, objects, events, or activities. All three children were using crawling as their predominant means of locomotion during the first observation session, and walking during the second.

Procedures

The children were videotaped in their respective homes 10 times over 12 months at approximately

Continued

EXCERPT 8.39   *Continued*

1-month intervals; each session lasted 1 hour. Table 2 indicates the age of the children at each videotaping session. The observations for two children extended from the prelinguistic vocalization period (11 months) to their beginning use of 2-word utterances, particularly agent + action, agent + object, action + object constructions. The observations for one of the children extended from his use of vocalization (11 months) to his use of successive single-word utterances. During each session the mother-child pair and the investigator were present.

The children were observed during each hour-long videotaping session under two conditions: a free-play situation and an elicitation situation. The tasks in the elicitation situation were designed to supplement the data obtained in the free-play situation by providing specific opportunities for agentive

behaviors to occur. They are described in detail in Appendix B. The basic structure of these agentive elicitation tasks remained the same over the 12-month period whereas specific objects within a task frequently changed from session to session. This provided some degree of structure and continuity across taping sessions and across subjects; it also allowed for more reliable observations of changes in agentive behavior (Greenfield & Smith, 1976; Schlesinger, 1974). During each session a minimum of 10 agentive elicitation tasks were presented—2 tasks for each of the 5 levels of behavior described below. These agentive elicitation tasks were interspersed throughout the free-play session. This format allowed for both freeplay by the children, as well as their elicited responses to particular tasks.

TABLE 2   Videotaped sessions per child; given are typical age (months) versus actual age (months:days)

Session	Typical Age	Actual Age		
		Denise	Michael	Christopher
1	11	10:24	10:23	11:6
2	12	11:26	11:23	11:30
3	13	12:29	12:28	13:3
4	14	13:28	13:27	14:1
5	15	14:24	14:22	15:12
6	16	15:30	15:28	16:11
7	17	17:10	16:24	17:20
8	18	18:22	17:27	18:20
9	20	20:16	19:17	20:8
10	22	22:4	22:1	22:20

The final example of a developmental study (Excerpt 8.40) is taken from a study by Wilder and Baken of respiratory patterns in infants and illustrates the use of a semilongitudinal design. The first paragraph of the excerpt provides a description of the ten subjects and serves to emphasize the point that the infants were developmentally normal and had normal hearing sensitivity. The second paragraph and Figure A in Excerpt 8.40 capture the essence of the semilongitudinal design. For instance, the measurement of Subject 1 began at two days of age and continued at various intervals until the child was about eighty days old. Subject 9, on the other hand, entered the study at 161 days of age and measurements ended when the child was 255 days old. Each subject was followed for about the same length of time (the longitudinal, within-subjects aspect), but subjects had different ages at the time of participation in the study (the cross-sectional, between-subjects aspect). Thus, the semilongitudinal design is a compromise between the cross-sectional and longitudinal designs that incorporates aspects of each one. Note, for example, that the number of subjects studied is neither as high as the cross-sectional example in Excerpt 8.38 nor as low as the longitudinal example shown in Excerpt 8.39. The semilongitudinal design tries to maximize the advantages of both the cross-sectional design and the longitudinal design while minimizing their disadvantages.

EXCERPT 8.40   Method: Subjects

The population for this study was composed of 4 male and 6 female infants who presented unremarkable pre-, peri-, and postnatal histories, and who had 5-minute Apgar scores of 8 or higher. Each child's development was monitored during the course of the study using selected items from Gesell's developmental scales (Gesell & Amatruda, 1947); the gross motor maturation of all subjects remained within normal limits. Hearing acuity was not formally assessed, but all infants responded appropriately to auditory stimuli.

The study used a semilongitudinal approach. The age of subjects at the time of entry into the pop-

ulation ranged from 2 to 161 days; each infant was observed over a period of approximately four months at intervals averaging 28 days. From the 62 individual observation sessions a statistical consultant selected four consecutive observations of each of the ten infants, providing a statistically useful sample of respiratory behavior over the age range in question (2–255 days). For data analysis these observations were grouped into eight 32-day age intervals, roughly representing age in months. Observation of each of the infants used in the analysis of data are summarized in Figure A.

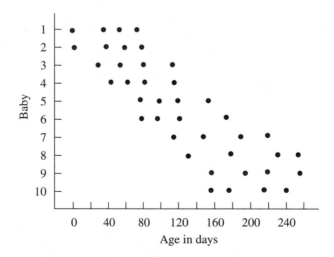

**FIGURE A   Distribution of the forty sample
observations among the study population**

From "Respiratory Patterns in Infant Cry," by C. N. Wilder and R. J. Baken, Winter 1974–75, *Human* *Communication,* No. 3, pp. 18–34. Reprinted with permission of the authors.

Correlational Research

Correlational research plays an important role in communicative disorders. Correlational studies are found in research on test reliability and validity, in factor analyses of large groups of variables, in studies aimed at predicting behavior from knowledge of certain variables, and in studies of the interrelations of many clinical variables. There is a broad spectrum of correlational research to be found in the field and no single example can typify correlational research. Nevertheless, a specific example would be helpful to illustrate briefly the manner in which a researcher might go about assembling important variables for correlational analysis.

Excerpt 8.41 is taken from a study of the relationship between speech and language impairments and reading disabilities. The basic goal of the research was to determine whether there was a relationship between specific language and articulation impairments and reading disabilities as assessed by word-identification and word-attack skills tests. The Subjects section of the Method section describes the subjects and their performance on several tests of speech and language (Table 1). The Reading Achievement section describes the reading skills tests that were used. Minimization of threats to internal and external validity is difficult in such a correlational study because the researcher does not have the ability to manipulate the independent (predictor) variables. That is to say, these predictor variables are attribute variables, the values of which depend on subject selection and careful measurement procedures. The author has described the subject selection and measurements carefully and the use of standardized tests helps reduce internal validity threats in the measurements of the predictor variables.

EXCERPT 8.41

Method

Subjects

Fifty-six children with speech-language impairments (S-LI) and 30 children with normal speech-language abilities participated in this investigation. In the S-LI group, there were 40 males and 16 females. At the beginning of the study, subjects in the S-LI group were in kindergarten and were an average age of 6 years, 2 months old. Each of the subjects in this group had been referred for a speech-language evaluation in one of two Midwest public school districts. In addition to the evaluation the children in this group received in the schools, a battery of standardized speech-language tests was administered for this investigation. This battery included three measures of receptive language abilities: Peabody Picture Vocabulary Test–Revised (Dunn & Dunn, 1981), Token Test for Children (DiSimoni, 1978), Grammatical Understanding subtest of the Test of Language Development-2 (Newcomer & Hammill, 1988), and three measures of expressive language abilities: Expressive One-Word Picture Vocabulary Test (Gardner, 1979), Structured Photographic Expressive Language Test-II (Werner & Kresheck, 1983), combined performance on the Sentence Imitation and Grammatical Closure subtests of the Test of Language Development-2, and a measure of articulation: Goldman-Fristoe Test of Articulation (Goldman & Fristoe, 1986). In addition, the Block Design and Picture Completion subtests of the Wechsler

Continued

EXCERPT 8.41   *Continued*

Preschool and Primary Scale of Intelligence (Wechsler, 1967) were administered.[1]

Children in the S-LI group had a variety of speech and language difficulties. The standardized test battery indicated that the majority of the subjects ($n = 41$) demonstrated a language impairment. A language impairment was operationally defined as performance of at least one *SD* below the mean on at least two of three receptive language measures and/or two of three expressive language measures. Nineteen subjects displayed impairments on both receptive and expressive language tests, 12 subjects showed language difficulties primarily on receptive measures, and 10 subjects displayed impairments primarily on expressive language tests. In some analyses for the present study, the above children with language impairments are referred to as the LI subgroup. The remaining 15 subjects in the S-LI group did not meet the criteria for a language impairment but demonstrated articulation problems and/or were enrolled in articulation therapy during the kindergarten school year (referred to as the AI subgroup). Twelve of these subjects performed below average on the Goldman-Fristoe Test of Articulation (mean percentile = 16.9 %, range < 1–33%). The other three subjects had been enrolled in articulation therapy throughout the kindergarten year and had resolved their articulation difficulties by the time of our assessment. Nevertheless, enrollment in articulation therapy was considered sufficient criterion for inclusion in this investigation. Some of the subjects in the Ll subgroup (37%) also had articulation impairments.

[1]For children older than 6-½ years, the Block Design and Picture Completion subtests from the Wechsler Intelligence Scale for Children–Revised (Wechsler, 1974) were administered. Testing was limited to the Block Design and Picture Completion subtests because of the time constraints and testing concerns imposed by the school systems. Previous researchers have also relied on the use of these subtests as a measure of nonverbal abilities (Bishop & Adams, 1990).

However, these subjects were included with the other subjects demonstrating language impairments (i.e., LI subgroup) when examining differences between subgroups. All subjects in the S-LI group demonstrated nonverbal abilities within the normal range. School records also indicated that children in this group had hearing and corrected vision within normal limits and no history of emotional disorders.

Thirty children without a history of speech-language impairments or a referral for such impairments also participated in this study. These children served as a comparison group to evaluate the performance of the S-LI group on measures of reading achievement. The normally developing subjects were enrolled in the same classrooms or schools as subjects in the S-LI group and were approximately the same age (6 years, 1 month at the beginning of the study). There were 18 males and 12 females in this group. Each of these children performed within normal limits on the battery of speech-language tests and measures of nonverbal ability.

The means and standard deviations for the normal and S-LI groups on the speech-language and nonverbal tests are presented in Table 1. Also shown in Table 1 are the means and standard deviations for the LI and AI subgroups within the S-LI group.

Reading achievement. Reading achievement was assessed in the first and second grades. The Word Identification (Word Id) and Word Attack subtests from the Woodcock Reading Mastery Tests—Revised (Woodcock, 1987) were administered to subjects in the spring of first and second grade. These subtests required subjects to read a list of words or pseudo-words presented in isolation, and as such, served as measures of written word recognition. In second grade, subjects were also given the Gray Oral Reading Test–Revised (GORT-R) (Wiederholt & Bryant, 1986). In addition to an oral reading quotient, this test provided a measure of speed and accuracy of word recognition in context and a measure of reading comprehension. The GORT-R was not administered in the first grade because the majority of the subjects with S-LI had limited reading abilities at that time.

Continued

EXCERPT 8.41   *Continued*

TABLE 1   **Mean standard scores (and standard deviations) on standardized tests in kindergarten for the normal and speech-language impaired (S-LI) groups and the language-impaired (LI) and articulation-impaired (AI) subgroups within the S-LI group**

	Normal $N = 30$	S-LI $N = 56$	LI $n = 41$	AI $n = 15$
PPVT	108.3	90.8	85.0	106.9
	(7.5)	(14.6)	(10.8)	(11.2)
Token	499.0	494.0	493.3	498.7
	(3.8)	(4.0)	(2.8)	(2.9)
TOLD-2	104.3	87.5	81.7	103.1
	(10.9)	(14.2)	(10.5)	(10.9)
EOWPVT	113.4	97.7	92.3	112.7
	(11.50)	(13.8)	(9.0)	(13.9)
SPELT-II	108.5	84.9	78.2	103.1
	(13.1)	(17.8)	(11.7)	(19.4)
Picture completion	12.9	11.5	10.8	13.3
	(1.8)	(2.4)	(2.2)	(2.2)
Block design	12.4	10.2	9.4	12.3
	(1.6)	(2.4)	(2.0)	(2.3)

Note. PPVT = Peabody Picture Vocabulary Test-Revised; Token = Token Test for Children; TOLD-2 = Test of Language Development-2, Syntax Quotient; EOWPVT = Expressive One-Word Picture Vocabulary Test; SPELT-II = Structured Photographic Expressive Language Test-II.

All subjects in the S-LI and normal groups completed the reading tests during first grade. Six subjects in the S-LI group and 1 subject in the normal group moved away and were unavailable for testing in the second grade. In addition, some of the subjects with S-LI repeated their kindergarten year ($n = 5$), whereas others were placed in developmental first grade classes prior to going to first grade ($n = 18$). Developmental first (D-1) classes have been instituted in some school districts to allow young or slowly developing children (often vaguely defined) an extra year of maturation before beginning first grade and formal reading instruction. Children in D-1 programs in our school districts repeated kindergarten classes during half of the school day and received primarily the nonacademic curriculum (e.g.,

art, music) of first grade during the other half of the day. In the case of the subjects repeating kindergarten or placed in D-1 classes, standardized speech-language tests and measures of phonological awareness and rapid naming were administered during the second year of kindergarten (or D-1 classes). The results of this testing served as these subjects' kindergarten data and were subsequently used for data analysis.

From "The Relationship between Speech-Language Impairments and Reading Disabilities," by W. H. Catts, 1993, *Journal of Speech and Hearing Research, 36,* pp. 948–958. Copyright 1993 by the American Speech-Language-Hearing Association. Reprinted with permission.

Another example of a correlational study can be seen in Excerpt 8.19, which was presented earlier in this chapter as an example of the selection of appropriate measures. As the text in Excerpt 8.19 indicates, the study attempted to correlate certain pretreatment variables with the outcome of stuttering treatment. Pretreatment variables were used as predictors of the relative degree of success in stuttering treatment. The correlational research in Excerpt 8.19 was aimed at verifying the prognostic value of different measures of stuttering severity, personality, and attitude by examining their correlations with, and their ability to predict, success in stuttering treatment.

Retrospective Research

In Part I, we cited some of the problems associated with retrospective research studies. Excerpt 8.42 presents two selections from the Method section of a study by Carhart and Porter on the relationship between pure-tone and spondee thresholds for subjects with various audiometric configurations. The first paragraph is important because it details subject-selection criteria that are significant for both internal and external validity. Note, for example, that satisfactory reliability during testing was one important criterion, that very young and very old patients were eliminated (probably because of the difficulty they present in testing), and that normal hearing persons were excluded. The sample ultimately chosen was large and included subjects with a variety of audiometric configurations (described in other parts of the Method section) that were probably reasonably representative of hearing-impaired patients seen in many audiology clinics.

The second paragraph is even more important because it directly addresses the main problem in retrospective research, namely, under what conditions were the data collected. In this brief paragraph, Carhart and Porter indicate the following steps that were taken to overcome the problems associated with retrospective research: (1) that the data were collected in sound-treated test environments, (2) that testing was performed by trained and qualified clinicians, (3) that calibration was checked frequently, (4) that the Carhart-Jerger technique was used to measure pure-tone thresholds and that a 2-dB bracketing method was used for all speech threshold measurements, (5) that tape-recorded spondee words were employed and that the speaker was Tillman, and (6) that the calibration values conformed or were made to conform to current reference standards. Only the authors' assurance that all of the data were collected under the conditions as described makes it possible for the critical reader to give any weight to the subsequent Results section. The evaluator of retrospective research, whether it be comparative or correlational, must be painstaking, indeed, when reading the Method section for such research may stand or fall on this section alone.

EXCERPT 8.42   Procedure

We explored the relationship between audiometric contour and threshold for spondees by performing a retrospective statistical analysis of records obtained in the Northwestern University Hearing Clinics between January 1966 and September 1968. Patients seen in these clinics were judged suitable

Continued

EXCERPT 8.42   Procedure   *Continued*

for inclusion in the study provided they (1) were between 10 and 80 years old, inclusive; (2) had exhibited satisfactory reliability during both pure-tone and speech testing; (3) did not have two or more thresholds better than 10 dB ISO 1964 in either ear; (4) had recordable thresholds from 250 through 4000 Hz for the better ear; and (5) yielded a measurable threshold when tested with spondees. Two thousand one hundred thirty-five cases satisfied these criteria. Every seventh record was then removed so as to yield an audiometrically heterogeneous pool for purposes of comparison with earlier studies. The audiograms for the better ears of the remaining 1823 persons were classified as to pattern into six groups.

· · · · · · · · · · · ·

Before considering the findings that emerged, a word must be said about the conditions in which the data under consideration had previously been gathered. All tests were administered in adequately sound-proofed booths. Testers were either full-time audiological clinicians or well-trained student clinicians working under the immediate supervision of full-time clinicians. All audiometers were monitored frequently with Bruel and Kjaer equipment to assure proper calibration. Pure-tone thresholds were obtained by the Hughson-Westlake method (Carhart & Jerger, 1959) with audiometers adjusted to the ISO 1964 standard. Speech thresholds were obtained by a bracketing method employing 2-dB steps. Test materials were spondee words spoken by Tillman and recorded on magnetic tape. The O-dB hearing level was set at 22 dB SPL as determined by a 1000-Hz calibration tone recorded to equal the frequent peaks for spondees as viewed with a VU meter. This setting conformed to the ASA 1953 standard for speech audiometers. However, for purposes of this paper, all spondee thresholds are reported re a reference level of 20 dB SPL because this value is specified for the TDH-39 earphone in the new ANSI standard for audiometers (1969). This change was made to bring the regression equations emerging from this study into conformity with current reference levels.

From "Audiometric Configuration and Prediction of Threshold for Spondees," by R. Carhart, and L. S. Porter, 1971, *Journal of Speech and Hearing Research, 14,* pp. 486–495. Copyright 1971 by the American Speech-Language-Hearing Association. Reprinted with permission.

Survey Research

We come next to the evaluation of survey research. Although there is an extensive body of literature on survey research methodology, questionnaire development, interview techniques, and the like (e.g., see Babbie, 1973; Davis, 1971; and Slonim, 1960), such research does not appear with much frequency in the literature. Thus, we will focus here on only a few selected issues that need to be identified by the critical evaluator of survey research and hope that the interested reader who wishes to delve more deeply into the area will consult the sources noted above.

The choice of a survey research design should be consistent with, and appropriate to, the purpose of the study. The first question the critical reader must raise, then, is whether the research reported was best conducted by means of a survey design or whether there were alternate, and perhaps better, research designs that could have been used to answer the research questions. Assuming that the survey design was appropriate, the next question deals with the adequacy of the sample surveyed. As we pointed out in Part I, it is difficult, if not impossible, to survey the entire population of interest (e.g., all speech pathologists in the United States, all speech and hearing facilities in the country). As a result, survey researchers often draw a sample of subjects that presumably is representative of the total population. On the surface, this may appear to be a relatively simple task; in reality, the task can be quite complex. Fortunately, there are a variety of sampling techniques that can be employed. These include random sampling, stratified sampling, cluster sampling, systematic sampling, and the like. We cannot address here the technical aspects of sampling or the advantages and disadvantages of various sampling techniques. Suffice it to say that the critical reader must address the issue of the adequacy of the sample used in survey research. It may not be readily apparent but the sampling issue in survey research is analogous to the differential-selection-of-subjects threat to internal validity, as well as the subject-selection threat to external validity.

The mortality threat to internal validity is a common problem in survey research. Mortality in this context is represented by the number of people surveyed who failed to respond to the survey instrument. Babbie (1973) points out that a response rate of at least 50 percent can be considered adequate for analysis and reporting purposes, that a response rate of 60 percent is good, and that a response of 70 percent or greater is very good. If the nonresponse rate is high, the researcher may have a biased sample, a sample that may not be representative of the population of interest, and a sample of responders who are quite different, on important dimensions, from individuals who failed to respond. It is for these reasons that survey researchers spend considerable time, effort, and money on attempts to enlist the cooperation of individuals who failed to respond to the initial request to participate in the survey. The careful reader of survey research must identify the mortality rate and determine whether the number of nonresponders poses a threat to both internal and external validity.

The instrumentation threat to internal validity is directly related to the adequacy of the survey instrument, be it a questionnaire or an interview. Good questionnaire development is a difficult and complex task, one not readily undertaken by the novice. Are the questions clear and unambiguous? Do the questions address the issues under study? Are the questions objective and nonthreatening? Do the questions lead to nonbiased responses? In an attempt to ensure the adequacy of a questionnaire, researchers often pretest the instrument. That is, a small sample of representative individuals is given a trial questionnaire for their reactions, their suggestions, and their comments. The pretest is an extremely important part of questionnaire development and the critical reader should be alert to the researcher's reference to the use of a pretest. It should be noted that the questionnaire itself is usually not available for the reader's inspection but should be made available to an interested reader if requested from the researcher. In longer articles or in books reporting the results of survey research, the questionnaire is usually included for the reader's inspection. Remember, a questionnaire survey is only as good as the questions asked.

The survey research interview has several advantages over the questionnaire format. Interviewing permits probing to obtain more or different data, allows for greater depth, and enables the interviewer to assess rapport and communication between interviewer and respondent and to determine whether these factors are affecting the data-collection process. On the other hand, interviews are costly and time-consuming, the interviewer needs to be trained, and the interaction between interviewer and respondent can have a strong influence on the data collected. In this context, of course, the interviewer and the interview format (e.g., structured vs. unstructured interviews) can pose an instrumentation threat to internal validity.

Excerpt 8.43 is from an article that reports Part I of a two-part survey of characteristics of hearing-impaired children in the public schools. The excerpt includes a two-paragraph introduction that explains the rationale for the survey and the specific purpose of Part I. The Method section outlines the areas covered in the survey questionnaire and how it was administered with the school audiologists. In addition, the Method section includes a description of the classification of the schoolchildren and how the random sampling was conducted within each classification. Also described is a procedure for follow-up on missing information and a statement regarding final missing data and the expected margin of error for all values reported for the random sample.

The random sampling within each classification is a procedure that ensures good external validity: consumers can be confident of generalizations made to subjects of the same kind in similar settings because of the random sampling within each classification that took place. Generalization to other kinds of settings or subjects, of course, would require replications. But the stratified random sampling used in this study is a strong procedure for improving external validity.

Also note that the entire questionnaire is available on request from one of the authors. This would enable interested consumers to review the questions and evaluate the instrument directly. The classification of subjects is quite detailed as indicated in the Method section and in the appendix. Internal validity is improved by using the strict criteria for defining subject groups and the subjects to whom generalization is appropriate is well specified. Note, too, the attempt to preserve the anonymity of the children, yet ensure the ability to follow up on missing data. In summary, this survey has included a number of steps to bolster both internal and external validity, yet deal with the practical realities of surveying thirteen Area Education Agencies spread over an entire state.

EXCERPT 8.43

Attempts by state and local educational agencies to implement Public Law 94–142 have highlighted the paucity of information on which educational programming is based for certain groups of handicapped children. Of particular concern at present are unserved and underserved populations, including children with hearing impairment. Although the educational and demographic characteristics of severely-to-profoundly hearing-impaired children are well-documented (Gentile, 1972; Balow & Brill, 1975; Moores, 1970; Trybus & Karchmer, 1977), less severely hearing-impaired children have not been studied systematically. Ross (1977) estimates that there are at least 20 times as many moderately hearing-impaired children as severely-to-profoundly hearing-impaired and that they can be found in every school building in the country. Many of them are unidentified or misdiagnosed (Ross, 1977), others are identified but do not have access to special support services (Davis, 1977), while others receive extensive educational support (Peterson, 1972). Unfortunately, little is known about the status and needs of moderately hearing-impaired children in general or the relations among important factors such as degree of hearing loss, hearing-aid use, classroom placement, and, in particular, psychoeducational status. The few studies in existence reporting educational achievement data on small numbers of moderately hearing-impaired children indicate that they are underachievers, delayed in academic skills, and in jeopardy regarding social relationships (Kodman, 1963; Quigley & Thomure, 1968; Davis,

Continued

EXCERPT 8.43   *Continued*

1974; Peterson, 1972). Although these studies provide helpful information, they are not designed to answer specific questions about the prevalence of patterns of hearing loss among school children, their use of amplification, educational placement, and special support services, or their psychoeducational status and needs. Without these types of demographic and educational data, it is unlikely that adequate educational programming will be developed and implemented for this population.

This study was designed to collect both demographic and psychoeducational data for a large number of randomly sampled hearing-impaired children enrolled in the public schools of Iowa. Only demographic data will be reported here. Psychoeducational data will be reviewed in a subsequent paper. The state's plan for providing services to hearing-impaired children has resulted in an unusually comprehensive identification and follow-up program, involving employment of about 70 audiologists, 500 speech-language pathologists, and 100 teachers of the hearing-impaired. The availability of so many special personnel makes it likely that moderately hearing-impaired children will be identified and evaluated, resulting in a pool of available data for a large number of children.

Method

A survey questionnaire was developed[1] that included inquiries about age, sex, onset of hearing loss, hearing status, educational placement and services, use and monitoring of amplification, and language and academic achievement. School audiologists were paid an hourly wage to perform the sampling and complete the questionnaires. All but two of the state's 15 Area Education Agencies (AEAs) participated in the study. The AEAs are multicounty agencies in Iowa charged with providing special support services to handicapped children within their geographic boundaries.

---

[1]The survey questionnaire is available on request from Julia M. Davis, Department of Speech Pathology and Audiology, University of Iowa, Iowa City, Iowa 52242.

A total of 1250 hearing-impaired children were included in the sample. On the basis of their most recent audiograms, the children were stratified into three main groups:

Group A consisted of those children with a bilateral or unilateral conductive hearing loss as defined by the existence of normal hearing by bone conduction and air-bone gaps greater than 10 dB. After the sampling was completed, children in group A were assigned to three subgroups based on degree of hearing loss, as shown in the Appendix.

Group B_1 consisted of those children with a bilateral or unilateral high frequency hearing loss. For sampling purposes, children were required to have air and bone conduction thresholds greater than 25 dB HL (ANSI, 1969) at frequencies only of 4,000 and/or 6,000 Hz and above.

Group C consisted of children with sensorineural or mixed hearing loss at more than one of the standard audiometric test frequencies, and not included in groups A or B_1. Within group C, children were assigned to six subgroups on the basis of the degree and configuration of their hearing losses, as shown in the Appendix.

In addition to the above predetermined major groupings (A, B_1, and C) and post-hoc subgroups (A_1, A_2, A_3, C_1, C_2, C_3, C_4, and C_5) three post-hoc classifications were made to allow for a more detailed analysis of high frequency hearing. As described in the Appendix, subgroups B_2, B_3, and B_4 represent high-frequency hearing loss with decreasing cutoff frequencies. When these three groups are viewed with the major group B_1, the result is a continuum of high-frequency hearing loss. That is, group B_1–B_4 represent a reduction in hearing sensitivity at increasingly lower frequencies. The three major groups, A, B_1, and C, are mutually exclusive. In addition, all of the A and C subgroups are derived solely from the A and C groups, respectively. In contrast, the B_2, B_3, and B_4 subgroups are derived from the major group C.

Each of the main groups in each AEA was randomly sampled; groups A and B_1 were sampled at a 5% rate and group C was sampled at a rate of 20%. Different sampling rates were employed to insure

Continued

EXCERPT 8.43   *Continued*

approximately equal numbers of children in each of the main groups. The AEA audiologists were provided with randomly generated numbers (between 1 and 20 for groups A and B₁ and between 1 and 5 for group C) for entry into their lists of children who exhibited hearing loss.

A questionnaire was then completed on each of the children sampled. The survey information was obtained from all available records on the children. Answers to all questions were not available for all children, however. Each child was coded with a 12 digit alphanumeric code that only the AEA employees could decipher. This code was used by the authors to request further clarification on individual children and yet preserve anonymity. The most recent copy of each child's audiometric evaluation

was included with each questionnaire. Questionnaire information was coded for computer analysis.

It was not unusual for data to be missing from a particular child's files, resulting in a variable n for many questions. Computation of an error prediction for a random sample indicated, however, that all demographic data are accurate to within ±6% for the total groups A, B₁, and C.

Case Study Research

Our last evaluation example concerns case study research, a type of descriptive research that is frequently found in the communicative disorders research literature. As we have pointed out earlier, case study research has both advantages and disadvantages. Case studies lay the groundwork for future research that will use larger groups of subjects by identifying variables that can or should be experimentally manipulated and by generating hypotheses that need to be tested. A case study obviously allows for intensive exploration of the phenomenon of interest and may shed light on rare phenomena or raise questions about the adequacy of well-established theoretical formulations (Hersen and Barlow, 1976). On the other hand, without replication, case studies may have limited generalizability. Also, case studies are especially vulnerable to subjective biases. A case may be studied because it fits the researcher's preconceptions or because it is especially dramatic. Whatever the advantages and disadvantages of case study research, the task that remains is to identify the evaluative criteria that can be used by the consumer of this research. It should be noted that case study research is the only descriptive design that is not altogether amenable to an analysis that incorporates the Campbell and Stanley evaluation framework, a framework we have employed throughout. In actuality, the factors that threaten internal validity in experimental research and in other descriptive research may be the factors that are the substance of the case study approach. As one example, history may be a contaminating influence in a variety of research designs. In case study research, a "history" event may provide considerable insight about the phenomenon under study. For instance, one of the child's parents separates from the household, producing a marked decrease (or increase) in the behavior being observed. Maturational influences, another contaminating variable, may, in fact, be the primary variable under investigation in case study research. Bias introduced by subject selection is inherent in case study research because subjects are selected for their uniqueness.

The evaluation of case study research revolves around the following considerations: (1) Is the approach appropriate to the purpose of the study? (2) Have methods been used to control for experimenter bias (videotaping the subject and allowing other clinicians or researchers to evaluate the behavior observed)? (3) Have careful measurements been made of the behavior or phenomenon under study? (4) Is sufficient detail provided about the procedures so that the procedures can be replicated by other interested parties? (5) Does the research lead to hypotheses that can be tested experimentally or to research questions that can be explored with other research designs? (6) Are the conclusions drawn by the researcher couched in appropriately cautious and conservative terms? and (7) Does, in fact, the case study reported contribute to our understanding of behavior, even if that behavior is restricted to a single subject? The evaluation of a case study must encompass the entire article from the introduction through the discussion. Space limitations prevent us from including an entire case study here. Instead, we have reprinted abstracts from two recent case studies in Excerpts 8.44 and 8.45. These abstracts describe briefly one speech pathology and one audiology case study. Readers are referred to the entire articles from which the abstracts are excerpted for further details regarding the specific cases and the methods used to study these cases.

EXCERPT 8.44

Palilalia is an acquired speech disorder characterized by reiteration of utterances in a context of increasing rate and decreasing loudness. The condition has been associated with bilateral subcortical neuropathology. The relationship of palilalia to other adult disfluency syndromes, aphasia, and motor speech disorders requires a thorough understanding of the nature of palilalic speech. To date no detailed description of the nature and severity of palilalic reiteration has appeared in the literature.

This case report systematically describes seven distinct types of reiteration, frequency (severity) of reiteration relative to seven types of speech tasks, and consistency and adaptation effects observed in a 29-year-old male.

From "Palilalia: A Descriptive Study of Pathological Reiterative Utterances," by L. L. LaPointe and J. Horner, 1981, *Journal of Speech and Hearing Disorders, 46,* pp. 34–38. Copyright 1981 by the American Speech-Language-Hearing Association. Reprinted with permission.

EXCERPT 8.45

A well-documented case report is presented in which the use of a high-output hearing aid over a 10-year period resulted in significant threshold shifts in the aided as compared to the unaided ear. At no time did the user experience loudness discomfort and she consistently wanted more gain from the hearing aid, indicating that there is no relationship between loudness discomfort levels and the sound pressure levels at which damage to the audi-

tory system occurs. Difficulties in detecting the cause of the threshold shifts and recommendations for case management are discussed.

From "Overamplification: A Well-Documented Case Report," by D. B. Hawkins, 1982, *Journal of Speech and Hearing Disorders, 47,* pp. 382–384. Copyright 1982 by the American Speech-Language-Hearing Association. Reprinted with permission.

EVALUATION CHECKLIST

Instructions: The four-category scale at the end of each part of the *Method* section checklist may be used to rate these parts of an article. The *Evaluation Items* help identify those topics that should be considered in arriving at the ratings. Comments on these topics, entered as *Evaluation Notes,* should serve as the basis for the ratings. An additional scale is provided to allow for an overall rating of the Method section.

Evaluation Items (Subjects)   *Evaluation Notes*

1. Sample size was adequate.

2. Subject selection and exclusion criteria were adequate and clearly defined.

3. Subjects were randomly selected and randomly assigned.

4. Overall or pair matching was employed.

5. Differential selection of subjects posed no threat to internal validity.

6. Regression effect controlled for subjects selected on basis of extreme scores.

7. Interaction of subject selection and treatment posed no threat to external validity.

8. General Comments.

Overall Rating (Subjects):

_____	_____	_____	_____
Poor	Fair	Good	Excellent

Evaluation Items (Materials)   *Evaluation Notes*

1. Instrumentation (hardware and behavioral) was appropriate.

2. Calibration procedures were described and were adequate.

3. Evidence presented on reliability and validity of hardware and behavioral instrumentation.

4. Experimenter and human observer bias was controlled.

5. Test environment was described and was adequate.

6. Instructions were described and were adequate.

7. There were adequate selection and measurement of independent (classification, predictor) variables.

8. There were adequate selection and measurement of dependent (criterion, predicted) variables.

9. General Comments.

Overall Rating (Materials):

Poor	Fair	Good	Excellent

Evaluation Items (Procedures)   *Evaluation Notes*

1. Research design was appropriate to purpose of study.

2. Procedures reduced threats to internal validity arising from:

    (a) history

    (b) maturation

    (c) pretesting

    (d) mortality

    (e) interaction of above

3. Procedures reduced threats to external validity arising from:

    (a) reactive arrangements

    (b) reactive effects of pretesting

    (c) subject selection

    (d) multiple treatments

4. General Comments.

Overall Rating (Procedures):

Poor	Fair	Good	Excellent

Overall Rating (Method):

Poor	Fair	Good	Excellent

References

Arndt, W. B. (1977). A psychometric evaluation of the Northwestern Syntax Screening Test. *Journal of Speech and Hearing Disorders, 42,* 316–319.

Babbie, E. R. (1973). *Survey research methods.* Belmont, CA: Wadsworth.

Barber, T. X. (1976). *Pitfalls in human research.* New York: Pergamon.

Barber, T. X., & Silver, M. J. (1968). Fact, fiction, and the experimenter bias effect. *Psychological Bulletin Monograph Supplement, 70* (6, Pt. 2).

Buros, O. K. (1972). *The seventh mental measurements yearbook.* Highland Park, NJ: Gryphon Press.

Christensen, L. B. (1988). *Experimental methodology* (4th ed.) Boston: Allyn & Bacon.

Darley, F. (Ed.). (1979). *Evaluation of appraisal techniques in speech and language pathology.* New York: John Wiley & Sons.

Davis, J. A. (1971). *Elementary survey analysis.* Englewood Cliffs, NJ: Prentice Hall.

Hersen, M., & Barlow, D. H. (1976). *Single case experimental designs: Strategies for studying behavior change.* New York: Pergamon.

Hipskind, N. M., & Rintelmann, W. F. (1969). Effects of experimenter bias upon pure-tone and speech audiometry. *Journal of Auditory Research, 9,* 298–305.

Lee, L. L. (1977). Reply to Arndt and Byrne. *Journal of Speech and Hearing Disorders, 42,* 323–327.

Levitt, H. (1983). Issue X: Advancing Technology. *Proceedings of the 1983 National Conference on Undergraduate, Graduate, and Continuing Education. ASHA Reports, 13,* 87–89.

Martin, R. R., & Haroldson, S. K. (1992). Stuttering and speech naturalness: Audio and audiovisual judgments. *Journal of Speech and Hearing Research, 35,* 521–528.

McCauley, R. J., & Swisher, L. (1984). Psychometric review of language and articulation tests for preschool children. *Journal of Speech and Hearing Disorders, 49,* 34–42.

Metz, D. E., Schiavetti, N., & Sacco, P. R. (1990). Acoustic and psychophysical dimensions of the perceived speech naturalness of nonstutterers and posttreatment stutterers. *Journal of Speech and Hearing Disorders, 55,* 516–525.

Orlikoff, R. F. (1991). Assessment of the dynamics of vocal fold contact area from the electroglottogram: Data from normal male subjects. *Journal of Speech and Hearing Research, 34,* 1066–1072.

Pedhazur, E. J., & Schmelkin, L. P. (1991). *Measurement, design, and analysis: An integrated approach.* Hillsdale, NJ: Lawrence Erlbaum Associates.

Perlman, A. L., VanDaele, D. J., & Otterbacher, M. S. (1995). Quantitative assessment of hyoid bone displacement from video images during swallowing. *Journal of Speech and Hearing Research, 38,* 579–585.

Plutchik, R. (1974). *Foundations of experimental research* (2nd ed.). New York: Harper & Row.

Read, C., Buder, E. H., & Kent, R. D. (1990). Speech analysis systems: A survey. *Journal of Speech and Hearing Research, 33,* 363–374.

Read, C., Buder, E. H., & Kent, R. D. (1992). Speech analysis systems: An evaluation. *Journal of Speech and Hearing Research, 35,* 314–342.

Rosenthal, R. (1966). *Experimenter effects in behavioral research.* New York: Appleton-Century-Crofts.

Rosenthal, R., & Rosnow, R. L. (Eds.). (1969). *Artifact in behavioral research.* New York: Academic Press.

Rosenthal, R., & Rosnow, R. L. (1975). *The volunteer subject.* New York: John Wiley & Sons.

Slonim, M. J. (1960). *Sampling.* New York: Simon & Schuster.

Titze, I. R., & Winholtz, W. S. (1993). The effect of microphone type and placement on voice perturbation measures. *Journal of Speech and Hearing Research, 36,* 1177–1190.

Zajac, D. J., & Yates, C. C. (1991). Accuracy of the pressure-flow method for estimating induced velopharyngeal orifice area: Effects of flow coefficient. *Journal of Speech and Hearing Research, 34,* 1073–1078.

Chapter 9

The Results Section

Basic terms, concepts, and procedures used in organizing and analyzing data derived from research in communicative disorders were described in Chapter 6. This chapter will consider the evaluation of the Results section of a research article through the use of examples that illustrate many of those basic terms, concepts, and procedures.

An important consideration in the evaluation of the Results section is the manner in which the results are related to the research problem. It is imperative that the Results section be organized in a clear fashion with regard to the general research problem and the various subproblems delineated under it. Without clear articulation of the results to the problem, even relatively simple data may be confusing and frustrating to the reader, whereas tight organization of the results around the research problem may make complex data comprehensible to most readers. Just as the writer has a responsibility to maintain the problem as the focus of the Results section, the reader must constantly bear the problem in mind while reading and evaluating the Results section.

Organization of Results

Upon completion of data collection, the researcher's first task is to organize the raw data to present a coherent picture of the results to readers. This section will present examples from the communicative disorders literature that illustrate some of the ways in which raw data have been organized for presentation. In reality, an author may have gone through several steps of organizing and reorganizing raw data on paper before arriving at a solution that enables him or her to present the results in as clear, complete, and efficient a manner as possible within the confines of a short journal article. What the reader eventually sees in print is usually a capsuled or boiled-down version of the raw data that renders them more palatable, yet still gives a clear indication of the general behavior or characteristics of subjects in the various conditions of the research design. The results may be organized for the reader by tabular or graphic presentation of the frequency distribution of the data or through the use of summary statistics that may describe the distribution more succinctly.

Frequency Distributions: Tabular and Graphic Presentations

It was stated in Chapter 6 that whenever variables are measured in a research study, the obtained values of the measurements form a distribution. The distribution may be in the form of category frequencies (for nominal data), ranks (for ordinal data), or score values (for interval or ratio data). Both tabular and graphic presentation of the frequency distribution may be effective means of data organization in order to begin making comparisons of results within subjects or between groups of subjects. Although any frequency distribution may be presented in either tabular or graphic form, there are some advantages unique to each type of illustration. In general, frequency distributions presented in graphic form (i.e., frequency histograms or polygons) give a more immediate overall picture of the distribution and have a more dramatic effect on the reader in showing the characteristics of the distribution. On the other hand, frequency distributions presented in a table are generally more convenient for inspection of specific values of the data or for making exact within-subjects and between-subjects comparisons. In some articles, authors have taken advantage of both types of presentations and included both a tabular and a graphic presentation of a frequency distribution.

Excerpt 9.1 shows the use of a table that includes both a frequency distribution and a cumulative frequency distribution of the scores of stutterers and nonstutterers on a scale of communication attitudes. Attitude scores are shown in the left-hand column, with the lower scores on the top of the table and the higher scores on the bottom of the table. The next column to the right (f) shows the number of nonstutterers who obtained each score. The next column (crf) shows the cumulative relative frequency (expressed as a decimal fraction of the number of subjects) of the nonstutterers obtaining each score on the attitude scale. The next two columns on the right-hand side show the data for the stutterers displayed in the same format. In addition, summary statistics (means and standard deviations) are shown at the bottom of the table for both groups of subjects. Inspection of the table reveals both the degree of separation and overlapping of the two groups in their scores on this communication attitude scale.

The next excerpt (9.2) shows a frequency distribution presented in the form of a histogram. This illustration shows the SICD Expressive Age posttreatment improvement (measured as proportional change relative to pretreatment development) of twenty children in a milieu language training program and twenty children in a communication training program. The bar heights in the histograms indicate the number of subjects in each group who achieved each of the SICD proportional change scores shown on the abscissa. The dark bars indicate the number of children in the milieu group who achieved each score change, and the light bars indicate the number of children in the communication training program who achieved each score change. Inspection of the two histograms reveals: (1) the distribution of milieu subjects' scores is close to a normal distribution in shape; (2) the distribution of communication training program subjects' scores is positively skewed; (3) the central tendencies are similar in the two groups (the means were 1.61 for milieu and 1.78 for communication training program); and (4) variability among subjects is smaller in the milieu group ($SD = 1.22$) and larger in the communication training program group ($SD = 2.14$).

EXCERPT 9.1

**TABLE 1   Frequency *(f)* and cumulative relative frequency *(crf)* distributions of
S-scale scores in the nonstuttering and stuttering groups**

Score	Nonstutterers (n = 144)		Stutterers (n = 120)	
	f	*crf*	*f*	*crf*
1	0	0.00		
2	7	0.05		
3	5	0.08		
4	11	0.16		
5	9	0.22	0	0.00
6	6	0.26	1	0.01
7	5	0.30	0	0.01
8	9	0.36	1	0.02
9	6	0.40	1	0.02
10	7	0.45	1	0.03
11	7	0.50	2	0.05
12	4	0.53	0	0.05
13	5	0.56	1	0.06
14	6	0.60	4	0.09
15	3	0.62	2	0.11
16	6	0.67	2	0.12
17	6	0.71	4	0.16
18	5	0.74	4	0.19
19	2	0.76	5	0.23
20	4	0.78	3	0.26
21	5	0.82	4	0.29
22	3	0.84	2	0.31
23	2	0.85	2	0.32
24	3	0.88	6	0.38
25	5	0.91	8	0.44
26	1	0.92	6	0.49
27	3	0.94	4	0.52
28	0	0.94	6	0.58
29	3	0.96	3	0.60
30	1	0.97	12	0.70
31	2	0.98	8	0.77
32	2	0.99	3	0.79
33	1	1.00	7	0.85
34	—	—	11	0.94
35	—	—	3	0.97
36	—	—	2	0.98
37	—	—	2	1.00
Mean	13.24		26.65	
SD	8.20		7.24	

EXCERPT 9.2

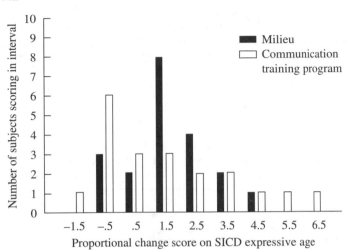

FIGURE 1   **Histogram of proportional change score for the SICD-E by treatment group**

From "An Exploratory Study of the Interaction between Language Teaching Methods and Child Characteristics," by P. J. Yoder, A. P. Kaiser, and C. A. Alpert, 1991, *Journal of* *Speech and Hearing Research, 34,* pp. 155–167. Copyright 1991 by the American Speech-Language-Hearing Association. Reprinted with permission.

The histograms in Excerpt 9.2 give a more immediate and dramatic picture of the overall results than does the table shown in Excerpt 9.1. On the other hand, closer inspection of the exact frequency of subjects obtaining each specific score is easier when inspecting the frequency table.

Excerpts 9.1 and 9.2 illustrate how tabular or graphic frequency distributions would appear in a journal article when the dependent variable data are scores at the interval or ratio level of measurement. The next two excerpts (9.3 and 9.4) show frequency distributions for data at the nominal and ordinal levels of measurements. In other words, they show the distribution of frequencies of categories (nominal level) or frequencies of rankings (ordinal level).

Excerpt 9.3 is from a study of conflict resolution abilities of children with normal language vs. children with specific language impairment. The excerpt illustrates the use of a frequency distribution table for displaying the number of older and younger subjects in each language group who used each one of a number of conflict resolution strategies during a role-playing exercise. The role-playing strategies are represented as the categories of a nominal dependent variable and are listed on the left side of the table. Younger and older children in each language group (*NL* = normal language; *SLI* = specific language impairment) constitute the four columns identified at the top of the table. The number in each cell indicates the number of children in the indicated group column who used the role-playing strategy indicated in the corresponding row. For example, seven young normal language children used the "physical" strategy (column 1, row 1) and fifteen older specific language impaired children used the "insistence" strategy (column 4, row 2). The Chi-square test in the footnote indicates that only the categories of "requests for explanation" and "reasons/moral persuasion" were used more by children with normal language than by children with specific language impairment. The Chi-square test will be illustrated with more in-depth discussion later in the chapter when we discuss examples of data analysis.

EXCERPT 9.3

TABLE 10   Number of children with normal language (NL) and children with specific language impairment (SLI) who used conflict resolution strategies with role-enactment tasks

Role Play Strategies	NL		SLI	
	Young	Old	Young	Old
Physical	7	3	8	7
Insistence	15	15	14	15
Threats/insults	7	4	8	5
Commands/demands	12	14	11	14
Assertions	15	15	15	15
Compliance	9	6	5	11
Counter	6	6	3	3
Mitigation/aggravation	7	5	4	7
Conditional	1	0	1	0
Compromise	1	4	3	2
Requests for explanation*	10	15	7	8
Reasons/moral persuasion**	9	13	8	6
Other	9	12	13	12

*$X^2 = 7.50$, $p < 0.01$; **$X^2 = 4.44$, $p < 0.05$.

Excerpt 9.4 illustrates the use of a frequency histogram to show the distribution of data for a dependent variable at the ordinal level of measurement. The example is from a study of quality judgments of speech transduced through hearing aids. The histogram shows the frequency of listeners' response rankings from best to worst (1 to 5 on the abscissa) of each of five different hearing aids (labeled *A* through *E*). The height of each bar represents the number of times each hearing aid was ranked at each position from best to worst by the listeners. Inspection of Figure 2 in Excerpt 9.4 reveals that hearing aid *E* was most often ranked as the best aid and hearing aid *D* was most frequently ranked as the

EXCERPT 9.4

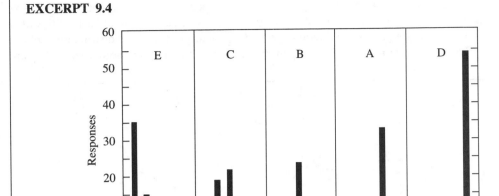

FIGURE 2   **Histograms representing frequency distributions of listener's response rankings of the aids, A through E. Each bar on the graph shows the number of times an aid was ranked in a given position, based upon the ratings across all listeners. Thirty subjects judged the aids on two different listening sessions, making 60 the total number of possible responses per aid. This figure is the responses for the female voice.**

worst aid. Hearing aids *C, B,* and *D* received more frequent rankings in the intermediate stages between best and worst.

The frequency histograms shown in Excerpts 9.2 and 9.4 and the frequency tables shown in Excerpts 9.1 and 9.3 all show the absolute frequencies at each score, ranking, or category. In addition, the table in Excerpt 9.1 shows the cumulative relative frequency. Readers may also expect to encounter frequency distributions that present all data as relative frequencies, expressed as a percentage or proportion of total cases in the distribution. Excerpt 9.5 shows the use of a relative frequency histogram to display voice onset time (VOT) data for the voiced plosive /b/ for three groups of subjects of different ages. The ordinates for the three histograms are labeled as Relative Frequency (%), and the abscissa of each histogram indicates VOT in milliseconds from − 5 on the left to + 30 on the right. The height of each bar in the histogram, then, does not represent the number of subjects at each VOT value, but rather the percentage of subjects in each group at each VOT value. These relative frequency distributions give a very clear picture of the distribution (central tendency and variability) of the data, but readers should be careful to note whether they are

EXCERPT 9.5

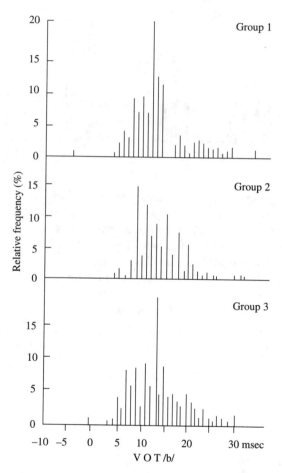

FIGURE 1   Relative frequency distribution for all productions of /b/ for three experimental groups. Group 1, aged 25 through 39; Group 2, aged 65 through 74; Group 3, over 75.

From "Voice Onset Time in a Normal-Aged Population," by P. M. Sweeting and R. J. Baken, 1982, *Journal of Speech and Hearing Research, 25,* pp. 129–134.

reading absolute number of subjects or relative number of subjects (e.g., percentage) at each score value.

As seen in the foregoing examples, frequency distributions can be a valuable addition to the Results section, because they provide a description of the overall distribution of the data. We noted in Chapter 6 that the selection of a format for organizing the data may depend partly on the author's style and partly on the requirements of the data. Nevertheless, the format chosen should: (1) present the data accurately, (2) be clearly labeled for easy reading and interpretation, and (3) relate well to the textual description of the data.

One other point should also be mentioned: the problem of accounting for missing data. Occasionally some data may be lost or not available for analysis, perhaps owing to equipment failure or failure of some subjects to complete all tasks (i.e., mortality). Authors should make a point of explaining to readers what happened in the particular study to account for any missing data. They should also comment on the implications (if any) of missing data for the validity of the study. Whenever the number of data entries in tables or figures varies from the number stated in the text or varies from condition to condition, the author should explain the reason for the discrepancy in the text or, perhaps, in a footnote. Some authors may offer an explanation of missing data or fluctuations in number of scores in the Method section, whereas other authors may wait and explain discrepancies as they arise in the Results section. Again, this is usually a matter of individual style, but all authors have a responsibility to their readers to explain number discrepancies or missing data somewhere in the article.

Summary Statistics: Central Tendency and Variability

A second way of organizing data in addition to, or instead of, the use of frequency distributions is the use of summary statistics. Summary statistics are parsimonious because they describe the overall distribution of a body of data in a simple numerical form that uses less space than does the presentation of the entire frequency distribution. Also, the summary statistics help to provide the foundation on which most analysis techniques are based, and, therefore, the selection of appropriate summary statistics is critical to appropriate analysis of the data. Most articles encountered in the communicative disorders literature present data that are organized through the use of summary statistics.

Summary statistics are used to describe the central tendency and variability of a distribution of data with a few numbers. The central tendency statistics describe what is "typical" or "average" in a distribution, and the variability statistics describe how the data spread out from the "typical" or "average" case in the distribution. In many articles, different conditions or groups of subjects are compared so that summary statistics are used to organize the data for each condition or subject group. Later, analysis of relationships or differences will refer to the summary statistics of each condition or group for the purpose of making comparisons.

Various summary statistics are available for describing distributions, and the selection of appropriate statistics depends on such factors as the level of measurement of the data, the number of observations, and normality or skewness of the distribution. Normal or nearly normal distributions of a fairly large number of interval or ratio measurements are usually summarized by reporting the mean and standard deviations of the measurements.

Lack of one or more of these data characteristics (i.e., small *N*, skewed distribution, or nominal or ordinal level of measurement) usually means that data should be summarized with the median or the mode as a measure of central tendency and some form of the range (e.g., total range or interquartile range) as a measure of variability.

In some instances, summary statistics may be included only in the textual narrative, especially if only a few numbers are presented. Excerpt 9.6 is an example from an article on sentence familiarity and lipreading that includes a small number of summary statistics. The authors apparently felt that the data were simple enough to include in textual presentation and that the use of tabular or graphic presentation was not warranted in this situation. Readers should have little or no difficulty digesting the summary statistics included in the paragraph.

EXCERPT 9.6   Results and Discussion

In analyzing the data obtained from the 102 hearing-impaired college students, familiarity values were computed for the 60 sentences. The sentence familiarity values covered nearly the total range offered the raters, 1.05 to 4.62, with a median of 2.67, a mean of 2.74, and a standard deviation of 0.88. These data indicate a relatively normal distribution of values. Although these data suggest a degree of construct (face) validity, it was decided that a follow-up study be conducted on a different class of students. One hundred thirty hearing-impaired college students enrolled in a freshman communication class served as raters. The testing procedure was identical to that used with the preparatory students. The familiarity values were computed for the 60 sentences. The sentence familiarity values ranged from 1.07 to 4.58 with a median of 2.91, a mean of 2.87, and a standard deviation of 0.82. These data for this freshman group are in general agreement with the preparatory group and indicate a normal distribution.

From "Sentence Familiarity as a Factor in Visual Speech Perception (Lipreading) of Deaf College Students," by L. L. Lloyd and J. G. Price. 1971, *Journal of Speech and Hearing Research, 14,* pp. 291–294. Copyright 1971 by the American Speech-Language-Hearing Association. Reprinted with permission.

The more usual case, however, involves presentation of summary statistics in tabular or graphic form, or, sometimes, in both forms. Graphic presentation (i.e., histograms, polygons) of summary statistics has the advantage of providing an easily viewed overall summary of results for different conditions or groups of subjects. Differences between subject groups, changes in dependent variables as a function of changes in independent variables, or differences in performances on different measures can often be immediately impressed on the reader by a well-formulated graphic presentation of summary statistics. On the other hand, graphic figures may suffer from a disadvantage: the difficulty in locating exact values of the summary statistics for each condition or group, especially when the ordinate or the abscissa is labeled with gross intervals. Some figures are labeled only at every tenth- or fifth-score interval and interpolation of exact scores between such gross intervals may be difficult. Tabular presentation of summary statistics may be less dramatic or immediately impressive to the reader, but it does have the advantage of allowing easier retrieval of exact values of summary statistics for any group or condition.

The process of graphical and tabular presentation of summary statistics is illustrated in Excerpt 9.7 which includes both a table and a figure presenting the same summary statistics on the effects of noise on speech intelligibility.

EXCERPT 9.7

TABLE 2   Mean, standard deviation, and range of scores obtained in experiment 1

| Group | Measure | Experimental Condition | | |
		Quiet	−4 S/N	−12 S/N
Normals	$\overline{X}$	99.2	94.8	92.4
	SD	2.5	3.0	4.4
	Range	92–100	90–100	82–96
High-frequency loss	$\overline{X}$	93.2	70.5	55.4
	SD	4.6	18.5	30.6
	Range	88–100	39–90	4–86
Flat loss	$\overline{X}$	94.6	85.4	80.5
	SD	6.4	6.9	12.3
	Range	80–100	74–96	54–94

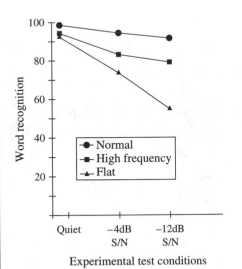

FIGURE 1
Test results of experiment 1 in which word-recognition scores are plotted as a function of the three experimental test conditions

From "Use of Low-Pass Noise in Word Recognition Testing," by R. L. Cohen and R. W. Keith, 1976, *Journal of Speech and Hearing Research, 19,* pp. 48–54.

Examination of the table and figure in Excerpt 9.7 reveals that the latter provides a more immediate overall picture of the general pattern of results. Normal subjects show better performance than either group of hearing-impaired subjects and only a small performance decrement from quiet listening to more difficult noise situations. Hearing-impaired subjects with flat audiograms perform better than do subjects with high-frequency hearing loss, and they show less dramatic performance decrement as noise level increases in the background. These conclusions are easily drawn from a brief perusal of Figure 1 in Excerpt 9.7. On the other hand, readers may wish to examine more closely the exact values of means and standard deviations of the word recognition scores of the different subject groups in the different listening conditions in order to make specific within-subjects or between-subjects comparisons. Readers will find such information more readily available in the table that displays in digital form the means, standard deviations, and ranges of word recognition scores of the three subject groups in each of the three listening conditions. By making the data available in both tabular and graphic form, these authors have judiciously organized their data in a fashion that allows readers the opportunity to view the overall pattern of results and to inspect exact values for within-subjects and between-subjects comparisons.

Excerpt 9.8 includes a bar graph that was used to display summary statistics (means) in a study of the influence of metrical patterns of words on phoneme production accuracy.

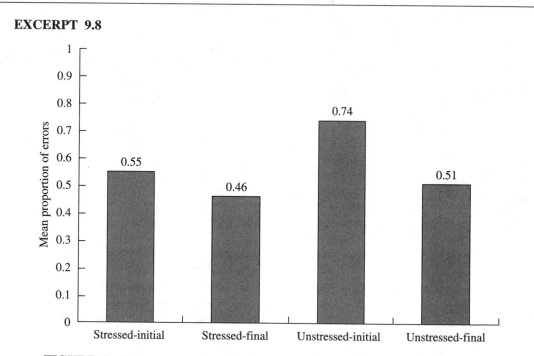

EXCERPT 9.8

FIGURE 3   Mean proportion of consonant errors according to syllable type

Mean proportion of production errors is indicated on the ordinate, and four different syllable stress patterns are indicated on the abscissa. The bar heights indicate the mean proportion of consonant errors made by twenty children for words with stressed vs. unstressed initial and final syllables. The presentation of results in the bar graph format provides readers with an overall picture of the influence of stress and syllable position on consonant errors. In addition, one unique feature of this bar graph is the inclusion of the actual mean above each bar (e.g., 0.55 for stressed-initial syllable type), which allows readers to see the exact values of the means as would be conveyed by a tabular format.

Excerpt 9.9 shows a bar graph displaying both the mean and standard deviation as summary statistics in a study of speech acquisition in children with prolonged cochlear implant experience. Mean score on the Fundamental Speech Skills Test (FSST) is indicated on the ordinate and age at the time of cochlear implantation is indicated on the abscissa. Total FSST score and three different FSST subtests are represented by the four different bar patterns indicated in the key in the graphic field. A cluster of these four bar patterns is shown for each of the three age groupings (2–4, 5–8, and 9–15 years) and for

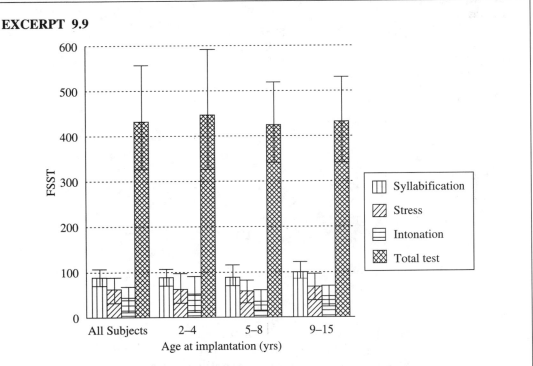

EXCERPT 9.9

FIGURE 3   Means and standard deviations from the FSST for total score and suprasegmentals subtests including: number of syllables produced, stress, and intonation contours

From "Acquisition of Speech by Children who have Prolonged Cochlear Implant Experience," by N. Tye-Murray, L. Spencer, and G. G. Woodworth, 1995, *Journal of Speech and Hearing Research, 38,* pp. 327–337. Copyright 1995 by the American Speech-Language-Hearing Association. Reprinted with permission.

all subjects combined along the abscissa. The bar heights indicate the mean FSST scores achieved by the children on each measure. In addition, an important feature of this bar graph is the inclusion of the standard deviation markers for each bar, which allow readers to see the values of the standard deviations of each measure for each age group relative to the means. For each bar, then, the height represents the mean, and the standard deviation markers (often called *error bars*) indicate the range within which approximately two-thirds (i.e., plus or minus one standard deviation) of the subjects fell.

Figure 1 in Excerpt 9.10 is an illustration taken from a study of audiometry with infants that uses a line graph to present *both* central tendency and variability data together

---

EXCERPT 9.10

Response Latency

Figure 1 shows the average response latency at each signal level for the two age groups. The graph illustrates three important features of the data. First, latency decreased systematically with increases in near-threshold SPL. Brackets on the graph represent one standard deviaton (SD) above and below mean thresholds. In general, the SDs show that intersubject variablity also decreased with increas-

ing signal level. Second, latency means and SDs in −10 trials were equivalent to the same measures in control (C) trials. Average latency in C trials, approximately 4 sec, was predictable based on random response over a period of 8 sec. Third, latencies were equivalent between age groups. In fact, the latencies were remarkably similar considering the variability often assoicated with infant behavior.

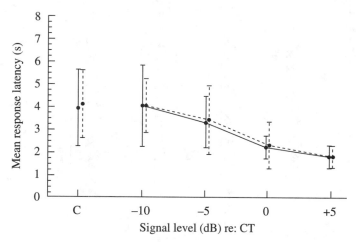

FIGURE 1   **Mean response latency values for 8-month-old (dotted line) and 12-month-old (solid line) infants under control and signal conditions. Brackets represent one standard deviation above and below mean latencies.**

in one graph. The independent variable on the abscissa is signal level in dB regarding the infant's clinical threshold (*CT*) with a control condition (no sound presented) indicated on the left. The dependent variable shown on the ordinate is the mean response latency in seconds of the infant's unidirectional head turn toward a loudspeaker and adjacent reinforcer during a visual reinforcement audiometry (VRA) task. The two lines indicate the mean performance of twenty eight-month-old infants (dotted line) and twenty twelve-month-old infants (solid line) under the control (no sound) and the signal (four intensity levels) conditions. The vertical bars connected to each line represent plus-or-minus one standard deviation above and below the mean for each age group at each value of the independent variable. The dotted vertical lines show the standard deviations for the eight-month-old infants, and the solid vertical lines show the standard deviations for the twelve-month-old infants. The accompanying text in the excerpt describes the pattern of data illustrated in the figure. Readers can compare the mean performance of the groups at each intensity level and also determine whether the groups differed in variability and central tendency. For example, not only does mean response latency decrease with intensity, but variability among infants does so as well.

As mentioned earlier, not all articles will contain data that would be organized with only means and standard deviations as the summary statistics. The summary statistics may be presented in the form of medians and ranges, either accompanying or replacing the means and standard deviations, because of reasons such as small sample sizes, skewed distributions, or unequal variances among subject groups or experimental conditions. Excerpt 9.11 presents a table from the Results section of a study of the durations of prolongations and repetitions of children who stutter. Nine dependent variables listed under the left-hand column are based on data gathered from recordings of fourteen children who stutter. The three data columns to the right show the mean, standard deviation (in parentheses), median, and range for each of the nine dependent variables. The medians were close to the means for some of the dependent variables, as is the case with normal distributions, but

---

EXCERPT 9.11

Data Analysis

Means (with standard deviations), medians and ranges were obtained for all eight measures of speech (dis)fluency. Further, Kendall rank-order correlation coefficients (T) were calculated to allow examination of possible relationships between and among these measures, along with age and interval from reported onset. Nonparametric analyses were chosen for several reasons, most notably to avoid violating assumptions of normalcy of distribution and homogeneity of variance. Further, differences in the absolute number of sound prolongations and sound/syllable repetitions contributed by each child

for analysis suggested the appropriateness of nonparametric procedures. It should be noted that prior to statistical analysis, the two measures expressed in percentage of frequencies of occurrence (i.e., frequency of disfluency and SPI) were submitted to arc-sine transformations.

Results

Table 1 shows the data obtained for each of the 14 children for all measures. Table 2 provides a summary of the group means (and standard deviations), medians and ranges for all measures of speech (dis)fluency.

Continued

EXCERPT 9.11 *Continued*

TABLE 2   Means (with standard deviations), medians, and ranges of measures of speech (dis)fluency obtained from 14 stuttering children

Measure	Mean (S.D.)	Median	Range
Duration of sound prolongation (in msec)	706 (296)	623	442–1063
Duration of sound/syllable repetitions	724 (145)	720	403–1003
Number of repeated units per instance of sound/syllable repetition	2.45 (.53)	2.25	2.0–3.8
Rate of repetition per instance of sound/ syllable repetition (in repetitions per sec)	3.48 (.923)	3.30	2.2–5.7
Frequency of speech disfluency per 100 words	19.9% (10.17)	16.0%	10–49%
SPI	46% (.20)	45%	3–79%
Overall speech rate (in words per minute)	107 (22.8)	107	51–142
Articulatory rate (in words per minute)	141.12 (22.7)	140.32	107–184.5
Articulatory rate (in syllables per second)	2.73 (.419)	2.72	2.09–3.4

From "Duration of Sound Prolongation and Sound/Syllable Repetition in Children who Stutter: Preliminary Observations," by P. M. Zebrowski, 1994, *Journal of Speech and Hearing Research, 37,* pp. 254–263. Copyright 1994 by the American Speech-Language-Hearing Association. Reprinted with permission.

were somewhat below the means for other dependent variables, indicating some positive skewness. As mentioned earlier, summary statistics help to provide a foundation for later use of data analysis techniques for examining differences and relationships. Means and standard deviations are usually used to summarize data that will be analyzed with parametric statistics, and alternate summary statistics such as the median and range are usually employed to summarize data that will be analyzed with nonparametric statistics. The accompanying text in the excerpt describes the author's rationale for choosing the nonparametric approach; this example will be referred to again in this chapter in the section on data analysis.

Some Characteristics of Good Data Organization

Results that are included in the text, table, and figures of an article should be organized in a manner that allows the reader to understand immediately the author's empirical statement regarding the problem posed in the introduction to the article. Readers should expect some of the following characteristics of good data organization when reading the Results section of an article.

First, table and figure captions should be brief but informative, and they should quickly convey the organization of the particular illustration. After reading the caption, the reader should know immediately where to find data entries for each subject group, experimental condition, or dependent variable that is included in the illustration. The caption should act as a clear road map to direct the reader through the illustration in the most efficient manner possible. Occasionally, a complex illustration may require a longer caption. There is nothing wrong with a lengthy caption *per se* as long as it is clearly written and the length is justifiable in helping the reader to understand the illustration. The Information for Authors page of every issue of *JSHR* emphasizes the importance of captions by stating:

> *Table titles and figure captions should be concise but explanatory. The reader should not have to refer to the text to decipher the information.*

Readers should expect the table titles and figure captions that they read to be prepared according to this statement.

One further point should be made with regard to figure captions. There should be a key either in the caption or in the field of a figure that identifies the meaning of the symbols used in the figure. For example, the figure in Excerpt 9.10 includes solid and dotted lines, and the figure's caption indicates which line refers to which age group. In Excerpt 9.9, a key is set in the field of the graph that identifies which bar refers to which dependent variable. Readers should expect to find such keys in either the caption or the field of a figure to provide ready understanding of the organization of the figure.

Second, each table or figure should be capable of standing alone as an illustration of the results. That is, the table should be sufficiently clear and complete so that the reader can spend some time studying it without having to refer constantly to the text to understand it. The text may summarize and analyze the results in the illustration, but the illustration should be well constructed so that it can act as an independent display of the results. If the reader has great difficulty understanding an illustration without constantly referring back to the text to make sense of the illustration, there is probably something wrong with its construction.

Third, a good illustration should dovetail with the description of the data in the text. The textual narrative should contain references to the illustrations, usually in consecutive order of presentation. This narrative will often summarize overall patterns of results and may mention specific values of data in the illustration. The text and illustrations should be parallel in the results presentation so that the reader does not have to jump back and forth in the Results section to understand the organization of the results in relation to the research problem. A good Results section contains a smoothly flowing narrative with tables and figures integrated into the text so that the flow of the narrative is not interrupted awkwardly by the references to illustrations.

A fourth point is that figures should be accurately proportioned so that the visual impression created for the reader actually reflects the data. Fortunately, the editorial boards of professional journals usually scrutinize figures to ensure accurate representation of results. Nonetheless, readers should be sure that values represented in tables or text are carefully presented in figures so that the overall effect is not a distortion of actual data values.

Finally, tables and figures should be as consistent and complete as possible. All available data or summary statistics should be displayed in similar manner for all groups or conditions to facilitate within-subjects and between-subjects comparisons. Consistency of tabular entries or graphic configurations are important for meaningful comparisons between such elements as experimental and control groups. Once a particular organization has been set up, readers should be able to follow it through different illustrations in an efficient manner. If it is necessary for an author to change the organization in presenting a large number of illustrations, the new organization should be clearly described so that readers are not confused by the change.

Many research articles present only descriptive statistics to organize the data with no further analysis included in the Results section. There may be a variety of reasons for an author's decision to exclude the analysis techniques. For example, the descriptive statistics used to organize the data may show such striking differences or lack of differences that further data analysis might only belabor the obvious. Or the research questions might have been phrased in such a way that descriptive measures of central tendency and variability would suffice for answering them. In any case, consumers of research should be aware that they may encounter articles that present only a descriptive organization of the data and that this may be entirely appropriate in many cases.

Analysis of Data

Once the data of a study have been organized so that readers may peruse them to grasp the pattern of results in relation to the original research problem, certain statistical procedures may be employed to analyze the results. These statistical procedures may be generally classified as the analysis of relationships and the analysis of differences, although these two kinds of analysis may overlap somewhat, as pointed out in Chapter 6. This section will begin with examples of data analysis using correlational statistics to examine relationships among variables and then proceed to examples of data analysis using inferential statistics (also called significance tests) to examine differences between subjects or conditions.

Correlational Analysis

Researchers often wish to examine (1) the strength and direction of relationships among two or more variables and (2) the manner in which performance on one variable may be predicted from performance on another variable. The first examination is accomplished through the calculation of correlation coefficients and the plotting of scattergrams (also called scatterplots), and the second examination is accomplished through the use of regression analysis. Correlation and regression are intimately related statistical procedures that are often completed together as one analysis package to examine relationships among variables. Some researchers, however, complete only one of the two analyses because they may be more interested in the strength and direction of the relationship than in predicting performance on one variable from another (or vice versa).

Correlation and regression analysis may be done in the relatively simple case of the relationship between two variables or it may be attempted for the more complicated case of the relationships among several variables. We will begin with examples of correlation and regression analysis of some simple bivariate examples to show how the results of such analysis could be presented in a journal article and then progress to some more complicated multivariate examples.

As mentioned in Chapter 6, the scattergram graphically depicts the relationship between two variables by showing the intersection point of the two measurements for each subject. If the two variables are positively correlated, subjects would tend to have high scores on both measures, medium scores on both measures, or low scores on both measures so that the pattern of dots on the scattergram slopes upward to the right of the graph. If the two variables are negatively related, subjects who score high on one variable tend to have low scores on the other variable so that the pattern of dots on the scattergram slopes downward to the right of the graph. Uncorrelated variables result in a scattergram that has dots spread around the graph in no particular order.

The strength of the relationship between the two variables can be roughly observed in the scattergram. A tight clustering of the dots around the center of an upward slopping pattern indicates a strong positive correlation, whereas a more diffuse pattern of dots spread around the center of an upward sloping pattern indicates a weaker positive correlation. By the same token, the clustering or dispersion of the dots around the center of a downward sloping pattern indicates the strength or weakness of a negative correlation.

Excerpt 9.12 includes two scattergrams that depict the relationship between objective and subjective speech intelligibility scores indexed with the relative arcsine unit (RAU) transform, a procedure often used to transform proportional or percentage scores into a format that is more suitable for statistical data analysis. Listeners' ability to understand speech was measured with an objective transcription procedure and a subjective scaling procedure, and each listener contributed multiple listening trials to the data pool with different listening passages.

The first scattergram in the excerpt (Figure 2) shows data from a group of twenty-eight normal-hearing subjects who listened to speech at several different signal-to-babble ratios in order to provide a range of speech intelligibility scores. Each filled circle represents a pair of intelligibility scores (one objective and one subjective). The diagonal line indicates where all circles would have fallen if the correlation were perfect (i.e., an r of +1.00) and if the regression equation had a slope of 1.00 and a y-intercept of 0, indicating the exact same score on both the objective and subjective intelligibility measures. This diagonal line is not the regression line of the actual data but is used for comparative purposes to show how close the score pairs are to being identical for each subject. The correlation is indicated in the field as $r = 0.82$, a strong positive correlation. Also note the authors' comments that all the data were clustered fairly close to the diagonal, except for one subject whose performance appeared to be aberrant (open squares in the scattergram); if that subject's scores were eliminated, the r would have been slightly higher (+0.87). The second figure in the excerpt shows the scattergram for a group of hearing-impaired listeners and includes the correlation coefficient (+0.85) and the actual regression line drawn in the scattergram for these data. The two scattergrams and correlations reveal that the strength and direction of the relationship between objective and subjective intelligibility scores were similar for the hearing-impaired and normal-hearing listeners.

EXCERPT 9.12

The data comprised two objective intelligibility scores and two corresponding subjective intelligibility estimates for 28 subjects. To homogenize the variances of these percentage data, all values were transformed into rationalized arcsine units (raus) before analysis as Studebaker (1985) described. The scale for rationalized arcsine units extends from –23 to 123. Values in the range from 20 to 80 are within about one unit of the corresponding percentage score.

Figure 2 illustrates the relationship between the objective and subjective intelligibility data for normal hearers. Each symbol depicts one pair of scores. There are two pairs of scores per subject. Despite some individual variation, and one aberrant subject shown by the open squares, these data are well described by the diagonal line, suggesting that objective and subjective intelligibility scores were essentially equal for these listeners. The linear correlation coefficient between subjective and objective scores was .82 (this correlation was .87 if the aberrant subject was excluded from the analysis).

. . . .

The speech intelligibility data consisted of 4–6 pairs of objective and subjective scores per subject. Figure 10 illustrates the relationship between subjective and objective scores. Each symbol depicts one pair of scores. The correlation between the two types of scores was .85; the regression line is shown.

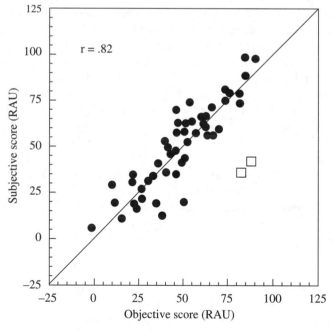

FIGURE 2   **Objective and subjective intelligibility data for 28 normal-hearing listeners. Each symbol depicts one pair of scores. There are two pairs of scores per subject.**

Continued

EXCERPT 9.12 *Continued*

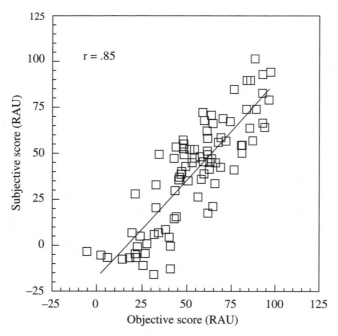

**FIGURE 10 Objective and subjective intelligibility data
for 15 hearing-impaired listeners, 13 of
them from the group depicted in Figure 4.
Each symbol depicts one pair of scores.**

From "Comparison of Objective and Subjective
Measures of Speech Intelligibility in Elderly Hearing-
Impaired Listeners," by R. M. Cox, G. C. Alexander, and
I. M. Rivera, 1991, *Journal of Speech and Hearing*
Research, 34, pp. 904–915. Copyright 1991 by the
American Speech-Language-Hearing Association.
Reprinted with permission.

Excerpt 9.13 shows the results of a detailed correlation and regression analysis of the
relationships among auditory and phonatory variables. The abstract explains the methods of
measuring and comparing the auditory and phonatory variables, and textual excerpt and figure show the detailed results of the regression analysis. Each panel in the figure is a scattergram demonstrating the relationship between a different auditory measure on each
abscissa and the two laryngeal reaction time measures (LRT) on the ordinate. The data
points for BLRT and an auditory measure are indicated in each scattergram by filled
squares, and the data points for MLRT and an auditory measure are indicated in each scattergram by open squares. Each scattergram has two regression lines drawn through it, one
for BLRT and one for MLRT prediction from each auditory measure. The dark lines are for
regression equations associated with correlations significantly above zero and the light lines
for a regression equation associated with a correlation not found to be significantly above
zero. The keys on the right of each panel show the regression equations for each prediction,

EXCERPT 9.13

Interaction between auditory and phonatory systems was explored in normal speakers by comparing laryngeal reaction time (LRT) with interpeak intervals from the auditory brainstem response (ABR) obtained using high and low stimulus presentation rates. Thirty-four subjects with no history of neurological or speech-language disorders and normal hearing sensitivity participated. Interpeak intervals were derived from ABR's recorded for each ear at rates of 21.1 and 91.1 clicks/s. LRT responses were obtained by instructing subjects to sustain an /s/ and then phonate an /a/ as fast as possible following visual cues. Two measures of reaction time performance were derived, Mean Laryngeal Reaction Time (MLRT) and Best Laryngeal Reaction Time (BLRT). Linear regression analyses were completed between each measure of reaction time performance and each ABR interpeak interval. Using either LRT

measure, two significant (p < .05) positive linear relationships were found. One involved the interpeak interval between Waves III and V and the other involved the interpeak interval between Waves I and V. Both were recorded at high stimulus presentation rates. These results support the small body of literature from normal speakers, stutterers, and spasmodic dysphonics suggesting interaction between the auditory and phonatory systems at the brainstem level.

. . . .

Figure 1 displays the following: (a) the individual data points ($n = 25$) for the dependent variables BLRT and MLRT and the independent variable IPI III–V L90, and the lines of best fit; (b) the individual data points ($n = 19$) for the dependent variables BLRT and MLRT and the independent variable IPI I–V L90, and the lines of best fit, and (c) the individ-

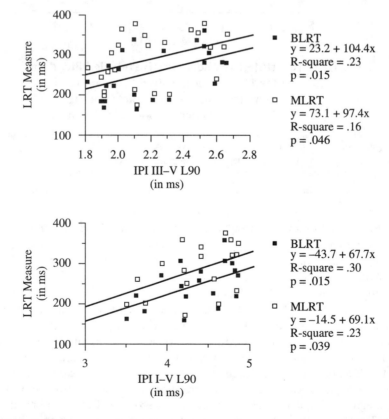

Continued

EXCERPT 9.13   *Continued*

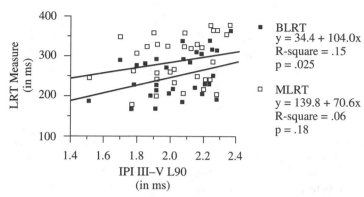

FIGURE 1   **The upper graph illustrates the lines of best fit for the individual data points (*n* = 25) of the dependent variables of BLRT (open squares) and MLRT (dark squares) in ms versus the independent variable of ABR interpeak interval IPI III–V L90 in ms. The middle graph illustrates the lines of best fit for the individual data points (*n* = 19) of the dependent variables of BLRT (open squares) and MLRT (dark squares) in ms versus the independent variable of ABR interpeak interval IP I–V L90 in ms. The lower graph illustrates the lines of best fit for the individual data points (*n* = 33) of the dependent variables of BLRT (open squares) and MLRT (dark squares) in ms versus the independent variable of ABR interpeak interval IPI III–V R20 in ms. The linear relationship between MLRT and the ABR measure did not reach statistical significance, so the line is lighter than for the relationship between BLRT and the ABR measure. The regression equation, the *R*-square value, and the level of significance between the two variables are written underneath the dependent variable name, to the right of each graph.**

ual data points (*n* = 33) for the dependent variables BLRT and MLRT and the independent variable IPI III–V R20, and the lines of best fit.

As can be seen from Figure 1, the slopes of the linear relationships were positive, meaning that longer ABR interpeak intervals predicted poorer LRT performance (i.e., longer BLRTs or MLRTs) and shorter ABR interpeak intervals predicted better LRT performance (i.e., shorter BLRTs or MLRTs).

From "Relationships between Selected Auditory and Phonatory Latency Measures in Normal Speakers," by S. V. Stager, 1990, *Journal of Speech and Hearing Research, 33,* pp. 156–162. Copyright 1990 by the American Speech-Language-Hearing Association. Reprinted with permission.

the *R*-square (percentage of shared variance), and the probability that the correlation is above zero. Note the detailed description presented in the figure caption, which is necessary because of the sheer volume of information presented in the figure.

Not all relationships are fit best with a linear regression equation. Sometimes the relationship between two variables is curvilinear and the regression equation that best fits the data and predicts the dependent variable from the independent variable is a formula for generating a curve such as a quadratic, logarithmic, or exponential function. Excerpt 9.14

EXCERPT 9.14

Figure 7 is a plot of the resulting fit for the regression equation along with unconnected plots for the age-shifted percentage of consonants correct data from Figure 6. The resulting equation accounts for a decisively high 93.3% of the variance, with a standard error of 6.83%. By traditional statistical criteria, it appears to be appropriate to claim that this equation and its corresponding fit provide a valid characterization of speech-sound normalization in both normal and speech-delayed children. The trend in Figure 7 is consistent with the position that there is a single course of normalization for both groups of children, differing only in temporal markers among the three speech-sound classes and between group assignment. This finding is markedly consistent with the first of the three hypotheses about speech-sound development proposed by Bishop and Edmundson (1987) and the findings of Curtiss, Katz, and Tallal (1992) for syntax.

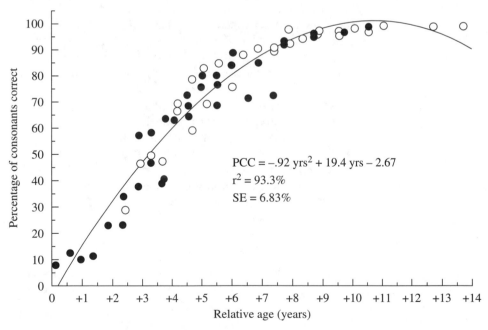

$$PCC = -.92 \text{ yrs}^2 + 19.4 \text{ yrs} - 2.67$$
$$r^2 = 93.3\%$$
$$SE = 6.83\%$$

FIGURE 7 **Regression analysis of the age-shifted percentage of consonants correct data in Figure 6**

shows data from a study of developmental phonological disorders, plotting percentage of consonants produced correctly by normally developing children (open circles) and delayed children (filled circles) against a normalized relative age measure. The ages of development for early-, middle-, and late-developing sounds for both groups were indexed relative to age of early-developing sounds for normal-developing children to derive a new independent variable called *relative age*. The figure shows the curvilinear regression equation for predicting percentage correct consonant production (dependent variable) from the relative age measure (independent variable) and also indicates the R^2 derived from the correlation between X and Y (i.e., the percentage of shared variance between X and Y) and the standard error of the prediction from the regression equation.

Excerpt 9.15 contains a table and three scattergrams that illustrate the use of the Spearman correlation with rank-order data in a study of vocal characteristics and male–female quality of the voice. Rank-order data were used in the analysis of the relationships among three variables: rating of male–female voice quality, fundamental frequency of the voice, and vocal tract resonance. Spearman rank-order correlations (rhos) are entered in the table for each of the three pairings of the variables: male–female voice quality with fundamental frequency, male–female voice quality with vocal tract resonance, and fundamental frequency with vocal tract resonance. These three relationships are indicated under the table heading "Comparison." The three columns of Spearman rhos include the correlations calculated for male speakers only, female speakers only, and male and female speakers combined. These same relationships are also depicted in the corresponding scattergrams. Male data are indicated by filled circles and female data are indicated by the open circles. The correlations for male and female data combined correspond to the entire scattergram for each variable pair.

The correlations of male–female voice quality with fundamental frequency are the highest ones, and the scattergram in Figure 2 depicts these correlations and shows the tightest clustering of the pattern of dots. In fact, the dot pattern clusters more tightly for the females than for the males, and the correlation for the female speakers only is higher than the correlation

EXCERPT 9.15

TABLE 1   Spearman rank-order correlation coefficients (RHOs) between degree of male-female voice quality (M-F voice quality), fundamental frequency (F_0), and vocal tract resonances (VTR)

	Rhos		
Comparison	Males and Females	Males Only	Females Only
M-F voice quality with F_0	0.94*	0.65*	0.88*
M-F voice quality with VTR	0.59*	0.00	0.27
VTR with F_0	0.56*	0.14	0.17

*$p < 0.01$.

Continued

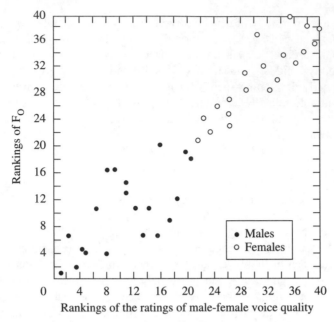

FIGURE 2 **Rankings of listener ratings of degree of male–female voice quality compared with rankings of fundamental frequency**

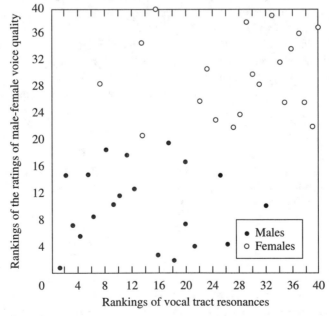

FIGURE 3 **Rankings of individual vocal tract resonances compared with rankings of listener ratings of degree of male–female voice quality**

Continued

EXCERPT 9.15   *Continued*

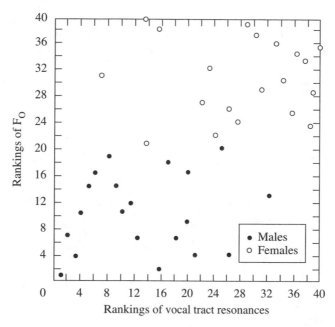

Rankings of vocal tract resonances

Rankings of F_O

• Males
○ Females

FIGURE 4   **Rankings of individual vocal tract resonances compared with rankings of fundamental frequency**

From "A Comparison of the Contributions of Two Voice Quality Characteristics to the Perception of Maleness and Femaleness in the Voice," by R. O. Coleman, 1976, *Journal of Speech and Hearing Research, 19,* pp. 168–180. Copyright 1976 by the American Speech-Language-Hearing Association. Reprinted with permission.

for male speakers only. The correlation for male and female data combined is highest of all because this correlation is based on a larger number of observations with a greater range of scores on both variables. The correlations of male–female voice quality with vocal tract resonance and of vocal tract resonance with fundamental frequency are much lower, and a more widely dispersed pattern of dots can be seen in Figures 3 and 4 in Excerpt 9.15 that are the corresponding scattergrams for these correlations. Significance of all the correlations is indicated by the asterisks in Table 1 that identify those correlations that were significantly different from zero at the 0.01 level. Readers should find it a relatively simple matter to compare the correlations and scattergrams for each pair of variables for each subject group because of the effective manner in which the correlational analysis has been displayed.

The Pearson correlations shown earlier were computed from interval- or ratio-level data, and the Spearman correlations (Excerpt 9.15) were computed from ordinal-level data. It was mentioned in Chapter 6, that correlational analysis may be performed with nominal-level data through the use of the X^2 statistic to evaluate the significance of the association between nominal-level variables. Excerpt 9.16 illustrates this use of X^2. In this example,

EXCERPT 9.16   Results

Table 1 shows the laryngeal behavior associated with each of the three types of stuttering. The association between the type of stuttering and laryngeal behavior was statistically significant ($X^2 = 22.4$; df = 4; $p < 0.001$). The nature of this association is considered for each of the three types of stuttering.

TABLE 1   Judgments of separation of the posterior aspects of the vocal folds associated with each of three types of stuttering*

	Type of Stuttering					
Laryngeal Behavior	Part-Word Repetition ($N = 55$)		Sound Prolongation ($N = 39$)		Broken Word ($N = 7$)	
	Number	%	Number	%	Number	%
Abduction	33	60	11	28	7	100
Adduction	15	27	28	72	0	0
Combination	7	3	0	0	0	0

*Number and percentage of the total instances of stuttering associated with a particular category of laryngeal behavior is given for each of the three types of stuttering. Nine of the ten subjects produced the 55 part-word repetitions, eight of the ten subjects produced the 39 sound prolongations, and three of the ten subjects produced the seven broken words.

From "Laryngeal Behavior during Stuttering," by E. G. Conture, G. N. McCall, and D. W. Brewer, 1977, *Journal of Speech and Hearing Research, 20,* pp. 661–668.   Copyright 1977 by the American Speech-Language-Hearing Association. Reprinted with permission.

Conture, McCall, and Brewer investigated the association between the occurrence of various laryngeal behaviors (adduction, abduction, and a combination of the two) and three different types of stuttering (part-word repetition, sound prolongation, and broken words). Table 1 in Excerpt 9.16 shows the frequency and percentage of occurrence of each laryngeal behavior during the occurrence of each of the three types of stuttering. In the text, the authors reported a X^2 value of 22.4 that was calculated from the frequencies of these nominal data and indicated that a significant ($p < 0.001$) association between type of stuttering and laryngeal behavior was evident. The authors used the remainder of the Results section to analyze the specific laryngeal behaviors observed for each type of stuttering.

Many studies examine the relationships among several variables simultaneously rather than just two at a time; that is, they are multiple correlation studies rather than bivariate. In this case, correlation coefficients are calculated for all possible combinations of two variables and are displayed in a correlation matrix that lists all variables down the vertical axis and across the horizontal axis of the table. The correlation coefficient for each pair is entered in the cell of the table that represents the intersection of the two variables, one from the vertical and one from the horizontal list. Discussion of the results may then center on the relative strength of the relationships among various pairs of variables. In addition, regression analysis may be done using various combinations of independent variables in a single regression equation to predict a given dependent variable listed in the matrix. A multiple correlation matrix and accompanying multiple regression analysis is exemplified by the study of the relationships among several acoustic measures and speech intelligibility that is shown in Excerpt 9.17. The excerpt displays text describing the correlational analysis, a table of regression data, and the intercorrelation matrix for a set of independent variables that are acoustic characteristics used to predict the dependent variable of speech intelligibility. The text describes how the regression analysis selected the four best independent variables for predicting the speech intelligibility variable, and Table 5 shows

EXCERPT 9.17

Analysis

All acoustic measures were incorporated into a multiple regression framework to determine which acoustic measures or combination of measures accounted significantly for the variance in the perceptual intelligibility measures. The potential predictor (independent) variables in the multivariate analysis were the seven acoustic measures (e.g., voice onset time, vowel duration). The criterion or predicted (dependent) variables were the intelligibility percentages. The intelligibility percentage scores were converted to arcsine values prior to the analysis. An all possible subsets regression analysis program was employed (Dixon, 1981). This regression analysis examines subsets of varying size (subset size is the number of independent variables

included in the equation), so that the "best" subset of predictor variables can be determined. In addition, this procedure allows the investigator to specify the identity and the ordering of predictor variables entered into the equation.

Results

By regression analysis, it was determined that 62.6% of the variance in the phonemic intelligibility scores was accounted for by four variables: fricative-affricative contrast, front-back vowel contrast, high-low vowel contrast, and lax-tense vowel contrast. Table 5 presents these subset data. Included are R^2, the square of the correlation between the dependent variable y and the predicted value of y, and adjusted R^2.

TABLE 5 **Multiple regression analysis: Squared multiple correlation (R^2), adjusted R^2, Mallows' Cp, coefficient of each variable, and t statistic for the best subset of predictor variables**

R^2	Adjusted R^2	CP
0.626155	0.490211	2.08

Variable	Coefficient	T statistic
fric.-affr.	0.520324	2.29
front-back	−0.172504	−2.80
high-low	0.0874958	1.38
tense-lax	−0.283510	−2.68
intercept	169.448	

Continued

EXCERPT 9.17   *Continued*

The inter-correlation matrix is given in Table 6. The four variables that comprised this "best" subset yielded a multiple correlation of 0.79 with the measured intelligibility scores.

The all-possible-subsets approach allowed a critical comparison of the data provided for subsets with combinations of one through seven variables. The addition of variables beyond four did not result in an appreciable increase in predictive efficiency. The subset containing all given acoustic variables (equivalent to the full equation multiple regression analysis with all dependent variables entered) accounted for 62.9% of the variance. Practical clin-ical and theoretical concerns did not warrant the addition of three contrast variables for an increase of only 0.3% of the variance.

The large multiple correlation between speech intelligibility and four acoustic aspects of speech, the fricative-affricate contrast and the three vowel contrasts, indicated that these four factors strongly influence intelligibility. A general conclusion of this research relating acoustic factors to word intelligibility is that the vowel parameters of duration and F1 and F2 formant locations, and the fricative-affricate durational parameters, are major predictors of the scored intelligibility of speech.

TABLE 6   Correlations between acoustic value for each contrast (voice-voiceless initial, voice-voiceless final, stop-nasal, fricative-affricate, front-back vowel, high-how vowel, tense-lax vowel, and intelligibility)

		vvic 1	vvfc 2	snc 3	fac 4	fbv 5	hiv 6	tiv 7	int 8
vvic	1	1.000							
vvfc	2	−0.223	1.000						
snc	3	−0.530	0.703	1.000					
fac	4	0.214	−0.080	−0.322	1.000				
bv	5	0.449	−0.456	−0.307	0.377	1.000			
hlv	6	−0.337	0.461	0.228	−0.309	−0.589	1.000		
tlv	7	−0.087	0.745	0.472	0.344	−0.153	0.263		
int	8	−0.238	−0.010	−0.187	−0.031	−0.574	0.408	−0.214	1.000

which variables were selected, the slope and intercept coefficients to be entered in the regression equation for each independent variable, and the resultant R^2 statistics. Table 6 shows the intercorrelation matrix, which presents the Pearson correlations for all the possible pairings of the variables.

Excerpt 9.18 shows a similar intercorrelation matrix, but the correlations entered in Table 3 of the excerpt are not Pearson correlations. Each correlation coefficient is a Kendall's rank-order Tau, a nonparametric correlation calculated from ordinal data that is very similar to the Spearman Rho illustrated in Excerpt 9. 15. The textual excerpt describes why a nonparametric approach was used and indicates that the discussion of the results will emphasize the relative strengths of the relationships among the disfluency measures

EXCERPT 9.18

Data Analysis

Means (with standard deviations), medians and ranges were obtained for all eight measures of speech (dis)fluency. Further, Kendall rank-order correlation coefficients (T) were calculated to allow examination of possible relationships between and among these measures, along with age and interval from reported onset. Nonparametric analyses were chosen for several reasons, most notably to avoid violating assumptions of normalcy of distribution and homogeneity of variance. Further, differences in the absolute number of sound prolongations and sound/syllable repetitions contributed by each child for analysis suggested the appropriateness of non-parametric procedures. It should be noted that prior to statistical analysis, the two measures expressed in percentage of frequencies of occurrence (i.e., frequency of disfluency and SPI) were submitted to arc-sine transformations.

Correlational Analysis

Table 3 presents Kendall rank-order correlation coefficients between mean age, interval between reported onset of stuttering and data collection, and eight measures of speech (dis)fluency for the stuttering children (N = 14) who participated in this study.

Eleven correlations were statistically significant at the .05 level or better. The main purpose of using correlational analyses with these data was to observe and describe relationships between and among specific (non)speech behaviors as a way of uncovering salient behaviors for future research. Therefore, because of the descriptive nature of this study, adjusted alphas were not used. The remainder of this section will be devoted to a discussion of the 11 correlations which reached significance.

TABLE 3   Kendall Rank-Order Correlation Coefficients (T) between age, interval from onset, and measures of (dis)fluent speech

	Age	Interval	SP	SSR	Units	Rate	FREQ	SPI	OVER	ARTIC
Age	—	.49*	.36	−.14	.23	.11	.24	.26	−.12	.17
Interval	—	—	.12	−.05	.26	.07	.25	.22	−.23	.01
SP	—	—	—	.05	.09	.01	.31	.45*	−.54**	−.42*
SSR	—	—	—	—	.18	−.42*	.02	.01	−.16	−.02
UNITS	—	—	—	—	—	.41*	−.15	−.15	.04	.20
RATE	—	—	—	—	—	—	−.23	−.07	.28	.12
FREQ	—	—	—	—	—	—	—	.47*	−.45*	−.24
SPI	—	—	—	—	—	—	—	—	−.49**	−.43*
OVER	—	—	—	—	—	—	—	—	—	.71**
ARTIC	—	—	—	—	—	—	—	—	—	—

Note. SP = Mean duration of sound prolongations; SSR = Mean duration of sound/syllable repetitions; Units = Mean number of repeated units per instance of sound/syllable repetition; Rate = Mean rate of repetition per instance of sound/syllable repetition; Freq = Mean frequency of speech disfluency in 100 words; SPI = Sound Prolongation Index; Over = Overall speech rate in wpm; Artic = Articulatory rate in sps.
*: $p < 0.05$
**: $p < 0.01$

and the age and onset interval data. The emphasis in this excerpt is on the strength and direction of the various relationships rather than on prediction of one variable from a combination of other variables.

In some cases, the emphasis in presenting the results of the correlational analysis is placed more squarely on the prediction equation, especially when an important practical implication of the research concerns the prediction of one variable from another. Excerpt 9.19 displays a table taken from Carhart and Porter's study of the relationships among

---

EXCERPT 9.19

TABLE 7   Coefficients of correlation and regression equations for prediction of speech reception threshold (SRT) from pure-tone thresholds (T's) for six groups classified according to audiometric pattern*

Classification	Coefficient	SRT = Regression Equation
Zero-Order	*r*	
Flat	0.975	$0.4 \text{ dB} + 0.94 \text{ T}_{1000}$
Gradual	0.931	$3.4 \text{ dB} + 0.84 \text{ T}_{1000}$
Marked	0.873	$12.0 \text{ dB} + 0.87 \text{ T}_{500}$
Rising	0.929	$0.0 \text{ dB} + 0.92 \text{ T}_{1000}$
Trough	0.951	$-10.6 \text{ dB} + 1.03 \text{ T}_{1000}$
Atypical	0.882	$4.8 \text{ dB} + 0.76 \text{ T}_{1000}$
First-Order	*R*	
Flat	0.978	$-0.3 \text{ dB} + 0.77 \text{ T}_{1000} + 0.19 \text{ T}_{2000}$
Gradual	0.952	$2.6 \text{ dB} + 0.39 \text{ T}_{500} + 0.53 \text{ T}_{1000}$
Marked	0.891	$7.3 \text{ dB} + 0.63 \text{ T}_{500} + 0.26 \text{ T}_{1000}$
Rising	0.955	$1.6 \text{ dB} + 0.60 \text{ T}_{1000} + 0.43 \text{ T}_{4000}$
Trough	0.962	$-12.5 \text{ dB} + 0.68 \text{ T}_{1000} + 0.41 \text{ T}_{2000}$
Atypical	0.927	$2.0 \text{ dB} + 0.37 \text{ T}_{500} + 0.51 \text{ T}_{1000}$
Second-Order	*R*	
Flat	0.979	$-1.1 \text{ dB} + 0.18 \text{ T}_{500} + 0.62 \text{ T}_{1000} + 0.18 \text{ T}_{2000}$
Gradual	0.956	$-0.1 \text{ dB} + 0.38 \text{ T}_{500} + 0.41 \text{ T}_{1000} + 0.16 \text{ T}_{2000}$
Marked	0.894	$3.0 \text{ dB} + 0.62 \text{ T}_{500} + 0.21 \text{ T}_{1000} + 0.11 \text{ T}_{2000}$
Rising	0.958	$1.7 \text{ dB} + 0.48 \text{ T}_{1000} + 0.21 \text{ T}_{2000} + 0.38 \text{ T}_{4000}$
Trough	0.966	$-10.9 \text{ dB} + 0.21 \text{ T}_{500} + 0.44 \text{ T}_{1000} + 0.45 \text{ T}_{2000}$
Atypical	0.937	$-0.5 \text{ dB} + 0.40 \text{ T}_{500} + 0.41 \text{ T}_{1000} + 0.11 \text{ T}_{2000}$

*The threshold for each frequency is designated by the appropriate subscript (for example T_{1000} = threshold for 1000 Hz). The right-hand section of each equation consists of a correction constant (first term) followed by one or more terms consisting of a beta coefficient multiplied by a threshold value.

thresholds at various pure-tone frequencies and speech reception thresholds (SRT). This table shows the correlations between predicted SRT and actual SRT (i.e., the multiple correlations) for each combination of predictor variables. The table also displays the regression equations for predicting SRT from each combination of pure-tone thresholds. A separate listing of these correlations and regression equations is made for each of six groups of hearing-impaired subjects with different audiometric configurations. Three sets of equations are included: zero-order, first-order, and second-order. The zero-order equations are used to predict SRT from the one pure-tone threshold that is most highly correlated with SRT. The first-order equations are used to predict SRT from the two pure-tone thresholds that are most highly correlated with SRT and the second-order equations are used to predict SRT from the three pure-tone thresholds that are most highly correlated with SRT. The prediction may become more accurate as more predictor variables are added to the regression equation, so several orders of equations are often run through in this fashion to find the most accurate prediction equation. Once the most accurate equation is found, it can be used to predict SRT from the pure-tone data of new patients who fall into the various categories of audiometric configuration. In the text of this article, the authors have suggested the best equations for making these predictions with patients having different types of audiometric configurations when various pure-tone data are available.

The focus in this last example is more on prediction of one variable from the others than on the analysis of strength and direction of the relationship among the variables. Both of these concepts are important and intimately related aspects of correlational analysis, but different authors may emphasize one of them over the other, depending on the purposes of a particular study. Traditionally, the analysis of the strength and direction of the relationship through presentation of correlation coefficients and scattergrams has been more prevalent in the research literature, but there has been more interest developing in the regression aspect of correlational analysis in recent years.

Analysis of Differences

Now that we have illustrated some of the typical formats in which correlational analysis may be presented in the Results section of a research article, we will present some examples of the use of inferential statistics to examine differences between subjects or to examine within-subjects differences between conditions. We will begin with cases of simple two-sample comparisons and progress to cases with more complicated comparisons of several samples.

The format for the presentation of inferential statistics to test the significance of differences may vary somewhat from article to article. Some authors prefer to include inferential statistics in a table that combines frequency distributions and summary statistics. The table may include values of central tendency and variability for the different groups or conditions that were compared and the values of the inferential statistics that were used to test the significance of the differences. The significance levels of the inferential statistics may be included in the table or may be placed in a footnote to the table. In other articles, the inferential analysis may be described in the narrative of the Results section, perhaps with the values of the inferential statistics and significance levels presented in parentheses. Such a narrative analysis may often make references to the summary statistics presented in a table of data organization. Some authors simply mention in the text that inferential tests were used and that differences were significant without specifically stating the values of the statistics or the significance levels that were reached. This latter alternative certainly provides less information than would be desirable for a complete evaluation of the article, but it has apparently come into vogue as a space-saving device because journal space is at such a premium.

The examples that follow will illustrate some of the diverse manners in which authors have presented inferential analysis in research articles in communicative disorders. Although these examples do not provide an exhaustive treatment of the possible formats that readers may encounter in the literature, they should enable consumers of research to appreciate the general manner in which statistical inference may be presented in journal articles and enable them to locate and examine inferential analysis in the articles they will read in the future.

As mentioned in Chapter 6, bivalent, or two sample differences may often be evaluated statistically. These might involve between-subjects comparison of two different groups or within-subjects comparison of the same group under two different conditions. The two samples, then, represent two different levels of an *independent* or *classification* variable. These two samples may be compared to each other on one or, in some cases, on more than one *dependent* variable. When the data used in such comparisons meet the requirements of the parametric statistical tests, the *t*-test (sometimes called the "Student's test" after the pseudonym of its inventor, W. S. Gosset) is used to make the bivalent comparison. When the data do not meet the requirements of the parametric model, nonparametric tests for the bivalent comparisons are used instead.

Whenever two *different* groups of subjects are compared, the particular *t*-test used is called an independent *t*-test or a *t*-test for unrelated measures or uncorrelated groups. In addition to this independent *t*-test, there is another *t*-test called the dependent *t*-test or the *t*-test for related measures or correlated groups. This dependent *t*-test is used for making within-subjects comparisons on the *same* group, such as comparison of scores on a test before and after treatment. As mentioned in Chapter 6, larger values of the resultant *t*-statistic indicate a more significant difference between groups or conditions (i.e., a larger value of *t* would have a lower probability of occurrence if the two samples were indeed the same under the null hypothesis). Conversely, small values of *t*-scores indicate less-significant differences.

Excerpt 9.20 shows an example of the use of the *t*-test to compare the means of two *different* groups of subjects (i.e., the independent *t*-test), and Excerpt 9.21 shows an example of the use of the *t*-test to compare the means of one group of subjects performing under two *different* conditions (i.e., the dependent *t*-test). In excerpt 9.20 a group of children with specific language impairment (SLI group) was compared to a group of children without language impairment who were matched to the SLI group in mean length of utterance (the MLU group). The dependent variable analyzed was number of unique noun stems. The independent *t*-test was used because the groups contained entirely different subjects; thus their scores were independent of each other, or uncorrelated. In excerpt 9.21 one group of children was tested in two different conditions: an interview context and a free play context. The dependent variable analyzed was number of utterances. The dependent *t*-test was used because there was only one group containing the same subjects tested twice; thus their scores in one condition were not independent of their scores in the other, or were correlated in the two conditions. Both excerpts present the analysis in a clear and straightforward com-

EXCERPT 9.20

Lexical productivity.   One way that youngsters can achieve a spuriously high percent of correct use is to rely heavily on only a few frequently used words that may be memorized forms. One way to evaluate this possibility is to count the number of different words that appear with the plural affix. Thus, the number of unique noun stems that appeared with regular plural inflection was tabulated for each child, and group means and standard deviations were calculated. Fixed forms, such as groceries, were excluded. The mean for the SLI group was 4.4, with an *SD* of 3.2; for the MLU group the mean was 5.1, and the *SD* was 2.4. The means for the two groups did not differ significantly ($t = -1.21$, $p = .231$). In these samples, the SLI group of children produced plural markings with a total of 100 different words; the MLU-matched children, 105. It is important to emphasize that these are unique noun stems, obtained in spontaneous utterances. Thus both groups of children generated a large number of unique and varied noun types that were marked for plurality, and the groups were not differentiated by the total number of different words. It does not appear, then, that the SLI group is differentiated from their MLU-matched controls on the basis of lexical productivity.

From "Morphological Deficits of Children with SLI: Evaluation of Number Marking and Agreement," by M. L. Rice and J. B. Oetting, 1993, *Journal of Speech and Hearing Research, 36,* pp. 1249–1257. Copyright 1993 by the American Speech-Language-Hearing Association. Reprinted with permission.

parison of the two means (and the two standard deviations in Excerpt 9.20) with the *t*-statistics and associated probabilities blended right into the text of the Results sections.

The *t*-test is most appropriate for comparing two means, but sometimes multiple *t*-tests are used either to compare two groups on a number of different dependent variables or to compare more than two groups. Caution should be exerted in making such comparisons, however, because the level of significance needs to be adjusted for the additional probability of making a Type I error associated with making multiple comparisons. A commonly used correction factor for multiple comparisons is the Bonferroni procedure, which takes the number of multiple comparisons into account in setting the correct alpha level. Excerpt 9.22 shows how the Bonferroni correction was applied to multiple *t*-tests in a

EXCERPT 9.21

Results

Approximately 3,650 child utterances were transcribed and scored. The structural and conversational characteristics of these utterances were examined for systematic variations between the freeplay and interview contexts. Pairwise *t* tests were performed when appropriate to facilitate statistically the interpretation of the data obtained. The results were as follows.

Structural Characteristics

Syntax.   The children produced more utterances within the interview context ($M = 226$ utterances) than the freeplay context ($M = 139$ utterances), as shown in Table 2. A pairwise *t* test indicated that the context differences were significant statistically [$t(9) = 8.75$; $p < .01$].

From "Language Sample Collection and Analysis: Interview Compared to Freeplay Assessment Contexts," by J. L. Evans and H. K. Craig, 1992, *Journal of Speech and Hearing Research, 35,* pp. 343–353. Copyright 1992 by the American Speech-Language-Hearing Association. Reprinted with permission.

EXCERPT 9.22

Based on pilot data commensurate with Steinsapir et al.'s (1986) study that indicated greater levels of perturbation in the voices of black speakers, independent (unpaired) one-tailed t-tests were used on each acoustic measure of vocal noise to test this hypothesis. Because the three measures (frequency perturbation, amplitude perturbation, and H/N ratio) are not independent, a Bonferroni adjustment to the .05 alpha level was made to control for error (Miller, 1981).

Mean relative jitter (RAP, in percent) for the black subjects averaged 0.40%, with a fairly large standard deviation (0.36%). The white subjects' RAP averaged 0.28%, with much smaller intersubject variability ($SD = 0.12\%$). Although the standard deviation for the black subjects was almost as high as the mean and three times greater than that for the white subjects, the mean RAP of both subject groups was lower than the 0.57% reported by Takahashi and

Koike (1975) for normal Japanese males. The standard deviation they report (0.13%), however, is similar to that of the white subjects in the present study. Despite greater frequency perturbation in the black voice samples, the difference between the two subject groups was not statistically significant.

The average shimmer measured in the black and in the white samples was 0.33 dB and 0.28 dB, respectively. The difference in mean shimmer was statistically significant ($t = 2.15$, $df = 98$, $p = .016$). Both means fall well within the ranges reported in the literature for healthy young adult men (e.g., Horiguchi, Haji, Baer, & Gould, 1987; Horii, 1980, 1982; Kitajima & Gould, 1976; Orlikoff, 1990a).

The mean harmonics-to-noise (H/N) ratio for the black voice samples was 14.77 dB, which was significantly lower than the mean H/N ratio of 16.32 dB for the white samples ($t = -2.58$, $df = 98$, $p = .005$).

TABLE 2   Means, standard deviations, and ranges for the mean vocal fundamental frequency (F_0, in Hz), first (F1) and second (F2) formant frequencies (in Hz), jitter (RAP, in percent), shimmer (in dB), and harmonics-to-noise (H/N) ratio (in dB) for the black and white vowel samples used in this study

	F_0	F1	F2	Jitter	Shimmer*	H/N* Ratio
Black Samples						
M	108.85	660	1181	0.40	0.331	14.77
SD	14.48	60	90	0.36	0.150	3.38
Range	84.91–141.04	560–797	1052–1501	0.14–2.33	0.110 – 0.662	6.68–20.96
White Samples						
M	107.55	662	1181	0.28	0.275	16.32
SD	15.11	72	88	0.12	0.111	2.56
Range	82.75–148.46	515 – 898	1030 –1411	0.17–0.89	0.095 – 0.704	10.49–21.45

*Level of significance = .02.

From "Speaker Race Identification from Acoustic Cues in the Vocal Signal," by J. H. Walton and R. F. Orlikoff, 1994, *Journal of Speech and Hearing Research, 37,* pp. 738–745. Copyright 1994 by the American Speech-Language-Hearing Association. Reprinted with permission.

study comparing black and white speakers on a number of different dependent variables. Means, standard deviations, and ranges are shown in the table for six dependent variables measured for the two independent groups of subjects. The textual excerpt shows the *t*-test analysis for the three dependent variables displayed in the right three columns of the table (jitter, shimmer, and H/N ratio). Excerpt 9.23 shows how the Bonferroni correction was applied to *t*-tests and correlations in a study comparing different pairs of speakers on a number of dependent variables. In addition, the study used an arc-sine transformation of the percentage scores, a commonly employed distribution normalization procedure used with proportion or percentage scores to make them more suitable for parametric statistical analysis. The table shows the means and standard deviations for the six dependent variables for the four different groups of speakers, and the excerpt shows the cautions used in approaching the multiple comparisons with the Bonferroni and arc-sine procedures.

EXCERPT 9.23

A commercial software package (SYSTAT, Wilkinson, 1989) was used to perform a series of *t* tests to compare characteristics of the language samples obtained, frequencies of disfluencies, speaking rates, interrupting behaviors, and response time latencies of the four speaker groups (stuttering children [C-St], nonstuttering children [C-Nst], mothers of stutterers [M-St], and mothers of non-stutterers [M-NSt]). Sets of six *t* test comparisons (four independent and two correlated) at an alpha level of 0.01 for each individual comparison and 0.06 for all six comparisons in each set as a family (i.e., Bonferroni adjusted for multiple comparisons) were performed for each of these variables. The four independent sample *t* tests in each set included comparisons of C-St and C-Nst, M-St and M-Nst, C-St and M-Nst, and C-Nst and M-St. The two correlated sample *t* tests in each set compared C-St and MSt, and C-Nst and M-Nst. For percentages of within-word and between-word disfluencies as well as the frequency of all disfluencies combined, arcsine transformations were performed to make differences in percent more suitable for subsequent parametric statistical analysis (Studebaker, 1985). Post hoc nonparametric Spearman rank-correlational coefficients with Bonferroni adjustments for multiple comparisons were determined to assess relations between speaking rate, interruptions, and RTL and between these three paralinguistic variables and children's disfluencies.

. . . .

Results

Characteristics of the Language Samples

Table 2 illustrates means and standard deviations for numbers of conversational turns, utterances, words, syllables, morphemes, and mean lengths of utterances (MLU) produced by stuttering children, nonstuttering children, mothers of stuttering children, and mothers of nonstuttering children. No significant differences were found in any of the *t* test comparisons for numbers of conversational turns, utterances, words, syllables or morphemes. Mothers of nonstuttering children were found to produce significantly longer MLUs ($M = 4.338$; $SD = 0.50$) than their own children ($M = 3.405$; $SD = 0.65$; $t = 3.454$; $p < 0.01$), and than the stuttering children ($M = 3.311$; $SD = 0.80$; $t = 3.816$; $p < 0.01$).

Continued

EXCERPT 9.23 *Continued*

TABLE 2   **Means and standard deviations for numbers of conversational turns, utterances, words, syllables and morphemes and mean lengths of utterances (MLU) for stuttering (C-St) and nonstuttering (C-NSt) children and their mothers (M-St and M-NSt)**

Measures	Speaker group							
	C-St		C-NSt		M-St		M-NSt	
	M	*SD*	*M*	*SD*	*M*	*SD*	*M*	*SD*
Conversational turns	57.2	17.6	61.9	17.9	55.1	16.8	62.0	18.6
Utterances	99.0	21.2	100.6	19.7	96.7	37.2	100.7	39.5
Words	301.3	13.5	302.6	2.8	338.4	145.4	410.4	196.5
Syllables	358.1	16.1	360.1	12.6	407.0	171.4	483.7	221.2
Morphemes	312.5	20.0	327.7	9.0	375.2	161.0	447.5	203.6
MLU	3.31	0.8	3.41	0.6	3.85	0.5	4.34	0.5

From "Speaking Rates, Response Time Latencies, and Interrupting Behaviors of Young Stutterers, Nonstutterers, and Their Mothers," by E. M. Kelly and E. G. Conture, 1992, *Journal of Speech and Hearing Research, 35,* pp. 1256–1267. Copyright 1992 by the American Speech-Language-Hearing Association.

The illustration in Excerpt 9.24 shows the use of the Mann-Whitney *U* test, a nonparametric test, to make a between-subjects comparison. The Mann-Whitney *U* test, as mentioned in Chapter 6, is often referred to as a nonparametric alternative to the *t*-test because it is used to make a two-sample comparison between subjects when the requirements for the *t*-test cannot be met by the data. In the example shown in Excerpt 9.24, two different groups of subjects are compared: a group of children who were beginning stutterers and an age- and gender-matched group of children who did not stutter. The Data Analysis section explains why the Mann-Whitney *U* was used in place of the *t*-test for five of the six dependent variables, and the Results section displays the text and figure for the analysis of one of these five variables, namely duration of sound/syllable repetitions. Note that the means of the two groups were fairly similar, that there was wide variability in both groups (more so for the stutterers), and that the Mann-Whitney *U* statistic indicated no significant difference between the groups.

As mentioned previously, the Mann-Whitney *U* test is often referred to as a nonparametric alternative to the independent *t*-test because it is used to make a bivalent between-subjects comparison. It should be noted, however, that the Mann-Whitney *U* statistic is calculated in a manner different from the manner in which the *t*-statistic is calculated. Smaller values of the Mann-Whitney *U* statistic indicate a more significant difference between groups and, conversely, larger values of Mann-Whitney *U* are nonsignificant.

When a nonparametric alternative to the *t*-test is used, the author may decide to include a central tendency measure other than the mean or a variability measure other than the standard deviation in the summary statistics table. This is because the mean and

EXCERPT 9.24

Data Analysis

As will be discussed, the stuttering and nonstutter-ing children in this study contributed unequal and/or small numbers of speech disfluencies of all types, including the disfluency types of primary interest, namely sound/syllable repetitions, sound prolongations, and whole-word repetitions. These unequal or small samples can be attributed to either low production of disfluent speech in general (as in the case of the nonstuttering children), or to speech disfluencies that were acoustically unmeasurable. In order to account for discrepancies in sample sizes and make appropriate between-group comparisons, the nonparametric Mann-Whitney U test (Siegel, 1956) was used to compare the stuttering and non-stuttering children in (a) duration of sound/syllable repetitions, (b) duration of sound prolongations, (c) number of repeated units per instance of sound/syllable repetition, (d) number of repeated units per instance of whole-word repetition, and (e) proportions of different speech disfluency types. In contrast, between-group comparisons of mean fre-quency of speech disfluency (that is, the average fre-quency of disfluency in three contiguous 100-word samples) were obtained through an independent-groups *t* test with adjusted degrees of freedom.

Results

Duration of Sound/Syllable Repetitions

The 10 stuttering children produced a total of 89 sound/syllable repetitions. Of these 89 sound/syllable repetitions, 5 were acoustically unmeasur-able either because of faint or indistinct acoustic energy as displayed on the video-sound spectro-graph or because of the investigator's inability to clearly observe either the beginning or end points associated with a particular speech disfluency (Zebrowski et al., 1985). As Figure 1 shows, the mean duration of the young stutterers' measurable ($N = 84$) sound/syllable repetitions was 556 ms ($SD = 370$ ms; range = 155–1878 ms).

Nine of the 10 nonstuttering children produced a total of 21 sound/syllable repetitions, 3 of which were unmeasurable. The mean duration of the non-stuttering children's measurable ($N = 18$) sound/syl-lable repetitions was 520 ms ($SD = 245$ ms; range = 187–967 ms). Results of Mann Whitney U analysis indicated no significant between-group dif-ferences (Mann Whitney U = 38, $C = 12$; $p > .01$) in the duration of sound/syllable repetitions.

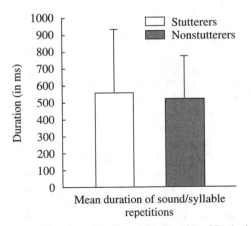

FIGURE 1
Mean duration (in ms) of acoustically measured sound/syllable repetitions produced by stuttering ($N = 10$) and nonstuttering ($N = 9$) children in one 300-word sample of conversational speech obtained from each child. Lines indicate one standard deviation above the mean.

From "Duration of the Speech Disfluencies of Beginning Stutterers," by P. M. Zebrowski, 1991, *Journal of Speech and Hearing Research, 34,* pp. 483–491. Copyright 1991 by the American Speech-Language-Hearing Association. Reprinted with permission.

standard deviation are usually associated with parametric statistics. In the example in Excerpt 9.24 the author included the mean as the measure of central tendency but used the range in addition to the standard deviation as a measure of variability.

The Mann-Whitney U test operates on the ranks of the subjects in the two groups rather than on their actual test scores. Thus, the level of measurement used for the dependent variable is ordinal. The Mann-Whitney U test would be an appropriate alternative to the t-test when the original dependent variable data are at the ordinal level of measurement or when interval- or ratio-level original data are transformed to the ordinal level of measurement for use with a nonparametric test because one of the other assumptions of a parametric test (e.g., normal distribution) cannot be met. The Wilcoxon Matched-Pairs Signed-Ranks Test (to be illustrated in the next excerpt) also makes use of ranks rather than actual scores, so that it is also appropriate for analyzing data at the ordinal level of measurement.

Excerpt 9.25 contains an illustration of the use of the Wilcoxon Matched-Pairs Signed-Ranks Test to make a bivalent within-subjects comparison. Wilcoxon's Matched-Pairs Signed-Ranks Test is often referred to as a nonparametric alternative to the dependent t-test because it is used to make a comparison of the performance of one group of subjects in two different conditions when the data are not appropriate for the use of parametric statistics. In the study by Adams and Moore, twelve stutterers were compared in two different conditions (with vs. without listening to masking noise) on four dependent variables: frequency of stuttering, vocal intensity, reading time, and palmar sweat anxiety. The Wilcoxon Matched-Pairs Signed-Ranks statistic (T) reported in the text showed significant differences only for frequency of stuttering and vocal intensity. Similar to the Mann-Whitney U test, a smaller value of the Wilcoxon statistic indicates a significant difference. Readers should observe that Adams and Moore (Excerpt 9.25) included the median and semi-interquartile range in their summary statistics as measures of central tendency and variability. The use of these descriptive statistics with a nonparametric inferential analysis is more consistent with the general practice of dealing with data for which parametric statistics are inappropriate.

EXCERPT 9.25

Statistical Analyses

Each of the four dependent variables (frequency of stuttering, palmar sweat anxiety, vocal intensity, and reading time) were compared across the two conditions. In every case, comparisons were conducted by using the nonparametric Wilcoxon Matched-Pairs Signed-Ranks Test (Siegel, 1956).

Results

Table 1 presents the median and semi-interquartile range values for the subjects' frequency of stuttering, vocal intensity, reading time, and palmar sweat anxiety in the two conditions.

First, the reduction in stuttering in the presence of noise was highly significant ($T = 0$, $N = 12$, $p < 0.005$). All 12 subjects had fewer dysfluencies in the presence of noise than in quiet. The increase in vocal intensity in the presence of noise was also significant ($T = 0$, $N = 12$, $p < 0.005$). Each of the 12 stutterers used greater vocal intensity while reading in noise than in quiet. Reading time did not differ appreciably across conditions. Six subjects took less time to read the passage in the masking condition, four took less reading time in quiet, and two exhibited no difference in reading time between conditions. The median palmar sweat measures for sub-

Continued

EXCERPT 9.25   *Continued*

TABLE 1   **Median and semi-interquartile range (Q) values for subjects' frequency of stuttering, vocal intensity, reading time, and palmar sweat anxiety in the masking and no-masking (control) conditions**

Condition	Frequency of Stutter	Vocal Intensity (dB)	Reading Time (secs)	Palmar Sweat Anxiety (microamperes)	
Masking	4.0	83.50	91.08	5.0	Median
	7.5	4.50	91.13	5.0	(Q)
No-Masking	19.0	74.50	85.83	4.5	Median
	17.5	3.50	132.83	5.5	(Q)

jects in the two conditions are almost identical. Five of the stutterers had no difference in their palmar sweat anxiety between conditions, four subjects had higher palmar sweat readings in the masking condition, and three individuals had lower palmar sweat readings with masking present. None of these previous four comparisons were influenced in any way by the order in which the subjects encountered the two conditions.

From "The Effects of Auditory Masking on the Anxiety Level, Frequency of Dysfluency, and Selected Vocal Characteristics of Stutterers," by M. R. Adams and W. H. Moore, 1972, *Journal of Speech and Hearing Research,* *15,* pp. 572–578. Copyright 1972 by the American Speech-Language-Hearing Association. Reprinted with permission.

As mentioned in Chapter 6, the X^2 statistic has a variety of uses. We have already seen it used as a measure of association in the example in Excerpt 9.16 in the correlational analysis section of this chapter. The example in Excerpt 9.26 shows the use of the X^2 statistic as an inferential test of the significance of the difference between two groups of subjects on nominal-level dependent variables that are dichotomized into two categories. The

EXCERPT 9.26

Type of Onset

Answers to the question "How did stuttering begin?" were classified according to two general types of onset, Sudden and Gradual. Sudden Onset included all responses that fell into one of three subcategories describing onset to occur with 1 day, 2–3 days, and 1 week. Gradual Onset included responses that fell into one of three subcategories describing onset to occur within 2 weeks, 3–4 weeks, and more than 5 weeks. Table 2 presents the distribution of subjects according to the two general types. One of the major results of this study, as shown in the table, is that 44% of the entire group reported what we defined as Sudden Onsets. As can be seen, males and females were similarly distributed according to the two onset types ($X^2 = 0.01$, $p = 0.92$) and the 2:1 male-to-female ratio observed for the entire sample was also maintained for each of the two types.

Continued

EXCERPT 9.26 *Continued*

TABLE 2 **The distribution of all subjects, and of males and females, according to reported onset type**

Group	N	Onset Type	
		Gradual	Sudden
All	87	49 (56%)	38 (44%)
Boys	59	33 (56%)	26 (44%)
Girls	28	16 (57%)	12 (43%)

Emotional and Physical Stress

The relationship between onset of stuttering and physical or emotional stress immediately preceding or at any time prior to onset was examined. Physical stress was identified in several questionnaire items pertaining to health history and current health status. Examples of physical stress were respiratory problems at birth, surgery or illness requiring hospitalization in infancy, asthma requiring continuing medical treatment, and acute illness shortly before stuttering onset. Examples of emotional stress were events such as divorce of parents, moving to another house, excessive sibling rivalry, or difficult day care arrangements, occurring within a few months preceding the onset of stuttering.

Table 3 shows that more subjects experienced onset without prior physical or emotional stress than with stress. Still, it is worth noticing that the reported histories of 43% of the subjects did contain indications of stress. The male-to-female ratio remained at 2:1 for with or without stress conditions. Statistical analysis yielded a Chi-square of 2.26 ($p = 0.61$) indicating that the presence or absence of stress was independent of gender. Relationships of stress to other factors will be evaluated later.

Familial Incidence

The presence or absence of family history of stuttering was also examined. Positive history was defined as at least one other first-degree (parent or sibling), second-degree (grandparent), or third-degree (blood-related aunt, uncle, or cousin) relative reported to have ever stuttered. One subject who was an adopted child was not included in this analysis.

Table 4 displays the familial incidence of stuttering data relative to gender. Although positive history was more common among males than among females, the Chi-square test indicated that the difference was not significant ($X^2 = 0.83$, $p = 0.32$).

TABLE 3 **The distribution of stuttering onset associated with emotional or physical stress**

Group	N	Stress	
		With	Without
All	87	37 (43%)	50 (57%)
Boys	59	24 (41%)	35 (59%)
Girls	28	13 (46%)	15 (54%)

Continued

EXCERPT 9.26   *Continued*

TABLE 4   **The distribution of all subjects, and of males and females, according to positive and negative familial history of stuttering**

		History	
Group	*N*	Positive	Negative
All	86*	57 (66%)	29 (34%)
Boys	58*	40 (69%)	18 (31%)
Girls	28	17 (61%)	11 (39%)

*No family history available for one adopted subject.

From "Onset of Stuttering in Preschool Children: Selected Factors," by E. Yairi and N. Ambrose, 1992, *Journal of Speech and Hearing Research, 35,* pp. 782–788. Copyright 1992 by the American Speech-Language-Hearing Association. Reprinted with permission.

X^2 statistic may also be encountered when more than two groups of subjects are compared or when groups are compared on a nominal variable that can be categorized in more than two ways. These comparisons can sometimes become somewhat cumbersome or difficult to interpret if there are too many categories but can be useful with a few categories. The X^2 statistic is similar to the *t*-test in the determination of its significance; that is, higher values of the X^2 statistic are needed to indicate statistical significance, and lower values indicate the lack of significant differences between the groups of subjects.

In the example in Excerpt 9.26, a comparison is made between males and females in three dependent variables: the type of onset of their stuttering, the presence of emotional or physical stress at onset, and their family histories of stuttering. Because the independent variable, gender, and the three dependent variables, type of stuttering onset, presence of stress, and family history of stuttering, were all measured at the nominal level of measurement, X^2 tests were used to test the significance of the difference between boys and girls first in type of stuttering onset, second in presence of stress at onset, and third in family history of stuttering. Table 2 in the excerpt compares boys and girls on type of stuttering onset, which was classified as gradual or sudden. Inspection of Table 2 in the excerpt shows a similar distribution of gradual vs. sudden onset for both boys and girls (note the percentages in parentheses in addition to the absolute frequencies, since the total number of boys and girls was different as would be expected in any sample of children who stutter). The X^2 statistic indicated in the textual excerpt was quite small (0.01), indicating no significant difference between boys and girls in the distribution of onset type. Table 3 shows a similar distribution of stress presence vs. absence for both boys and girls, and the X^2 statistic indicated in the text was low again (2.26), indicating no significant difference between genders. Finally, Table 4 shows the family history data, which are similar for boys and girls, and the X^2 statistic in the text was 0.83, indicating no gender difference as well.

The bivalent statistical inference tests previously discussed were used for making comparisons between two different groups of subjects in a between-subjects research design or for comparing the same subjects' performances in two different conditions in a within-subjects research design. However, when more than two samples are compared simultaneously (as in multivalent or parametric research studies), these two-sample comparison statistics are usually replaced by a statistical procedure for making simultaneous comparisons of more than two samples of data. The analysis of variance (ANOVA) was described in Chapter 6 as an appropriate statistical test for analyzing differences among three or more groups of subjects or among three or more conditions. For example, a multivalent between-subjects experiment might have three different groups of subjects representing three levels of the independent variable; a multivalent within-subjects experiment might have one group of subjects measured under three different conditions that reflect three levels of the independent variable. A parametric experiment might have two groups of subjects (representing two levels of a between-subjects independent variable) performing under two different conditions (representing two levels of a within-subjects independent variable).

The ANOVA allows the researcher to test the main effect of each independent variable and the interaction effects among the independent variables. The number of independent variables tested in an ANOVA is usually referred to as the number of *ways* of the ANOVA (e.g., a one-way ANOVA tests only one independent variable, a two-way ANOVA tests two independent variables simultaneously, a three-way ANOVA tests three independent variables simultaneously). As indicated in Chapter 6, ANOVAs are available for making between-subjects comparisons, within-subjects comparisons (sometimes called *repeated measures* comparisons because the measurement with each subject is repeated in each condition), and a combination of a between-subjects comparison on one independent variable and a within-subjects comparison on another independent variable (called a *mixed model* ANOVA).

Excerpt 9.27 illustrates the use of a one-way ANOVA making a between-subjects comparison in a study of age differences in auditory/articulatory correspondences. Forty-five children were measured, fifteen each in the age groups five, six, and seven years old, on metaphonological tasks designed to study their knowledge of auditory and articulatory correspondences. Table 1 in the excerpt shows the means, standard deviations, and ranges of the performances of the three age groups on a nonverbal matching task in which children had to match an auditory and a visual stimulus without using a verbal response. As can be seen from the table, the mean performances increased from the younger to the older children. The results of the one-way, between-subjects ANOVA are described in the textual excerpt. The overall F indicated significant difference across the age variable, and specific Sheffe contrast tests indicated that the two younger groups were different from the older group but not from each other (i.e., groups aged five and six differed from children aged seven). A one-way between-subjects ANOVA is the simplest, most straightforward version of this statistical procedure and more complex designs build upon this concept of simultaneous statistical inference with one test.

Results

Nonverbal Matching

The mean number of correct responses on the non-verbal matching task was computed for each age group (see Table 1 for descriptive statistics). The results of a one-way analysis of variance (ANOVA) revealed significant differences among group means $(F(2, 42) = 34.22, p < .001)$. A Scheffe post-hoc comparison (Weinberg & Goldberg, 1979) revealed significant differences between ages 5 and 7 $(F = 32.66, p < .001)$ and between ages 6 and 7 $(F = 16.00, p < .001)$.

TABLE 1 Number of correct responses on nonverbal matching task by three age groups

Age group	*M*	*SD*	Range
5 (*N* = 15)	10.93	1.751	8–14
6 (*N* = 15)	12.67	2.664	8–17
7 (*N* = 15)	16.73	1.223	14–18

From "Children's Knowledge of Auditory/Articulatory Correspondences: Phonologic and Metaphonologic," by H. B. Klein, S. H. Lederer, and E. E. Cortese, 1991, *Journal of Speech and Hearing Research, 34,* pp. 559–564. Copyright 1991 by the American Speech-Language-Hearing Association. Reprinted with permission.

The next example in Excerpt 9.28 shows a two-way ANOVA design with a between-subjects comparison made on each independent variable. The first independent variable was fluency, with two levels represented by two different groups: the stuttering vs. non-stuttering children. The second independent variable was age, with five levels represented by the five different groups: seven, eight, nine, ten, and eleven-plus years of age. The dependent variable was a thirty-five-item Dutch version of the Communication Attitude Test (CAT-D), in which a higher score indicates a more negative attitude toward speech and a lower score indicates a more positive attitude toward speech. Table 1 displays the means and standard deviations of stuttering and nonstuttering groups (further subdivided by gender, which was not analyzed in the ANOVA because of the small number of female stutterers—see textual excerpt for an explanation of this), and Table 2 displays the means and standard deviations of different age groups. Table 3 is the ANOVA summary table and indicates a significant F-ratio for group and group by age interaction, but an insignificant F-ratio for age as an independent variable main effect. Figure 1 shows the obvious difference in means between stuttering and nonstuttering children at each age level; notice also that standard deviations show some overlap at the younger ages but almost no overlap at the older ages. The figure also shows how the stuttering and nonstuttering groups diverged as age increased: stuttering children's CAT-D scores increased with older ages and non-stuttering children's CAT-D scores decreased with age. Table 4 displays the contrast tests comparing fluency groups at each age and the mean squares and F-ratios all show greater

EXCERPT 9.28

One of the purposes of the present study was to compare the speech attitudes of stuttering and nonstuttering children at different age groups. Toward this end, both subject groups were subdivided into five age levels (7, 8, 9, 10, and 11-plus years). The sample size in each of these five age groups for the stutterers was 24, 13, 10, 9, and 14, respectively, and for the nonstuttering controls, 62, 40, 42, 41, and 86, respectively. A two-way analysis of variance was used to evaluate whether the CAT-D scores of the stuttering and the nonstuttering children differed statistically across the five age levels and whether there was a significant group × age interaction.

Results

The mean CAT-D scores, and their standard deviations, for the stutterers and the nonstuttering children are presented in Table 1. The stuttering children obtained notably higher mean test scores than did their controls; indeed, the overall CAT-D score for the stutterers was almost twice that of the nonstuttering children.

Also shown in Table 1 are the mean scores for the male and the female subjects. The descriptive difference between the groups was present also for the sexes. Both the boys and the girls who stuttered scored higher on the CAT-D than did their nonstuttering peers. Interestingly, within the group of stutterers, the females obtained a notably higher CAT-D score than did the males. This sex difference was not apparent among the nonstuttering children (see also Brutten & Dunham, 1989). This finding may suggest the presence of gender differences in speech attitudes among stutterers. However, because the number of female stutterers studied in the present investigation was so small, a separate analysis of their scores was not justified.

Another purpose of the present study was to analyze whether the differences in CAT-D scores of the two subject groups were influenced by the age level of the children. In this respect, the data summarized in Table 2 show that the average CAT-D score of the stuttering children was descriptively higher than that of their nonstuttering peers at each of the five age levels studied.

A two-way analysis of variance (BMDP4V) was used to test whether the observed difference between the CAT-D scores of the two subject groups across all age levels was statistically significant, and whether a significant group × age level interaction existed (Table 3).

A significant main effect was found between the CAT-D scores of the stuttering and the nonstuttering children, $F(1, 331) = 97.66$; $p < 0.05$. In other words, the stuttering children, as a group, obtained significantly higher scores on the CAT-D than did the control subjects. The ANOVA also revealed a significant group × age level interaction, $F(4, 331) = 2.71$; $p < .05$. Thus, the difference in the

TABLE 1   Descriptive statistics of the CAT-D scores for the stuttering and the nonstuttering children as a group and subdivided by sex

Group	N	M	SD
Stutterers			
Male	63	15.95	7.28
Female	7	23.29	2.69
Total	70	16.69	7.29
Nonstutterers			
Male	134	8.57	5.22
Female	137	8.85	5.84
Total	271	8.71	5.53

Continued

EXCERPT 9.28   *Continued*

TABLE 2   Descriptive statistics of the CAT-D scores for the stuttering and the nonstuttering children at each of five age levels

Group	N	M	SD
Stutterers			
7 years	24	14.79	6.62
8 years	13	17.23	9.86
9 years	10	17.60	6.35
10 years	9	18.56	6.80
11 years +	14	17.57	6.93
Nonstutterers			
7 years	62	9.98	5.57
8 years	40	10.35	4.49
9 years	42	10.62	5.92
10 years	41	8.20	5.17
11 years +	86	6.34	5.12

TABLE 3   Two-way analysis of variance of the CAT-D scores of the stuttering and the nonstuttering children at five different age levels

Source	SS	df	MS	F	p
Group	3228.93	1	3228.93	97.66	.00
Age	146.05	4	36.51	1.10	.35
Group × age	358.06	4	89.52	2.71	.03
Error	10943.97	331	33.06		

CAT-D scores of the two subject groups was dependent upon the age level of the children. A simple effects analysis (BMDP4V), the results of which are summarized in Table 4, was used to examine this interaction effect in more detail.

The between-group difference in CAT-D scores was found to be statistically significant at each of the five age levels. That is to say, the stuttering children at each level scored significantly higher on the CAT-D than did their nonstuttering peers. However, as the significant group × age level interaction indicated (Table 3), the magnitude of the between-group difference at the various age levels was not equal. This finding is consistent with the descriptive data, summarized in Table 2, that show that the

between-group difference in the mean CAT-D scores was larger at the older age levels than at the younger ones. Closer inspection of the scores in Table 2 suggested that this growing discrepancy between the two groups was due to a differential trend in CAT-D scores among the subjects at the different age levels. The stuttering children tended to show somewhat higher CAT-D scores with increasing age, a trend which was most apparent at the younger age groups. An opposite trend could be observed among the nonstutterers. The mean CAT-D scores of the nonstuttering children decreased after age 9. Figure 1 makes this trend difference in the performance of the two subject groups apparent.

Continued

EXCERPT 9.28 *Continued*

TABLE 4 **Simple effects analysis of the CAT-D scores of the stuttering and the nonstuttering children at five different age levels**

Source	SS	df	MS	F	p
Group—7 yrs	399.94	1	399.94	12.10	.00
Group—8 yrs	464.52	1	464.52	14.05	.00
Group—9 yrs	393.62	1	393.62	11.90	.00
Group—10 yrs	792.16	1	792.16	23.96	.00
Group—11 yrs+	1519.54	1	1519.54	45.96	.00
Error	109343.97	331	33.06		

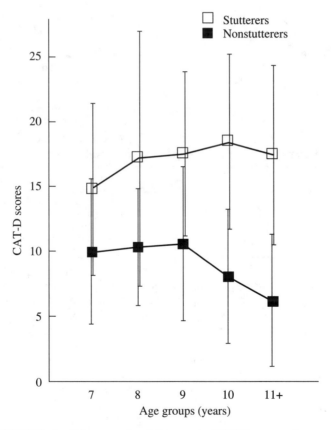

FIGURE 1 **Line graph of the mean CAT-D scores (squares) and their standard deviations (extensions) for the stuttering and the nonstuttering children at five different age levels**

group differences at the older ages. This divergent age pattern for the two groups resulted in an averaging of CAT-D scores for ages across groups that made age a nonsignificant factor: in other words, CAT-D scores averaged across groups did not vary significantly as age increased. The text explains the ANOVA results quite clearly and thoroughly and makes careful reference to the tables and figure in presenting each difference.

Excerpt 9.29 illustrates the use of an analysis of variance for the comparison of two groups of subjects (children with normal articulation vs. children with impaired articulation) performing under three different conditions (responding to digits, random words, and words in sentences). A mixed model ANOVA was used to compare the performances of the two groups of children (between-subjects comparison) as the first main effect. The second main effect examined was the difference between the three stimulus presentation conditions (within-subjects comparison). Finally, the interaction effect between subject groups and stimulus conditions was evaluated. The results of these three parts of the analysis of variance are shown in the figure, table, and text included in the excerpt.

Figure 1 in Excerpt 9.29 is a bar graph depicting the mean number of stimuli correctly recalled by the two groups of children in each of the stimulus conditions. The table is a

---

EXCERPT 9.29

Results

Number of Items Recalled

Figure 1 is a graph of the mean number of items recalled correctly by the two groups of children for the three types of stimulus material. A groups-by-stimulus-material-type analysis of variance (ANOVA), with repeated measures on material type (Winer, 1962), was performed on the number of

items recalled to determine which of the recall performance differences were statistically significant. Results of the ANOVA (summarized in Table 1) were that the groups-by-stimulus-material interaction was significant ($p < 0.01$), as were each of the main effects. Because of the significant interaction, group means for each of the stimulus-material-type conditions were analyzed. The group with good articulation recalled significantly more items than

TABLE 1   Summary of ANOVA to test for differences in mean number of items recalled for 28 children with poor articulation and 28 children with good articulation for three stimulus material types

Source	df	MS	F	p
Between Subjects	55	2.22	—	—
Groups (B)	1	36.21	22.77	<0.01
Error (S within B)	54	1.59	—	—
Within Subjects	112	10.11	—	—
Stimulus material (A)	2	338.04	206.11	<0.01
Stimulus material × groups (A × B)	2	9.13	5.57	<0.01
Error (A × S within B)	108	1.64	—	—

Continued

EXCERPT 9.29 *Continued*

did the group with poor articulation when the word items were cast as sentences ($F = 29.61$; df 1,108; $p < 0.01$). The two groups did not perform differently on the digit or random-word tasks. Both groups were found to recall significantly ($p < 0.01$) more items on the sentence task than on the digit or random-word tasks. (See Figure 1.)

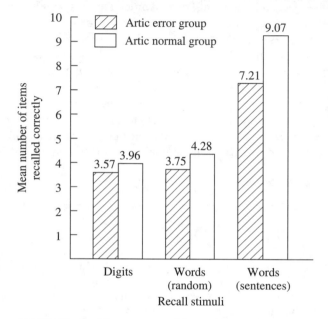

FIGURE 1   **The mean number of items (string length) recalled correctly by the articulation-error ($N = 28$) and articulation-normal ($N = 28$) groups for each of the three types of stimulus material**

From "Short-Term Memory and Language Skills in Articulation-Deficient Children," by J. H. Saxman and J. F. Miller, 1973, *Journal of Speech and Hearing Research, 16,* pp. 721–730. Copyright 1973 by the American Speech-Language-Hearing Association. Reprinted with permission.

complete ANOVA summary table similar to the one described in Chapter 6. The between-subjects and within-subjects main effects and the interaction effect are listed in the left column and the degrees of freedom, mean squares, F-ratios, and significance levels are listed in the other columns for each main effect and interaction. In such an ANOVA, significant differences are indicated by large F-ratios and nonsignificant differences are indicated by smaller F-ratios, although the absolute value of a significant F depends on the number of degrees of freedom associated with each comparison.

The F was significant for the main effect of the between-subjects comparison, indicating that the normal and articulation-impaired children performed differently on the recall task. The within-subjects F for the comparison of the effects of the different stimulus materials was also significant, indicating that recall performance was not the same for the different stimuli. The stimulus material by groups interaction was also significant, indicating that the two groups of children performed differently on the different types of material. This interaction effect is further explored in the text with references to the figure. Saxman and Miller indicated in the text that follow-up comparisons with contrast tests of specific pairs of means (e.g., normal vs. articulation-impaired children on recall of words in sentences) revealed that the two groups of children did not perform differently on recall of digits or random words but that they did perform differently on recall of words in sentences. This finding is the essence of the interaction effect and the most important result of this analysis of variance.

Inspection of Figure 1 in Excerpt 9.29 confirms the notion that the two groups of children were different in their recall of words in sentences but not in their recall of either digits or random words. A greater separation of the means of the two groups can be seen for the words in sentences than for the digits or random words when the figure is inspected closely. In this example, a rather thorough recounting of the analysis of variance was provided that included the ANOVA summary table, the figure, and a narrative description of the comparisons.

Some Characteristics of Good Data Analysis

The analysis of data in a Results section should present a clear picture of the strength and direction of relationships or of the significant differences that were found. Readers should expect some of the following characteristics of good analysis of data.

Illustrations that are used in the analysis of relationships or differences should conform to the same standards that were discussed earlier in the section on organization of data. Table and figure captions should be brief but informative. Tables and figures should be capable of standing alone in presenting the analysis, and the narrative should dovetail easily with the illustrations in the discussion of the data analysis.

The analysis of relationships should employ statistical techniques that are appropriate to such factors as the level of measurement of the data and the number of observations. Readers should be aware of the general appropriateness of indices such as the Pearson and Spearman correlation coefficients, the X^2, and the contingency coefficient that are used in the analysis of relationships. The significance levels of the correlations that are reported should be included when necessary, and consumers may also expect authors to comment on the practical meaning of correlations, as well as their statistical significance. This may often be accompanied by reference to the index of determination (R^2) in discussing the overlap of variance among variables.

The evaluation of intercorrelation matrices or of multiple regression analyses may be particularly difficult for novice consumers. Authors may aid consumers in this task through careful presentation and discussion of these analyses, especially in the integration of the narrative with the illustrations. Despite this, evaluation of multiple correlation and regression analyses will usually require more time and effort from consumers. Frequent exposure to multiple correlation studies should serve to sharpen the reader's evaluative skills in this area.

The analysis of differences should employ statistical techniques that are appropriate to the level of measurement used, the number of observations, the number of comparisons, and so forth. Readers should be aware of the appropriateness of parametric and nonparametric inference tests. Readers should also be cognizant of the appropriate uses of two-sample comparison statistics and of the need for analysis of variance techniques for simultaneous comparisons. These analyses should present a clear and consistent summary of significant and nonsignificant differences and of main and interaction effects when necessary. Such analyses often include reference to both a table and a figure to clarify the narrative explanation of the differences found. Multiple comparisons with complex interactions may present some difficulty to novice consumers; once again, authors may aid these readers through careful integration of tables, figures, and text.

EVALUATION CHECKLIST

Instructions: The four-category scale at the end of this checklist may be used to rate the *Results* section of an article. The *Evaluation Items* help identify those topics that should be considered in arriving at the rating. Comments on these topics, entered as *Evaluation Notes,* should serve as the basis for the overall rating.

Evaluation Items   *Evaluation Notes*

1. Results were clearly related to research problem.

2. Tables and figures were integrated with text.

3. Summary statistics were used appropriately.

4. Organization of data was clear.

5. Statistical analysis was appropriate to:

    (a) level of measurement

    (b) number of observations

    (c) type of sample

    (d) shape of distribution

6. There was appropriate use of correlational and inferential analysis.

7. There was clear presentation of significant and nonsignificant correlations.

8. There was clear presentation of significant and nonsignificant differences.

9. General comments.

Overall Rating (Results):

_____	_____	_____	_____
Poor	Fair	Good	Excellent

Chapter *10*

The Discussion and Conclusions Section

The last section of an article, usually titled *Discussion* or *Conclusions* or both, is written with somewhat more license than are the other sections, and readers may often notice more variation among authors in the organization of this section. In fact, consumers of research may encounter shorter articles that combine the results and conclusions into one section. Nevertheless, there are some general topics that are usually addressed at the end of an article, and consumers of research should be aware of the importance of these in the culmination of a research article. Five general topics will be included in our evaluation checklist for the Discussion and Conclusions section:

> Relationship of Conclusions to Preceding Parts of the Article
> Relationship of Results to Previous Research
> Theoretical Implications of the Research
> Practical Implications of the Research
> Implications for Future Research

Each of these general topics will be discussed separately in the next five sections.

Relationship of Conclusions to Preceding Parts of the Article

The discussion section should contain some material that relates the conclusions directly to the *Problem, Method,* and *Results* of the investigation and that unites the preceding sections into a coherent whole.

The Research Problem

The conclusions of a research article should be directed clearly toward the *research problem* that was presented in the first section of the article. Complete restatement of the problem and rationale would be cumbersome at this point in an article, but in many of the better articles in the literature, the discussion commences with a brief reminder of the problem and a general statement of the conclusion of the investigation regarding the problem or research questions.

Excerpts 10.1 and 10.2 present introductory paragraphs from two Discussion sections that neatly remind readers of the research problem and quickly summarize the results in relation to the problem. The conclusions of both studies reflect clearly and directly on the research problems and set the stage for further discussion of the limitations and implications of the research.

Some of the longer research articles that include several specific research questions or subproblems may devote a section of the Discussion to a more complete review of the research questions and results as an overall summary. This is particularly appropriate when

---

EXCERPT 10.1 Discussion

The aim of this study was to determine if children with SLI and no history of neurological disease demonstrate evidence of an absent or depressed cortical evoked potential to frequency-modulated tones. The results obtained were unequivocal. Averaged cortically evoked responses to these complex acoustic stimuli were obtained in all children regardless of whether they were normal language learners or children with SLI. These results therefore provide strong evidence against this physiological response characteristic serving as a phenotypic marker for SLI.

From "Auditory Evoked Responses to Frequency-Modulated Tones in Children with Specific Language Impairment," by J. B. Tomblin, P. J. Abbas, N. L. Records, and L. M. Brenneman, 1995, *Journal of Speech and Hearing Research, 38,* pp. 387–392. Copyright 1995 by the American Speech-Language-Hearing Association. Reprinted with permission.

EXCERPT 10.2 Discussion

It will be recalled that this study was conducted to see if the reduction in stuttering during singing is related to altered vocalization as suggested by Wingate (1969) or to the familiarity of the lyrics of the song being sung, or both. The results of the present investigation clearly indicated that during singing altered vocalization in the form of extended utterance duration and the familiarity of the lyrics being sung are both associated with significant decrements in stuttering frequency.

From "Factors Contributing to the Reduction of Stuttering during Singing," by E. C. Healey, A. R. Mallard, and M. R. Adams, 1976, *Journal of Speech and Hearing Research, 19,* pp. 475–480. Copyright 1976 by the American Speech-Language-Hearing Association. Reprinted with permission.

the results are lengthy, complex, or concern several related issues. Excerpt 10.3 shows how Folkins summarized four research questions and the manner in which his data addressed each of them in a separate conclusion section at the end of a lengthy article on muscle activity involved in jaw closing during speech.

EXCERPT 10.3 Conclusions

The following is a review of the above data in relation to the four issues raised in the introduction:

1. How is elevation of the mandible during speech divided between the muscles? Based on the data presented here medial pterygoid seems to be involved in all jaw-closing movements, but masseter and temporalis often play a role, especially for larger movements. Recordings from lateral pterygoid differed substantially between subjects and tasks. In future studies it will be important to develop techniques to specify whether recordings are from the inferior or superior heads of lateral pterygoid.

2. Do timing parameters vary between different muscles? As illustrated in Figure 3, no consistent differences in the timing of peak EMG activity were found between muscles. The duration of medial pterygoid activity tended to be longer than temporalis or masseter, as shown in Figure 4.

3. Are there relations between the timing of muscle activity and jaw-closing movements? In some instances peak EMG activity tended to occur later when displacement was increased, but this usually was not so.

4. Are the relative levels of involvement between muscles kept in the same ratio relations or are the relative levels of activity variable? When jaw-closing movements were repeated for a train of syllables, the muscles were sometimes maintained at similar levels from syllable to syllable, but in many instances the relative amounts of EMG activity changed dramatically for similar jaw movements.

From "Muscle Activity for Jaw Closing during Speech," J. W. Folkins, 1981, *Journal of Speech and Hearing Research, 24*, pp. 601–615. Copyright 1981 by the American Speech-Language-Hearing Association. Reprinted with permission.

The Method of Investigation

The Discussion section should also present some remarks concerning the *method* of the investigation and how it relates to the conclusion of the study. Any limitations of the research imposed by the particular method should be considered. Qualifying remarks may be found concerning the subjects, materials, or procedures employed and how they may have limited the conclusions that may be drawn from the data.

Of particular concern is the manner in which the author discusses the potential threats to internal and external validity in the investigation and how these threats may have been reduced in the design of the study. As readers will have surmised, every empirical investigation may be subject to some threats to internal and external validity, and the better studies are those that minimize these threats. Minimization implies, however, that there is usually some residue of jeopardy to internal and external validity. This residue should be addressed in the Discussion section in order to qualify the conclusions and, perhaps, to suggest future research possibilities to improve or extend the findings of the investigation.

The better studies in the literature, then, are those that not only reduce the threats to internal and external validity but also discuss the residue of jeopardy with some candor in qualifying the results. Of course, if an inordinately large number of research design limitations are discussed, readers may question the wisdom of the journal editor for publishing the study in the first place. In other words, as the limitations become more extensive and significant, the value of the research is reduced accordingly.

The next four excerpts from Discussion sections illustrate the ways in which authors have considered various limitations of the method of investigation and discussed appropriate qualifications of their conclusions based on these limitations. Excerpt 10.4 is taken from a Discussion subsection, entitled Some Qualifications, and considers some problems of internal validity associated with "transitory factors" that could affect children's performances and instrumentation and the problem of sample size related to external validity.

EXCERPT 10.4   Discussion

Some Qualifications

The sampling procedure employed in this study was utilized as a means of insuring that the subjects' utterances would be directly comparable. Since this study examined semantic relations reflected in language usage, it was critical that utterances in response to the same stimuli be obtained from each subject. On the other hand, it is recognized that a complete set of proposition rules could not be written with a 50-utterance corpus. The proposition rules written merely represented some of the child's semantic relation system. The small sample size no doubt made the acquired data more likely to be altered by moods or other transitory factors affecting a child's linguistic performance. The questions asked of the child were quite open ended, however, and judging from the Morehead and Ingram (1973) finding that children's spontaneous and "response" utterances did not differ, we believed that the use of such questions would have benefits over comparisons of language samples in a setting with no controls. It appears that unless one can acquire utterances numbering in the several hundreds as seen in normative studies (Bloom, 1970; Brown, 1973)

such "purely" naturalistic samples might be risky for comparative purposes. Nevertheless, the use of specific questions does leave the possibility that the child's language usage was influenced by his ability to comprehend the questions. It would also be difficult to dismiss the possibility that the experimenter's questions affected to some extent the form and content of the child's sampled language.

Though the language-disordered children in this study represented a random sample of children requiring language intervention, the number of disordered children employed (20) was not sufficiently extensive to rule out the exclusion of disordered children demonstrating language usage quite dissimilar to the usage described in this investigation. Caution should therefore be taken in interpreting the present data as representative of all language-disordered children's usage.

From "An Examination of the Semantic Relations Reflected in the Language Usage of Normal and Language-Disordered Children," by L. B. Leonard, J. G. Bolders, and J. A. Miller, 1976, *Journal of Speech and Hearing Research, 19,* pp. 371–392. Copyright 1976 by the American Speech-Language-Hearing Association. Reprinted with permission.

Excerpt 10.5 is from a study of physical and perceptual measures of hypernasality and discusses two limitations in method. The first limitation concerns the problem of using a perceptual measure of hypernasality as an outside criterion for validating physical measures of hypernasality, and the second problem concerns the use of simulated hypernasality instead of samples of speakers who were actually hypernasal. Despite these admitted

EXCERPT 10.5

An inherent problem in establishing the validity of a method of measuring physical correlates of hypernasality stems in part from the fact that perceptual measures themselves are not highly reliable. The less-than-desirable reliability of hypernasal ratings, in turn, appears to result from the fact that the percept of hypernasality in speech is multidimensional in nature, being influenced by such factors as nasal emission noise, misarticulation, compensatory substitutions, loudness, and pitch, in addition to acoustic consequences of velopharyngeal incompetence. Observer bias and the amount of experience with the hypernasal speech of cleft palate, deaf, dysarthric speakers, and so forth, are also known to influence listener reliability of nasality ratings.

In view of the problem, it was encouraging to find a reasonably high correlation between the N/V ratio and the perceived hypernasality scores derived from naive listeners. The paired-comparison paradigm undoubtedly helped to reduce the difficulty of the lis-teners' task in rating hypernasality in the speech samples. Admittedly, the use of simulated hypernasality weakens the conclusion of this study, although all the speech samples were judged by three speech-language pathologists experienced in voice evaluation as representative of hypernasal speech of various degrees. Further investigation is needed to examine how the N/V ratio would correlate with mechano physiological measures such as velar height, velopharyngeal wall distance, velopharyngeal orifice size, and so forth. Compilation of normative data on the N/V ratio for children and adults also needs to be made for the method to be used as an aid to diagnostic and therapeutic procedures.

From "An Accelerometric Measure as a Physical Correlate of Perceived Hypernasality in Speech," by Y. Horii, 1983, *Journal of Speech and Hearing Research, 26*, pp. 476–480. Copyright 1983 by the American Speech-Language-Hearing Association. Reprinted with permission.

limitations, reasonable correlations were found between physical and perceptual measures of hypernasality and the author makes some valuable suggestions for collection of normative data with the physical measure.

Excerpt 10.6 presents a caveat regarding a possible carry-over sequencing effect that could not be controlled by counterbalancing or randomizing conditions or using a between-subjects design. Notice how the author tries to entertain three possible explanations for the

EXCERPT 10.6

Before offering possible explanations for these results, a caveat is in order. This experiment required that the subject perform the speech task first to increase the possibility that stuttering samples would be obtained in addition to the fluent tokens. It is possible that the state of excitability for the speech task carried over into the finger counting task. Thus, we must view our conclusions with caution. We are left with at least three possibilities: (a) a *radiation effect:* discoordination of fine motor control in severe stutterers that includes not only speech muscles but hand muscles, (b) a *generalized* arousal effect: carry over effects of performing the speech task before the finger task, and/or (c) a *speech mediation effect:* greater execution time for the finger task not due to difficulties in hand coordination but possibly because subjects were "speaking to themselves" as they counted on their fingers. Further research is needed to test these possibilities.

From "Initiation versus Execution Time during Manual and Oral Counting by Stutterers," by G. Borden, 1983, *Journal of Speech and Hearing Research, 26*, pp. 389–396. Copyright 1983 by the American Speech-Language-Hearing Association. Reprinted with permission.

results in light of this problem and suggests that future research is needed to examine these possible explanations.

Excerpt 10.7 is from a study of communication between infants with hearing loss and their hearing mothers and concerns the subject-selection threat to external validity. This excerpt shows how it may be difficult to generalize to mother-child pairs that were less advantaged in regard to the provision of early intervention services. In addition, it is pointed out that conclusions could be drawn about maternal attempts to communicate but not about the perception of maternal language by the infants.

EXCERPT 10.7   Discussion

Findings from the current study should be interpreted in light of the relatively advantaged status of the participating families of infants with a hearing loss compared to many other such families. In addition to potential benefits from early identification of infant hearing loss and early provision of intervention services, these families were advantaged by the relatively high educational levels of mothers and the absence of potentially disabling medical or cognitive-motor conditions in the infants. Therefore, findings may not be generalizable to other portions of the population of infants with hearing loss.

In this study, hearing mothers directed as much language toward infants with hearing loss as toward hearing infants. No estimate was made regarding the amount of maternal language that could actually

be perceived by the infants with hearing loss, so no claim is made here that the language model available to the two groups of infants was the same. However, the fact that the two groups of mothers did not differ in frequency of production of language suggests that the mothers of infants with hearing loss had not "given up" trying to communicate with them and were continuing to interact with their infants in verbal as well as nonverbal ways.

From "Communication Behaviors of Infants with Hearing Loss and Their Hearing Mothers," by P. E. Spencer, 1993, *Journal of Speech and Hearing Research, 36*, pp. 311–321. Copyright 1993 by the American Speech-Language-Hearing Association. Reprinted with permission.

The Results of the Investigation

The conclusions in the Discussion section should be drawn directly and fairly from the results. Although the Discussion section should not be merely a rehashing of the results, authors often refer to the data to support their conclusions. Occasionally, authors may even include a table or figure in the Discussion section to summarize their own results and, perhaps, the results of other studies to aid in the presentation of the conclusions. The important point is that the conclusions should be tied directly and fairly to empirical results, and comments that are not empirically based should be labeled as speculations, not as conclusions. Speculations are often important in the generation of new research and contribute to the creativity that is important in designing new research, but authors and readers alike must be aware of the difference between solid conclusions drawn directly from empirical data and intuitive speculations about the nature of phenomena.

Excerpt 10.8 is the entire Discussion section from a study that compared adult normal language users with a group of adults with well-documented histories of specific language impairment and presents some obvious conclusions regarding differences between the two groups. The results are discussed directly with regard to the original motivation for the

EXCERPT 10.8   Discussion

The primary motivation for this study was the need to identify a set of valid measures and associated decision criteria for the diagnosis of specific language impairment in adults that can then be used for family pedigree studies. When this study was initiated, it was not known whether it would be possible to detect any residual signs of language impairment in adults with histories of SLI, because there had been little previous research describing the language characteristics of such individuals. The data from this study, however, indicated that adults with histories of SLI in childhood continue to present language behaviors that allow them to be differentiated from a group of similar individuals who do not have such a history of communication impairment. Two different sets of language and cognitive measures, one that could be used in a face-to-face setting and one that could be administered over the telephone, yielded predicted classification error rates of .03 and .05, respectively. These results suggest that very accurate diagnoses of adults with SLI should be possible, enabling us to construct accurate family pedigrees. A cautionary note should be raised, however. The data obtained from these subjects was not obtained under blind circumstances where the examiner was not aware of the subject's diagnostic status. To the extent that this knowledge could influence the scores obtained by these subjects, the diagnostic accuracy reported could be inflated. However, the measures employed were primarily standardized with objective scoring standards, and two of them, temporal processing and confrontation naming, were under computer control. Thus, it was unlikely that there was much room for bias in these data.

For each test battery, the classification errors produced by the discriminant analysis all involved the placement of SLI cases in the class of normal-language subjects. All normal-language individuals were correctly classified; that is, their sensitivity was 1.00. This slight bias toward classifying language-impaired subjects as normal results from the fact that all subjects were given an a priori prob-

ability of .80 of having normal language skills. The resultant tendency to classify language-impaired individuals as normal will introduce a bias against a genetic pattern being discovered in the pedigrees generated with this system. This tendency therefore makes this a conservative instrument for genetic hypotheses.

It should also be pointed out that the test batteries evaluated in this study, as well as the discriminant functions, provide information on the language status of adults, but this must be supplemented with hearing and nonverbal intelligence information in order to determine the person's status with respect to SLI. Thus, only those people identified as language impaired by the discriminant function who also have normal nonverbal intelligence and normal hearing as children would be considered specifically language impaired.

The levels of diagnostic accuracy obtained in future samples tested with these batteries will deviate from these predicted values to the extent that the population of people with language impairment differ in the nature or severity of the language problem and to the extent to which the prevalence of language impairment deviates from .20. The population used in this study consisted of young adults; however, most of the adults in a pedigree will be the parents and grandparents of language-impaired children and, therefore, will be older than the subjects in this study. It was necessary to use young adults in this study because of the need to have people with documented language impairment. The systematic assessment of language with standardized assessment instruments did not become common in the clinics we sampled until the early 1970s; therefore, clients who were older than our subjects usually had very limited data in their clinical files on their language status and could not be used.

The fact that our subjects were younger than those who would typically be the adult relatives in a pedigree study required that we be concerned that a decrement in performance associated with age on the measures to be used for diagnosis could lead to

Continued

EXCERPT 10.8   Discussion   *Continued*

an over-identification of SLI in older adults. Because of this, we attempted, whenever possible, to use measures in this study that had been normed or studied with older adults. The MAE provides for age and educational adjustment of scores on each test for clients between 16 and 69 years; therefore, the sentence imitation, written spelling, and word association tasks, which were three of the eight different measures in the final test batteries, can be adjusted for age effects. The PPVT–R has norms for adults up to 40 years, allowing standard scores to be used up to this age level. Further, Bayles, Tomoeda and Boone (1985) have reported no change in PPVT–R scores from age 20 to 79. Ramig (1983) and Duchin and Mysak (1987) have reported significant differences in speaking rate between young adults, middle-age adults, and older adults, suggesting that adjustments in this measure may be necessary. However, these studies did not use the same method of computing speaking rate as that used in this study. Specifically, this study measured words per minute rather than syllables per minute and it did not include words produced in mazes. Preliminary work by us, using 34 subjects ranging in age from 30 to 90, has not shown any significant changes in speaking rate between 30 and 70. This preliminary work has also indicated that there are no changes in the Modified Token Test performance until age 80. Further work is needed to confirm these results, but at this time it does not appear that performance on the tasks used in these batteries is strongly associated with age until age 80.

The language-impaired subjects in this study were not only different from the control subjects in language ability, but also differed with respect to their performance IQ as measured by the WAIS–R. The language-impaired subjects had an average performance IQ of 90, whereas the controls averaged nearly 99. We might expect that if these people are specifically language impaired, they should have an average IQ of 100. However as Leonard (1987) and Johnston (1988) have noted, there is considerable evidence that SLI is not in fact limited to linguistic

functions and usually extends to deficits in nonverbal cognitive domains as well. In addition, the SLI subjects in this study have performance IQs that are very similar to those reported by Aram and Nation (1975) and Schery (1985). Thus, it is likely that our subjects are representative of the language-impaired population in general. We have also noted (Tomblin, Freese, & Records, 1991) that WISC–R performance IQs from childhood were available for 20 SLI subjects in this study and that the mean was 98.5, which represented average ability. In contrast, this group obtained an average WAIS–R performance IQ of 89.75 as adults. This decline in performance IQ is not consistent with other research on the stability of performance IQ scores of normally developing people; rather, these studies reported consistency between these two measures of nonverbal IQ (Sattler, 1988; Zimmerman, Covin & Woo-Sam, 1986). Nevertheless, these results do support the original determination of normal performance IQ based upon the clinic file records of these subjects when they were children. The decline in performance IQ between childhood and adulthood should be investigated further to determine whether this is a common feature of SLI and, if so, why this occurs.

In addition to providing a diagnostic system for SLI in adults, the results of this study also provide valuable information about the language and cognitive status of young adults with histories of language impairment. The manifestation of SLI in adults has received very limited attention. Weiner (1974) and Aram, Ekelman, and Nation (1984) demonstrated that adolescents with histories of language impairment continue to present language problems. Further, Hall and Tomblin (1978) reported that the majority of adults who presented specific language disorders as children continued to be viewed by their parents as having some form of language disorder. In particular, these difficulties were described as those involving grammatical errors and word-finding problems. Likewise, patterns of persistence into adulthood of language and

Continued

EXCERPT 10.8   Discussion   *Continued*

cognitive deficits in people who are learning disabled have been reported (Buchanan & Wolf, 1986; McCue, Shelly, & Goldstein, 1986; O'Donnall, Kurtz & Ramanaiah, 1983; Sarazin & Spreen, 1986). These studies allowed us to predict that most individuals with SLI may be expected to present at least subtle signs of continuing difficulties in language usage into adulthood. The results of this study provide support for this prediction and indicate that, at least for many people with rather clear signs of language impairment in childhood, we can expect the language difficulties to be persistent throughout the person's life.

All of the language-impaired subjects in this study received at least some clinical services for their language impairment, and several had been clients at the University of Iowa Summer Residential Program in which they received intensive language intervention during a 6-week period. However, these data should not be used as evidence for the absence of efficacious intervention, because there was no untreated control group in this study. It is very possible that these people did benefit from these services. Nonetheless, these data do suggest that we may not be able to completely "normalize" the language performance in such people, thus supporting the view of Wallach and Miller (1988, p. 4) that "language disorders persist through the school years and through adulthood."

Inspection of Figures 1 and 2 also provides evidence that the language deficits of these individuals extend over a wide range of language and cognitive behaviors. Although differences were found on all tasks, the Sentence Repetition task in the telephone setting and the Modified Token Test in the face-to-face setting resulted in substantial differences between the two groups. Interestingly, each of these tasks involves the use of sentences and each places considerable demand on the retention of sentential information; thus, each task appears to place substantial demands on information processing. It is also likely that speaking rate, a measure retained in both test batteries, also is affected by this linguistic

information processing demand. Deficits in information processing capacity and/or the allocation of these resources within children with SLI recently has been proposed by several authors (Gathercole & Baddeley, 1990; Kirchner & Klatzky, 1985). As suggested by Johnston (1988), it is possible that such processing limitations serve as early contributors to the development of the language-learning deficit. Likewise, these information processing limitations may continue to impede language usage even when language learning has probably reached its peak, as it had in the young adults of this study.

The difficulties that individuals with SLI have with reading and spelling have been well documented (Maxwell & Wallach, 1984), and, therefore, it is not surprising that our adult subjects also demonstrated significantly poorer performance in these areas when compared with the control subjects. The fact that written spelling differentiated the two groups, and thus was included in the final face-to-face battery, is consistent with prior research concerning the presence of spelling difficulties in people with language and learning disabilities as well as the persistence of these problems into adulthood (Spreen, 1987). Thus, similar to information-processing problems, our results suggest that phonological difficulties appear to be a constant feature of SLI.

Overall, the data from this study suggest that signs of SLI persist into adulthood for most people who had clear histories of this condition during childhood. These signs can be measured at sufficient levels to permit rather accurate identification using language measures that place demands upon information processing and phonological performance. The presence of these persistent signs is not necessarily evidence that these people are significantly handicapped by these language difficulties. A companion study with the same subjects as this study (Records, Tomblin, & Freese, 1990) has shown that these people do not view the quality of their lives differently than the control population. However, this study focused upon the subject's self-perceptions of

Continued

EXCERPT 10.8   Discussion   *Continued*

their lives and, therefore, it is not clear how others would view these people as communicators, nor to what degree their life activities are limited by their language skills. Now that we know that SLI does exist in adulthood, further efforts need to be made to learn more about the nature and character of this condition in these individuals.

study, and clear conclusions regarding this motivation are stated immediately. A cautionary note regarding the lack of a blind method of data collection is exerted, and the authors took steps to explain why this methodological issue probably had a minimal effect, if any, on the results. In addition, the authors pointed out a problem in subject age selection necessitated by practical circumstances and explained the implications of this for their conclusions. They also pointed out very clearly why, in the absence of a control group, these results could not be used to make inferences about the effects of earlier treatment when these adults were younger and they limited very clearly their conclusions to the persistence of signs of SLI from childhood into adulthood.

Excerpt 10.9 is from the study of factors contributing to reduction of stuttering during singing that Excerpt 10.2 came from. Again, the conclusions are drawn directly from the results, which were reasonably straightforward.

EXCERPT 10.9

Taken alone, our finding that subjects significantly extended utterance durations during song provides a measure of support for Wingate's "modified vocalization" hypothesis. At the same time, certain of our results indicate that extended utterance duration, and by implication, modified vocalization, can only account for part of the reduction in stuttering during singing. It appears as though the familiarity of the melody and lyrics of the song being sung also has an important effect on stuttering frequency. More specifically, our subjects experienced the greatest decrement in stuttering when they sang the melody and lyrics of a song with which they were familiar. Consequently, the construct of "familiarity" should

be added to Wingate's formulation so that we can more completely specify the variables that are associated with the diminution of stuttering during singing.

In this experiment, familiarity was defined by the stutterer's ability to reproduce from memory the melody and lyrics of one of three songs well known to him. Such familiarity is most likely to develop with repeated practice or exposure to the songs. The fact that all of our subjects were able to correctly produce from memory the melody and lyrics of at least one test song is important. This observation strongly suggests that each of these individuals was indeed familiar with both the vocal patterns and

Continued

EXCERPT 10.9   *Continued*

articulatory gestures associated with the conventional lyrics of the material he sang in Condition 2. Evidently, the stutterers had repeatedly practiced, prior to the experiment, the requisite physiologic maneuvers essential for the production of the melody or words, or both, of one of the test songs. That this type of repeated motor practice could promote a decrease in stuttering should not be surprising in view of the results obtained in three earlier

studies by Wingate (1966), Besozzi and Adams (1969), and Bruce (1974).

From "Factors Contributing to the Reduction of Stuttering during Singing," by E. C. Healey, A. R. Mallard, and M. R. Adams, 1976, *Journal of Speech and Hearing Research, 19,* pp. 475–480. Copyright 1976 by the American Speech-Language-Hearing Association. Reprinted with permission.

Results are not always clear-cut, however. Occasionally the researcher may run into puzzling results that are difficult to interpret or that may not reflect a valid measure of what the researcher sought in the original problem statement. In that case, the researcher is faced with the dilemma of trying to explain a difficult result and may need to speculate on the problem of interpretation of results and suggest future research for solving the dilemma. Excerpt 10.10, from a study of auditory speech perception of hearing-impaired children, shows how the author tried to grapple with a puzzling result that accompanied a number of other, more interpretable results. Note how he has offered several possible explanations for the result and suggested future research to clear up the issue.

EXCERPT 10.10

Experiment 2 was also designed to provide information on the perception of pitch and intonation. Subjects in the 75–89 dB HL and 90–104 dB HL groups had little difficulty identifying talker sex, but the mean score of the 105–114 dB HL group failed to reach the 1% level of significance. All subject groups performed at chance levels on the intonation subtest. There are, however, several reasons for believing that this subtest did not provide a valid measure of perceptual ability. Many of the subjects, for example, exhibited natural intonation patterns in their own speech, strongly suggesting that they had auditory access to intonation. Moreover, the ease of access shown by many subjects to the 0.6 octave difference of average fundamental frequency between the male and female talkers is inconsistent with their failure to perceive the 1.26 octave range

of fundamental frequencies in the natural intonation contours. It seems probable that the poor performance of all subjects on the intonation subtest was due to their lack of experience in making conscious judgments about intonation patterns and in interpreting those patterns in terms of emotional state. It may also have been that the monotone was confusing because it is not a normal intonation pattern. The issue of the perception of intonation contours by subjects with sensorineural hearing loss clearly requires further research.

From "Auditory Perception of Speech Contrasts by Subjects with Sensorineural Hearing Loss," by A. Boothroyd, 1984, *Journal of Speech and Hearing Research, 27,* pp. 134–144. Copyright 1984 by the American Speech-Language-Hearing Association. Reprinted with permission.

Relationship of Results to Previous Research

The Discussion section should relate the results of the investigation to the findings of previous research. Scientific research is a cumulative endeavor that relies on the results of many studies for a broad understanding and explanation of phenomena. One research study cannot cover sufficient territory to answer completely all of the relevant questions regarding a given topic. Therefore, it is important for a researcher to inform consumers of research about the relationship of his or her findings to other research findings in the literature.

The Discussion section should provide both completeness and accuracy of references to previous research. Completeness demands that the author be aware of the literature in the area of his or her investigation and that he or she relate the findings to as many relevant studies as possible within the space limitations of the journal article format. In some cases, reference to certain previous research may have to be omitted if the manuscript is too long, and only the most directly related articles can be covered. References to previous research findings should also be accurate. Occasionally, an author may seriously misinterpret the findings of a previous study and go awry in discussing the relationship of his or her findings to that study. If such errors go undetected, the development of knowledge on a given topic may become confusing and misleading to consumers of research.

It is also important for authors to provide an objective and balanced account of both the agreements and disagreements of their results with those of previous research. Sometimes the findings of a particular article dovetail nicely with previous results in the research literature. For example, the results of a study with children may show evidence of an orderly developmental trend in some behavior or characteristic when compared with the results of studies with children of other ages. On the other hand, an article may present results that are at odds with previous research. For example, a replication study may find a pattern of results different from those that have been previously reported. Or a study employing a new procedure to study a well-researched phenomenon may reveal that previous data can be obtained only with a certain procedure and that procedural changes may yield conflicting answers to the same question.

Those points on which there is agreement may provide material for the discussion of theoretical and practical implications of the research, as we will see in the next section of this chapter. When there is disagreement, however, the author has a special responsibility to the readers to try to explain *why* there were disagreements between his or her results and those of previous research. For example, there might have been methodological, subject, or statistical differences between two investigations that could explain the discrepant results and such differences should be explored in the Discussion section. Often, the author may suggest avenues for future research that may help to explain why two studies show discrepant results.

Occasionally, the discussion of the relationship of results to previous research must cover some difficult territory. Subtle differences between studies must be analyzed to determine if the differences found are really meaningful or if they represent small fluctuations in human performance due to sampling or measurement errors. Also, obvious differences between studies may involve controversial topics that are subject to theoretical bias. The important point is for consumers to look for an objective attitude on the part of an author who is discussing discrepancies between the results of various studies. The writer of a research article has a responsibility to readers to present a balanced and objective analysis of the discrepancies and agreements between his or her findings and the body of research in existence on a particular topic. The writer should also be certain to identify the theoretical bias in the field on *both* sides of the issue at hand to indicate the merits of *each* side in the interpretation of a cumulative body of research data.

How can the reader determine if previous research has been completely and accurately described and if the discussion of agreements and disagreements has been fairly and objectively treated? First, consumers need to be aware of the important research that already exists on the topic covered in an article they are reading. Students and clinicians new to the field will develop this awareness over time as they read and assimilate more and more research. Second, for consumers who have questions about previous research, the best course of action is to find the references cited in the article's bibliography or reference list (that is one reason for appending a bibliography to an article) and read the original references (and the articles listed in those bibliographies) to check an author's interpretation of previous research.

The next three excerpts are taken from Discussion sections that illustrate balanced and objective approaches to the consideration of agreements and disagreements of the results with previous research results.

In Excerpt 10.11, Maske-Cash and Curlee discuss the results of research on speech initiation times of children who stutter and children who do not stutter. The excerpted text indicates how their results agree with the data trends shown in previous research but points out some differences in the absolute values of the means and standard deviations. Note that they offered some explanations for the differences in the data and ruled out age as a factor that could account for the differences. In addition, they pointed out how a theoretical model could be applied to their data.

EXCERPT 10.11 Comparisons of These Findings with Other Studies

Overall, the results of this study indicate that stuttering children are slower than nonstutterers when initiating speech in response to a visual cue. This is consistent with the findings of most studies comparing the speech initiation times of stuttering and nonstuttering children and adults.

The main differences among the studies were mean reaction times and standard deviations. The mean speech initiation times of the children in this study ranged from approximately 50 milliseconds slower (Till et al., 1983) to 100–500 milliseconds faster (Cross & Luper, 1979; Cullinan & Springer, 1980; and McKnight & Cullinan, 1987) than those reported in previous studies. The standard deviations in the present study are similar to those in the Till et al. (1983) study; however, other studies with similarly aged children (Cross & Luper, 1979; Cullinan & Springer, 1980; McKnight & Cullinan, 1987) reported standard deviations that were approximately 100 milliseconds smaller. The age range of the children in the present study was similar to that in earlier studies (Cross & Luper, 1979; Cullinan & Springer, 1980; McKnight & Cullinan, 1987); therefore, age should not account for the differences found among the studies. The differences in speech reaction times among these studies likely result from differences in the types of responses and procedures employed and in such subject variables as stuttering severity, which characterize samples of this population. It should be noted that despite the differences found, the pattern of findings of the above studies is consistent for the stuttering

Continued

EXCERPT 10.11   Comparisons of These Findings with Other Studies   *Continued*

children to exhibit slower reaction times than the nonstuttering children.

The pattern of results after the stuttering-only and stuttering-plus regrouping is consistent with the findings of Cullinan & Springer (1980) and McKnight & Cullinan (1987). The stuttering-plus group was slower than the stuttering-only group, which was slower than the nonstuttering group. Cullinan & Springer (1980) hypothesized that the slower performance of their entire stuttering group appeared to be related to the high incidence of other speech or language problems in this population. McKnight & Cullinan (1987) stressed that such differences demonstrate the importance of subgrouping stuttering children when comparing them with nonstuttering children. The pattern of findings of this study are also not unlike the study of Watson et al. (1991) who subgrouped stuttering adults into "linguistically-impaired" and "linguistically normal" groups, before comparing them with linguistically normal nonstutterers in a laryngeal reaction time paradigm. The consistency of the findings of the present study with those reported by others strengthens the external validity of the current findings.

The "Demands and Capacities" model of stuttering (Adams, 1990) could be applied to the results of this study. Adams stated that "fluency breaks down when environmental and/or self-imposed demands exceed the speaker's cognitive, linguistic, motoric and/or emotional capacities for responding" (page 136). Perhaps, in the present study, the environmental demands (the use of utterances of different lengths and meaningfulness and the instructions of the examiner to respond as quickly as possible) and self-imposed demands (subjects' responses to these environmental demands, e.g., increased attention, motivation, and/or apprehension) resulted in reaction times that reflected capacity and/or self-demand differences among the three groups. If so, either the self-imposed demands were greater for the stuttering-plus group and/or their capacities were lower than the stuttering-only and nonstuttering groups.

From "Effect of Utterance Length and Meaningfulness on the Speech Initiation Times of Children Who Stutter and Children Who Do Not Stutter," by W. S. Maske-Cash and R. F. Curlee, 1995, *Journal of Speech and Hearing Research, 38,* pp. 18–25. Copyright 1995 by the American Speech-Language-Hearing Association. Reprinted with permission.

Excerpt 10.12 is from the same study of auditory evoked responses in children with and without SLI that was used in Excerpt 10.1 and illustrates an attempt to explain a sharp contrast between their findings and those of a previously published study. Note how the authors needed to do some extra follow-up research in the literature to find the unpublished dissertation upon which the journal article was based in order to ascertain information about the subjects that might explain the differences between the findings of the two studies.

EXCERPT 10.12

The results of this study contrast rather sharply with those obtained by Stefanatos et al. (1989). There are several possible explanations for these differences. It is possible that these differences in outcome are due to differences in method; however, there were very few differences in the methods of the two studies. A more likely reason for the differences between our results and those obtained by Stefanatos et al. has to

Continued

EXCERPT 10.12   *Continued*

do with the subjects used. In his unpublished dissertation, Stefanatos noted that the children with receptive language impairment "corresponded roughly to the syndrome described by Landau and Kleffner (1957)" (Stefanatos, 1984, p. 71). Some of these children presented histories of seizures, and most of them had histories of normal language development followed by a regression in language. Stefanatos also included a group of children with SLI who did not have receptive language impairment. This group of children did not present signs of Landau-Kleffner Syndrome, and they showed normal evoked potentials to the frequency-modulated tones. The children with SLI who participated in the current study were similar to Stefanatos' group of children with expressive SLI in that they did not show signs of Landau-Kleffner Syndrome; however, they did present evidence of a receptive language impairment as well.

It may be, therefore, that the absence of cortical evoked responses to frequency-varying tones is associated with the cortical neuropathy associated with Landau-Kleffner Syndrome, rather than being a property of SLI. To support this hypothesis, Stefanatos (1993) reported that children having Landau-Kleffner syndrome did not show a cortical evoked response, whereas those children with expressive developmental language impairment showed a response similar to that of the control group of children.

From "Auditory Evoked Responses to Frequency-Modulated Tones in Children with Specific Language Impairment," by J. B. Tomblin, P. J. Abbas, N. L. Records, and L. M. Brenneman, 1995, *Journal of Speech and Hearing Research, 38,* pp. 387–392. Copyright 1995 by the American Speech-Language-Hearing Association. Reprinted with permission.

Excerpt 10.13 illustrates an extended effort to compare the results of a study of tympanometric estimates of ear canal volume to previously published data. The first paragraph summarizes the influence of different measurement procedures and calculations on resulting admittance values. In the next paragraph, the authors point out the difficulties that procedural and computational differences cause in trying to compare the results of different studies and indicate that their data will only be compared with the data of two previous studies that were directly comparable regarding measurement and computational procedures. The data of the three studies are compared in the excerpt's Table 4; in addition, the recalculated data in the excerpt's Table 5 are compared to the Table 4 data. Note the last two sentences in the excerpt caution readers regarding specification of procedures when comparing values among studies in the literature.

EXCERPT 10.13

In summary, the data in Figure 3 show that different tympanometric estimates of ear canal volume produced admittance values at 0 daPa ranging from .804 acoustic mmhos (1312 acoustic ohms) to .484 acoustic mmhos (2187 acoustic ohms) for the 220-

Hz probe tone and from 2.473 acoustic mmhos (461 acoustic ohms) to 1.750 acoustic mmhos (691 acoustic ohms) for the 660-Hz probe tone. For identical conditions encountered in the plane of the tympanic membrane, a difference in the assumptions

Continued

EXCERPT 10.13   *Continued*

made regarding the immittance characteristics of the ear canal volume produced a difference in the calculated admittance of 40% (impedance of 67%) at 220 Hz and of 29% (impedance of 50%) at 660 Hz.

As the data in Figure 3 demonstrate, static immittance values corrected to the plane of the tympanic membrane will vary substantially depending on whether the values are calculated at 0 daPa or at MAX and on the assumptions made regarding the immittance characteristics of the ear canal volume. These procedural and computational differences across studies make a direct comparison of admittance values with previous data difficult. In addition, most clinically available instruments measure only the magnitude of immittance and express this value in terms of an equivalent volume of air, which is dependent on altitude and barometric pressure (Lilly, 1973; Van Camp et al., 1976; Wiley & Block, 1979). The present admittance data, however, were directly comparable with data presented by Porter and Winston (1973) and by Margolis and Smith (1977). These investigators clearly specified the measurement and computational procedures used in

their respective studies. Table 4 shows the mean and standard deviations (in parentheses) for conductance and susceptance (in acoustic mmhos) at 220 Hz and at 660 Hz obtained in these two studies compared with the results obtained in the present study. In all studies, ear canal volume was estimated from the tympanograms at high negative ear canal pressures (–200 to –400 daPa); ear canal conductance was assumed to be greater than 0 acoustic mmhos. The data from the three studies are in agreement, although the susceptance values corrected to the plane of the tympanic membrane in this study are slightly larger than those reported in the other two studies. This difference is understandable when one considers the ear canal pressure used to estimate the ear canal volume. The ear canal pressure used in the current study was –400 daPa, which produces a slightly smaller ear canal volume estimate than would be obtained at –200 daPa (Porter & Winston, 1973) or at –300 daPa (Margolis & Smith, 1977).

Static admittance then was recalculated both at 0 daPa and at MAX using the recommended

TABLE 4   **The means (standard deviations) for the maximum conductance (*Cond*) and susceptance (*Susc*) values (in acoustic mmhos) at 220 Hz and at 660 Hz reported in three investigations. The number of subjects and the ear canal pressure used for the tympanometric estimate of ear canal volume in each investigation are shown in parentheses.**

Investigation	220-Hz Probe				660-Hz Probe			
	Cond		Susc		Cond		Susc	
Porter & Winston (1973) (*n* = 16; –200 daPa)	.40	(.19)	.78	(.31)	2.41	(1.59)	1.62	(.51)
Margolis & Smith (1977) (*n* = 17; –300 daPa)	.30	(.12)	.73	(.27)	2.11	(1.33)	1.58	(.54)
Present investigation (*n* = 8; –400 daPa)	.31	(.16)	.80	(.35)	2.13	(1.46)	1.67	(.38)

Continued

Chapter 10 The Discussion and Conclusions Section

EXCERPT 10.13   *Continued*

TABLE 5   Static immittance for 220-Hz and 660-Hz probe tones calculated at 0 daPa and at MAX using the recommended procedure (–400 daPa at 660 Hz) to correct for the immittance characteristics of the ear canal volume. Static values are expressed in admittance and impedance both in rectangular and polar notation.

Static Values	220-Hz Probe				660-Hz Probe			
	MAX		0 daPa		MAX		0 daPa	
Admittance (acoustic mmhos)								
G_a	.36	(.15)	.27	(.06)	2.53	(1.59)	1.88	(.71)
jB_a	.93	(.37)	.75	(.18)	1.67	(.38)	1.54	(.37)
Y_a	.99	(.40)	.80	(.18)	3.09	(1.51)	2.45	(.74)
e	68.70	(3.12)	69.82	(3.87)	37.88	(11.31)	41.17	(8.54)
Impedance (acoustic ohms)								
R_a	407	(142)	456	(149)	289	(99)	326	(92)
$-jX_a$	1042	(329)	1235	(354)	260	(172)	313	(198)
Z_a	1121	(353)	1320	(374)	394	(186)	458	(205)
−e	69	(3)	70	(4)	38	(11)	41	(9)

procedure to correct for the immittance characteristics of the ear canal volume. Table 5 shows the results of these calculations expressed in admittance and in impedance in both rectangular and polar notations. Ear canal volume was estimated from the 660-Hz susceptance tympanograms at an ear canal pressure of –400 daPa. This susceptance value divided by 3 was used to correct the 220-Hz data to the plane of the tympanic membrane. For both probe frequencies, ear canal conductance was assumed to equal 0 acoustic mmhos. Comparing these data with those in Table 4 again shows the importance of specifying the procedure used to correct for ear canal volume. Failure to do so undoubtedly has contributed to the variability in static immittance values reported in the literature.

From "An Evaluation of Tympanometric Estimates of Ear Canal Volume," by J. E. Shanks, and D J. Lilly, 1981, *Journal of Speech and Hearing Research, 24,* pp. 557–566. Copyright 1981 by the American Speech-Language-Hearing Association. Reprinted with permission.

Theoretical Implications of the Research

It is important for the author of a research article to state clearly the theoretical implications of findings with regard to past and current thinking in the field. In the last section, we discussed the relationship of the results to previous research. The theoretical implications of the results are closely tied to this relationship because the results of a single article are often juxtaposed with those of previous research to form the nomothetic network developed for any particular topic.

Implications may be drawn regarding the validity of a previously stated theory. Research results of a particular article may be supportive of an existing theory and further support may be gleaned from the agreement of that research article with previous research. Through the accumulation of more data in agreement with the predictions made by a particular theory, the theory gradually develops more plausibility as a valid explanation of the phenomenon under study. On the other hand, results of a particular study (and, possibly, other previous research) may be in disagreement with a particular theory. In such a case, the theory may need revision to account for discrepancies between the predictions made by the theory and the empirical evidence. In fact, so many data in disagreement with the theory may accumulate over the years that a theory may eventually be discarded because of its failure to find empirical support.

Theoretical implications are not limited to the discussion of previous theories in light of the data of a research article. The author may take the public opportunity to generate a new theory or to modify an old one so radically that it would no longer be recognizable in its revised form as a relative of the old theory. The data of a new article may be so provocative as to require new and original thinking for the explanation of the phenomenon under study. Readers will recall that two types of theory were mentioned in Chapter 1: those that are advanced before research is executed and await empirical confirmation and those that synthesize the existent empirical data. Both types of theory may be entertained in the Discussion and Conclusions section when the theoretical implications of the research are discussed.

Where can the reader expect to find the discussion of the theoretical implications in the research article? This depends on the style of the particular author. Some authors prefer to combine the discussion of the relationship of results to previous research with the discussion of theoretical implications at the beginning of the Conclusions section. This especially makes sense if the results of a particular investigation are to be combined with those of previous research in commenting on a theory. Others prefer to separate the discussion of theoretical implications from the discussion of relationship of results to previous research. Some authors even give considerable attention to theoretical issues in the introduction, literature review, or rationale before reporting data and refer back to this material in the theoretical implications portion of the conclusion. The important point is that the author needs to lend theoretical perspective to the empirical data and to articulate the theoretical implications of his or her findings so that readers understand where the research fits in the nomothetic network regarding the particular topic.

Excerpt 10.14 is from a study of age-related changes in phonation and illustrates the discussion of theoretical implications of research. The authors made references to both previous research results and the male–female coalescence model of aging in discussing a reasonably clear-cut theoretical explanation of why duty cycles may have increased with aging in males. As the last two paragraphs of the excerpt show, however, the shorter duty cycles in older than younger women were more difficult to explain, and the authors exerted caution with the suggested theoretical interpretations.

EXCERPT 10.14   Duty Cycle Measurements

One of the most interesting findings of this investigation was that duty cycle measures increased with aging in men and decreased with aging in women. As a result, the aged men in the study had longer duty cycle measures than the aged women for all but the high-pitch condition. Titze (1989) and Holmberg et al. (1988) reported longer duty cycles in females than males. Longer duty cycles for females than males were apparent for the young adult subjects in the current investigation as well. It appears, however, that this gender difference is reversed with aging.

Hollien (1987) proposed a male-female coalescence model of aging. Hollien suggested that hormonal changes at menopause reduce some of the gender differences in laryngeal behaviors that occurred because of hormonal changes at puberty. Hollien noted that this model was consistent with fundamental frequency data. The findings of the present investigation indicate that the model also is consistent with duty cycle measures.

Increased duty cycle measures have been associated with less vocal fold contact and a shorter period of contact (Childers & Krishnamurthy, 1985; Fourcin & Abberton, 1971; Lecluse, Brocaar, & Verschure, 1975; Rothenberg & Mahshie, 1988; Wechsler, 1976). Longer duty cycles for old than young men indicate that there is less complete vocal fold closure for males with aging. Degeneration of the vocal ligament and mucosa, cartilage ossification, and vocal fold bowing have been reported as part of the process of normal aging (Honjo & Isshiki, 1980; Kahane, 1987; Morrison & Gore-Hickman, 1986; Mueller et al., 1984). In addition, laryngeal neuromuscular control may be affected by aging (Bach, Lederer, & Dinolt, 1941; Bondareff, 1985; Horii & Weinberg, 1979; Malmgren & Ringwood, 1988; Segre, 1971). One or more of these age-related changes could impede complete vocal fold approximation and result in longer duty cycles for elderly than young males.

Some of the age-related changes that could impede complete vocal fold approximation are more prominent in males than females. Hirano et al. (1982) and Hirano et al. (1983) reported that age-related tissue changes in the vocal folds were more evident in males than females. Honjo and Isshiki (1980) reported, on the basis of laryngoscopic examination, that 67% of aged men and 26% of aged women had vocal fold atrophy. Kahane (1980) reported that age-related ossification/calcification of laryngeal cartilages begins earlier and is more extensive in males than females. Given the evidence of more marked age-related vocal fold atrophy, tissue degeneration, and cartilage ossification for males than females, it is likely that reduced vocal fold contact with aging is more prevalent for males than females. Changes in the vocal folds and laryngeal cartilages of healthy aged women may not be significant enough to reduce the degree of vocal fold contact. Therefore, it is not surprising that the males and not the females in this investigation showed a pattern of increased duty cycles with aging.

It is harder to explain the finding of shorter duty cycles in elderly than young women. Although gender differences in the magnitude of age-related changes in vocal fold behaviors were predicted, differences in the direction of change were not. One possible explanation for this finding relates to reports of edema formation on the vocal folds of aged women (Honjo & Isshiki, 1980; Linville, Skarin, & Fornatto, 1989). Titze (1989) described gender differences in vocal fold shape, tissue properties, and patterns of vocal fold closure and speculated that these differences contribute to longer open quotients in females than males. Vocal fold edema may alter the shape and tissue viscoelasticity of the vocal folds of aged females, making the manner in which the vocal folds close more similar to that of young males. As a result, duty cycle measures could become smaller.

The finding of smaller duty cycles in aged than young women should be interpreted cautiously. There are few data that would support or predict this finding. Also, the magnitude of the differences between young and old women's duty cycles was smaller than that seen for the male groups. Further investigation and replication of this finding should be done before shorter duty cycles are considered a characteristic of the aged female voice.

Excerpts 10.15 and 10.16 present examples from Discussion sections that illustrate two of the many ways in which theoretical implications of the results of a study may be discussed. The first excerpt is taken from an article on augmentative communication input to youth with mental retardation using the System for Augmenting Language (SAL). The authors discuss implications of their results relative to previous theories concerning input from the environment in language acquisition. The second excerpt, from a study of intelligibility and phonetic contrast errors in speakers with amyotrophic lateral sclerosis (ALS), discusses the implications of the results regarding dysarthric status and gender of subjects for possible physiological explanations of observed error patterns. The authors suggest the need for further research to clarify the issue of potential gender differences in susceptibility to particular neurological speech impairments.

EXCERPT 10.15   Discussion

The primary objective of this study was to characterize the augmented input that home and school adult partners provided to youth with mental retardation as they began to use the SAL. Three major aspects of augmented input, frequency, style and manner, and presence of teaching strategies, were examined.

Partners' input to youth with beginning achievement patterns contained a higher percentage of augmented utterances than did the input of partners of youth with advanced achievement patterns. One explanation could be that the SAL was too difficult for the youth with a beginning achievement pattern to learn. It is important to note, however, that all youth who participated in this longitudinal study learned to use the SAL for adult- and peer-directed communication at varying levels of sophistication (Romski & Sevcik, in press; Romski, Sevcik, Robinson, & Bakeman, 1994; Romski, Sevcik, & Wilkinson,1994). Another, perhaps more feasible, explanation may be that partners of youth with beginning achievement patterns discovered that greater amounts of augmented input were needed to model SAL use and to focus the youth's attention on the SAL.

The relatively modest amounts of partner-augmented input appears pertinent to theories of the role of environmental input in language acquisition. Nelson (1977, 1987, 1989) and colleagues (Nelson, Bonvillian, Denninger, Kaplan, & Baker, 1984; Nelson, Carskaddon, & Bonvillian, 1973) have posited a Rare Event Learning Model of language acquisition (RELM) in which they suggest that a limited amount of exposure to salient, meaningful, and appropriately tailored input can be sufficient to promote youth's language learning. Further, such input only infrequently leads to change in the child's linguistic system; in order for learning to occur, appropriate input must be paired with "uptake" of information (Kuczaj, 1982) on the child's part. At present, this Rare Event Learning Model has been applied only to the language learning process of nondisabled youth. The current study, however, suggests that relatively infrequent but salient input is effective in assisting youth with mental retardation in the process of mastering initial linguistic skills. It may be that the use of the SAL heightened the youths' attention to and awareness of the symbols and thereby promoted the likelihood of their learning.

EXCERPT 10.16

Additional insights into the nature of speech deficits observed in the present study also arose from a consideration of analyses in which subgroups based on dysarthric status and gender were considered. In the present study, the clinical diagnosis of dysarthria was substantiated by significantly poorer performance of dysarthrics than nondysarthrics on numerous measures related to bulbar and subsystem involvement, overall speech intelligibility, and diadochokinetic rate. Analyses on the most frequent contrast errors revealed that dysarthric subjects made significantly more errors than nondysarthrics for the Fricative versus affricate and the Alveolar versus palatal fricative contrasts and that dysarthric status was involved in interactions with gender in two other cases—Initial voicing and Vowel duration. Additionally, a simple examination of errors made *only* by dysarthrics includes four errors that were not among the most frequent errors made by the entire group, but were among those that have been previously reported as frequently occurring in speakers with ALS (Kent et al., 1990, 1992)—Stop versus affricate, Stop versus nasal, Final consonant versus null, and Initial consonant cluster reduction.

Although the male and female subjects were *not* found to differ in bulbar and subsystem involvement, results of analyses including gender and dysarthric status as factors suggested a particular vulnerability in male subjects for increased errors on the Alveolar versus palatal fricative contrast. In addition, men with dysarthria appeared to be particularly affected in their error rates for two of the contrasts that were more frequently in error: Initial voicing and Vowel duration contrasts.

Gender differences in initial voicing have been reported previously by Kent and his colleagues (1992). Those researchers suggested that male-female differences in overall levels of errors on this contrast may be due to a greater susceptibility of males to the loss of laryngeal motor neurons, either because of physiological differences in the degenerative process (Weismer & Fromm, 1983) or because of preexisting differences in the relative size of laryngeal structures that result in differential susceptibility to the effects of comparable neuronal losses (Weismer & Liss, 1991b). Alternatively, inherent gender differences in speech production prior to the onset of ALS, such as extent and slope of F2 transitions (Weismer, Kent, Hodge, & Martin, 1988) could also result in differing error patterns or compensatory strategies in response to the disease. Additional research comparing speech production between the genders for both normal and dysarthric speakers is needed to clarify this issue and is particularly needed to rule out sampling error as an explanation associated with the small number of dysarthric male subjects available to the present study.

Excerpt 10.17 is an extended example of a thorough discussion of the theoretical implications of a cineflourographic study of kinematic aspects of speech during stuttering adaptation. The rather lengthy excerpt is included because it illustrates so well the schemapiric interplay of theory and data. The first part of the discussion concerns the negative impact of these data on previous theory and offers reasons why the previous theory may have been incorrect. An alternate explanation is then offered that may account for the data of the article, and predictions are made from the alternate explanation that can be tested with future research. It is interesting to note that the original speculations that were not supported by the data of this article were put forth by one of the authors, yet he was

EXCERPT 10.17   Discussion

These results show that practice may have certain effects on the kinematic parameters of the articulators as practice with a manual task has on limb kinematics. Specifically, practice, at least initially, seems to be associated with an increased velocity of the articulators. For both nonstutterers and stutterers the most consistent change was the increase in the peak velocities of the tongue tip between Trials 1 and 2—four of the five subjects showed increased velocities for this gesture.

The results, however, indicate clearly that the speculations of Zimmermann (1980c) and Zimmermann et al., (1981) are not supported. That is, the hypothesis that decreased velocities and displacements and increased movement duration are necessary conditions for fluency enhancement does not hold. The results show that the adaptation effect does not directly depend on a particular pattern, though an increased velocity of the tongue tip between Trials 1 and 2 seems to be a relatively consistent finding.

The hypothesis that the specific changes in the kinematics (velocity, displacement, and transition time) are necessary conditions for fluency in stutterers may have been, from the onset, naive. As mentioned, the speculations arose from the kinematic descriptions reported by Zimmermann (1980a, 1980c) and the premise that kinematic differences between stutterers and nonstutterers may be related to a compensatory sensory-motor strategy for aberrantly tuned pathways. The underlying premise was that movements of lower velocities, decreased displacements, and longer durations would have fewer and less disruptive afferent effects on the speech output process. Though our results do not disprove this position, they make the speculations less feasible.

The speculations of Zimmermann (1980a, 1980c) may have suffered from the implicit assignment of causal status to the surface (kinematic) descriptors of a system. Rather than viewing these descriptors as controlled variables (somehow represented and controlled in the brain), it may be more appropriate to view these parameters as "emergent qualities" of the speech production system, or the result of underlying control processes. This distinction arises from a dynamic perspective on movement systems rather than a model in which each parameter for each movement is programmed (Kelso, in press; Kelso, Holt, Kugler, & Turvey, 1980; Kugler, Kelso, & Turvey, 1980).[3] Hence, to afford causal status to these descriptors may have been a critical error. What level of analysis, then, can be used to understand better the principles of motor systems which must be related to the adaptation effect?

A Dynamic Perspective

A dynamic perspective on movement control has been developed that does not assume that the products of motor function are isomorphic with the underlying processes from which those products derived. Thus, as Kelso et al. (1980) pointed out, the surface (kinematic) descriptors do not attain ontological status. It is not necessary to assign causal status to kinematic descriptors; instead, the surface descriptors can be viewed as an a posteriori fact of the system and not as an a priori reference signal coded and stored in the brain and imposed on the system. In other words, the spatial-temporal organization is the result of the physical processes involved in movement control. A discussion of these principles is found in Werner (1977) and is reiterated in relation to movement control systems by Kugler et al. (1980).

The critical point to be made regarding the data presented is that a different approach toward stuttering and the control of movement may change the initial hypothesis. More heuristically valuable hypotheses may be developed by viewing stuttering—and speech in general—in terms of a physical analogue. This account of movement suggests that the final position of a limb, or other structure, is determined

[3]Much of the following discussion arose from discussions with J. A. Scott Kelso.

Continued

EXCERPT 10.17   Discussion   *Continued*

by the dynamic parameters of the system. While we observe the kinematic consequence of movement, the kinematic details are merely consequences of the system's dynamics and are determined by those dynamics (Fitch & Turvey, 1978; Kelso, 1981; Kugler et al., 1980).

Mass spring analogues of limb movements have been helpful in conceptualizing movement processes (Fel'dman, 1980; Kelso, Holt, & Flatt, 1980; Polit & Bizzi, 1978). If the articulators are viewed as a mass-spring system, certain predictions about the effect of fluency-enhancing conditions on movement arise. Zimmermann et al. (1981) suggested that stuttering behavior may be related to a variable background activity, tonic muscle action in the muscles involved in speech. Variable background activity in the muscles involved in speech may be depicted as continuous variation of the stiffness of a spring in a mass-spring system. Instantaneous velocities may be affected directly by variations in spring (muscle) stiffness.[4] If it is suspected that the adaptation effect is associated with a decrease in the magnitude and variability of tonic muscular activity, then one would predict that the variability of instantaneous velocities would decrease from Reading 1 to Reading 2. All three stutterers reduced the variability of the instantaneous velocities between Trials 1 and 2, whereas one of the nonstutterers remained the same while the other increased variability.

This directional change is consistent with the hypothesis that fluency enhancement in an adaptation procedure may be associated with the stabilization of background activity in the speech musculature. Furthermore, the data suggest that the oscillatory model approach may have at least heuristic value in the investigation of speech and its pathologies.

[4]*Instantaneous velocity* refers to the velocity of movement between two points on the displacement-by-time graphs. These points are 10 msec apart at the filming speed of 100 fps. The mean is calculated by summing the instantaneous velocities between each pair of points and dividing by the number of pairs in the utterance /cæt/.

The data and the inferences from this post hoc analysis are consistent with hypotheses about the processes underlying the adaptation effect. The stabilization of background activity in the muscles of the articulators may be associated with a decrease in arousal. Thus, the kinematic variable that may be most appropriate for indexing psychophysiological factors (Wingate, 1966) may be that which indexes variations in tonic background activity of the muscles. The association between muscle activity and arousal makes this perspective compelling for accounting for the fluency enhancement in stutterers. That the reduction in the variability in instantaneous velocities is most consistent between Trials 1 and 2 agrees with the long-held belief that the greatest reduction in arousal occurs between Trials 1 and 2 in the adaptation procedure.

Practice also may play a role in the changes in motor organization that take place in the adaptation procedure. The increase in the velocity of the tongue tip for four of the five subjects between Trials 1 and 2 is consistent with the finding of Landa (in press), who studied the effects of practice on kinematic parameters in learning a simple manual task. Landa also found that the velocity of movement consistently increased with practice on this task.

That only the stutterers show a consistent reduction in the variability of instantaneous velocities may suggest differences in the processes underlying the adaptation effect in stutterers and nonstutterers. The adaptation effect in stutterers may be associated with (a) the stabilization of tonic muscle activity, which may be associated with a decrease in arousal, and (b) the effects of practice. For the nonstutterers, however, the most important variables may be the kinematic reorganizations associated with practice rather than the stabilization of tonic activity, that is, a reduction in arousal.

It may be misleading to suggest an "either/or" situation. Instead, the appropriate question can be phrased in terms of how much each of these variables accounts for the adaptation effect in any given

Continued

EXCERPT 10.17 Discussion *Continued*

subject. The most valuable perspective may be to view practice and arousal reduction as interacting or overlapping processes considered in terms of their relative weightings in a formula that may predict the outcome of an adaptation procedure. Stutterers and nonstutterers may simply fall on opposite ends of the continuum of values for the arousal coefficient.

The issue of relevant factors (e.g., psychomotor vs. motor-linguistic) in the adaptation process may be reduced to two questions suggested by Zimmermann et al. (1981): (a) How are inputs to motoneuron pools changed? and (b) What are the direct and indirect events leading to these changes? While each process must manifest its influence on the motoneuron pools associated with the muscles involved in speech, changes associated with practice and with arousal may be differentiable in terms of their effects on the pattern of muscle activity (at the motor unit level) and in terms of the variables affecting the different patterns.

It may be predicted then that stutterers and non-stutterers will show differences in the patterns of change in the motor unit behavior of speech muscles between Trials 1 and 2. The patterns for the nonstutterers would be associated with changes more connected with practice (i.e., changes in the patterning of phasic units) than with changes in arousal (fewer changes in the behaviors of small tonic motor units). The motor unit patterns of stutterers, on the other hand, would be associated with changes in both. Such speculations are open to empirical test.

From "A Cineflourographic Investigation of Repeated Fluent Productions of Stutterers in an Adaptation Procedure," by G. N. Zimmermann and J. M. Hanley, 1983, *Journal of Speech and Hearing Research, 26,* pp. 35–42. Copyright 1983 by the American Speech-Language-Hearing Association. Reprinted with permission.

able to criticize his own previous hypothesis in light of his new data and embark on a different path of reasoning. Good science demands this kind of candor in examining the relation between theory and data for the advancement of knowledge in any field. This example is a paragon of scientific excellence.

Practical Implications of the Research

In addition to the consideration of theoretical implications, the discussion and conclusions often address the question of practical implications of the results. As we mentioned earlier, it is often difficult to draw a true dichotomy between purely basic and applied research. Rather, there is usually a continuum along which research may fall with regard to its basic or applied orientation and with regard to whether practical implications are immediate or further off in the future. What some may consider to be pure research today may, surprisingly, turn out to have a practical implication tomorrow. The transistor, for example, was developed by scientists engaged in basic research in physics rather than by an inventor whose primary goal was to patent an invention for immediate sale.

In some cases an author may have no immediate practical application in mind because the research may have been more basic in its orientation or because applied considerations may have been reserved by the author until the accumulation of sufficient research to make judicious practical decisions. In such a case, the author may eschew the opportunity to discuss practical application if it is believed that such premature speculation would be unjustified or would be misconstrued by readers. On the other hand, the author might speculate about practical implications if he or she believed that appropriately cautioned speculation could be justified. For instance, the author might hope that this speculation would provoke readers with more practical inclinations to read his or her research or, perhaps, to begin applied research of their own. Readers should be careful to discern that such speculation is accomplished in a prudent and reasonable fashion. Consumers should also be cognizant of the need for patience in the anticipation of future practical applications when more research is necessary before a particular concept can be applied clinically in an ethical and professional manner.

Some research is undertaken with more immediate practical goals in mind and the author then has a special responsibility to delineate for the audience the implications of the research for assessment and management of communicative disorders. General suggestions for clinical practice may be offered in a few sentences or the author may feel that a more thorough didactic presentation is necessary. Sometimes the author may even write a separate article on the clinical implications of the research, especially at the culmination of a series of related research articles on a particular topic.

Direct practical application of the results of research should be advocated only when the accumulated research has demonstrated the reliability and validity of techniques for assessment and management of communicative disorders. In addition, the limitations of these techniques should be delineated in appropriate caveats to the readers. Unfortunately, some techniques have fallen into disfavor and have been abandoned because practical applications were proffered before sufficient research was completed to ensure clinical success. In such cases, researchers may have suggested clinical application before they had collected sufficient data to warrant immediate use, or clinicians may have attempted to apply techniques that research had not yet confirmed as suitable for clinical use. In some cases *both* researchers and clinicians may have been guilty of overzealous and premature application of inchoate techniques that were destined to fail without extensive research into their proper development. Therefore, it is imperative for both producers and consumers of research to be aware of the limitations inherent in any technique and of the need for cautious clinical application during the development of new techniques.

The next four excerpts, taken from Discussion sections, illustrate the reasonable and cautious discussion of practical implications of research. Excerpt 10.18 contains paragraphs that discuss the development of a program for standardization of judgments of

---

EXCERPT 10.18

The ultimate purpose of the research program that includes this study, finally, is to develop some means by which judgments of stuttering behavior may be standardized across researchers and across clinicians. One possible solution might be the development of an audiovisually recorded library of agreed exemplars of stuttering (see Cordes & Ingham, 1994a; Curlee, 1993). Such exemplars could eliminate the confusion caused by conflicting written descriptors of stuttering (see Conture, 1990; Ham, 1989). They could also form the basis of training programs, such as those used effectively in

Continued

EXCERPT 10.18   *Continued*

two preliminary studies (Cordes & Ingham, 1994c; Ingham, Cordes, & Gow, 1993), that could teach judges to identify stuttering consistently and accurately in clinical and experimental judgment situations. The most important finding of the present study, then, may be that 261 of the 720 intervals were agreed by 10 researchers and clinicians, on two occasions, to represent stuttered or nonstuttered speech; these intervals might now become the focus of training programs and other attempts to standardize behavioral measures of stuttering.

Many difficulties remain to be solved, of course, before time-interval exemplars and measurement procedures can be widely adopted. The particular characteristics of agreed intervals that make them useful and/or definitive exemplars of stuttered or nonstuttered speech must be determined, but these characteristics might never be adequately described in currently available terms. It is already clear that neither traditional descriptors such as disfluency types and severity ratings, nor more recent constructions such as the division between within-word and between-word disfluencies, can account for the differences between agreed and disagreed intervals. Subjectively, for example, it simply does not appear to be true that intervals containing severe stuttering are agreed to be stuttered and all others are disagreed. Many intervals agreed by the expert judges include stuttering that the present authors would describe as quite mild (but nevertheless unequivocally abnormal). Similarly, agreed stuttered intervals do not appear to share some standard topographical feature such as multiple repetitions or long prolongations; in fact, many of the agreed

intervals seem to contain behaviors that are clearly between words, that are visible but not necessarily audible, that would be classified as normal disfluencies according to schemes that define between-word interjections as normal, and that nevertheless are agreed by the authors and by all 10 of the current judges to be stuttered.

The ongoing research that has followed from these expert identifications of exemplar intervals appears to have demonstrated that training with between 12 and 44 expert-agreed intervals can increase the accuracy with which undergraduate students judge other speakers. This result provides one answer to the question of how expert-agreed intervals might earn the status of exemplars of stuttering: Useful exemplars will be those that are functional in developing measurement and training systems that can overcome current concerns about the validity (see Adams & Runyan, 1981; Perkins, 1990; Ryan, 1974; Smith, 1990) and the reliability (see Cordes & Ingham, 1994a; Young, 1984) of observer judgments of stuttering and/or disfluency. A system that can provide accurate and reproducible data must be developed, by some means, if the results of behavioral and physiological research about stuttering are to continue to depend on observer identifications of stuttered and nonstuttered speech.

stuttering behaviors by different persons in different settings. Note how the authors drew on their own results and previous research for specific suggestions to incorporate into training programs for improving judgments of stuttering behavior.

Excerpt 10.19 is from the Discussion section of an article by Tye-Murray and Kirk on vowel and diphthong production by children with cochlear implants in which the children's spontaneous speech production was compared to their performance on the Phonetic Level Evaluation (PLE) procedure. Note the authors' strong cautions about the use of the PLE with this particular population and their attempts to explain why the PLE may not have provided results that correlated well with spontaneous speech production. In addition,

EXCERPT 10.19   Discussion

This investigation examined the vowel and diphthong production of eight young cochlear implant recipients over time and related measures from the PLE to measures of spontaneous speech performance.

The results speak to the appropriateness of using the PLE as an indicator of speech development and as a guide for speech remediation. The overall correlation between the PLE and the spontaneous speech measures was significant when all test sessions were combined. However, Figure 7 indicates that this relationship was nonetheless weak. This interpretation is further borne out by the correlations performed for each of the five test dates. Only one test session, 12 months, yielded a significant relationship. This had only a modest predictive power, accounting for 36% of the variance (Figure 11). The PLE appears to be a particularly poor predictor of how well diphthongs can be produced during spontaneous speech. One reason for this might relate to the dynamic nature of diphthong production: Movement from one steady state posture to another is required. The PLE requires subjects to sustain each sound at three different intensity levels, and diphthongs may not be amenable to these tasks.

In sum, the present results suggest that performance on the PLE has low predictive value for vowel and diphthong production during spontaneous speech. The reasons for this poor correspondence cannot be deduced with the present data. At least three reasons are plausible. First, the present results might reflect the fundamental difference between spontaneous and imitative speech tasks. Second, they may indicate that the hierarchy of tasks proposed by Ling (1976) does not follow typical developmental trends. Finally, they may indicate that the PLE should only be used as Ling originally intended: only parts of the evaluation administered at any one time, for the purpose of determining the next speech treatment objective. Regardless of these reasons, it is recommended that measures in addition to the PLE be taken into account when designing speech treatment objectives for a talker who is severely or profoundly hearing impaired. Moreover,

some caution should be exercised in using a summation of the PLE vowel and diphthong scores as an indicator of communication aid benefit or in evaluating performance over time.

A recent investigation by Shaw and Coggins (1991) presents another reason to exercise caution. These investigators determined interrater reliability of the PLE by asking five judges to score the PLE of 10 children who were hearing-impaired. They concluded that the interrater reliability was unacceptable, usually below 0.80. This finding led them to conclude that "The instrument relies on a complex coding system that appears to compromise the accuracy of the observer's scoring. . . . That the PLE may have unacceptably low levels of interrater agreement presents a strong challenge to the accuracy of this clinical instrument" (p. 997).

The interrater reliability for the PLE was better in this study than in the study by Shaw and Coggins (1991): 0.92. Similarly, high reliability is reported by Tobey et al. (1991). Shaw and Coggins (1991) found that reliability was better for subjects whose articulatory proficiency was either very good or very poor, rather than in the midrange. This may account for the different reliability estimates. Whereas the subjects studied by Shaw and Coggins represent a range of articulatory proficiency, subjects in this investigation generally had poor articulation.

Recently, Ling (1991) has developed his own numerical system for quantifying performance on the PLE and the Phonologic Speech Evaluation, called the Phonetic-Phonologic Speech Evaluation Record. This system creates a combined inventory of phonetic and phonologic speech skills. For the evaluation of vowels and diphthongs, the inventory of sounds has been reduced to [a, u, i, ʌ, æ, I, aI, aʊ, ɝ, ɔI], to expedite testing. Items are assigned a value ranging from a scale of "0" to "4". Any vowel or diphthong incorrectly produced or one that cannot be stimulated receives a score of "0". An item that is produced habitually with good breath control and natural voice quality receives a score of "4". For the phonetic level evaluation, the child is asked to produce an item in repeated and alternated sylla-

Continued

EXCERPT 10.19   Discussion   *Continued*

bles, although the scoring system does not distinguish between the two tasks, as in Kirk and Hill-
Brown (1985). The child need no longer produce
pitch-varied syllables, as in the original PLE. An
overall vowel and diphthong score is computed by
summing the individual scores. A similar analysis is
performed on vowel and diphthong items recorded
during spontaneous speech. The summation of
scores yields a phonologic level numeric summary.
The phonetic and phonologic summary shows "the
overall extent to which the various stages of speech
acquisition have been mastered and indicate
whether the bulk of problems lie at the phonetic or
phonologic level of production" (p. 9).

Ling's numerical scoring procedure (1991) accords
with the present suggestion that more emphasis be
placed upon the Phonologic Level Evaluation and that
measures in addition to the PLE be used for determining treatment objectives. It remains to be determined
how this revised PLE will relate to measures of spontaneous speech and other test measures and whether
the Phonetic-Phonologic Speech Evaluation Record
will yield acceptable interrater reliability.

---

they indicated some implications of their results for future research on the recent revision
of the PLE.

Excerpt 10.20 is from the article by Cox, Alexander, and Rivera that was used in
Excerpt 9.12 to illustrate the use of scattergrams for describing relationships. The practical implications discussed in Excerpt 10.20 are derived from their results concerning the
correlations between objective and subjective intelligibility for elderly hearing-impaired
listeners shown in Figure 10 of that article which is included in Excerpt 9.12. Note the
authors' attempts to balance the relative advantages of objective and subjective measures
in their discussion of the potential clinical use of speech intelligibility measures.

EXCERPT 10.20   General Discussion

In this work, we undertook to evaluate the relationship between an objective measure of speech intelligibility and a corresponding subjective intelligibility estimation procedure. The overall purpose was
to determine whether hearing aid benefit assessments for elderly hearing-impaired listeners would
be likely to give the same results when the two measurement procedures were used. The results suggested that, despite differences in absolute scores, a
comparative hearing aid evaluation using subjective
intelligibility estimates would usually produce
essentially the same result as a comparative evaluation using the objective intelligibility measurement
procedure.

This is an auspicious outcome because subjective
measurements have many practical advantages over
objective ones. However, it is important to note that
the critical differences for subjective estimates were
substantially larger than those for objective scores.
Furthermore, the CDs obtained in these studies for

Continued

EXCERPT 10.20   General Discussion   *Continued*

both normal-hearing and hearing-impaired listeners were in close agreement with analogous CDs drawn from several other investigations. Thus, it appears that the objective measurement procedure used here is considerably more reliable than the subjective procedure. The result would be that the subjective procedure is less sensitive to benefit differences across hearing aid conditions, and larger differences between conditions would be required to produce a significant outcome. This situation could be remedied by obtaining more subjective estimates to gen-

erate the final score in each tested condition. However, this would diminish the administration-time advantage associated with the subjective procedure.

From "Comparison of Objective and Subjective Measures of Speech Intelligibility in Elderly Hearing-Impaired Listeners," by R. M. Cox, G. C. Alexander, and I. M. Rivera, 1991, *Journal of Speech and Hearing Research, 34,* pp. 904–915. Copyright 1991 by the American Speech-Language-Hearing Association. Reprinted with permission.

Excerpt 10.21 is from a study of acoustical characteristics of syllabic stress in esophageal speakers and includes two paragraphs from the Introduction and two paragraphs from the Discussion sections to illustrate how well part of the rationale and the problem statement integrated with the practical implications drawn at the end of the study. The first two paragraphs show part of the authors' rationale for studying prosodic variables in esophageal speech and the general purpose and specific research questions of the study. The next two paragraphs of the excerpt briefly summarize some of the results, suggest some possible physiological mechanisms, and indicate the direct clinical implications of the results regarding treatment with esophageal speakers.

EXCERPT 10.21

Because it appears that esophageal speakers exhibit reduced ability to manipulate fundamental frequency, sound pressure, and duration, clinical expectations for perfecting esophageal speech may be limited. Speech clinicians sometimes assume that esophageal speakers will be unable to approximate normal prosodic patterning associated with syllable stress and intonation.

The present study was designed to explore the production of intended syllabic stress by excellent esophageal speakers. More specifically, do excellent esophageal speakers and normal speakers characterize primary syllabic stress with similar patterns of fundamental frequency, sound pressure, and duration? Further, are excellent esophageal speakers able

to produce normal patterns of stress-associated acoustical characteristics irrespective of stress position within syllables and within sentences?

. . . .

In general, the results of this study suggest that some laryngectomees are able to manipulate f_0, SPL, and duration in a manner reasonably comparable to normal speakers. The physiological factors contributing to these abilities are unknown at this time, but the amount of remaining musculature and the integrity of its neural innervation as well as the nature of the surgical reconstruction may be relevant (Simpson, Smith, & Gordon, 1972). Precise tension control of the neoglottic folds combined with optimal tissue viscoelasticity would facilitate rapid

Continued

EXCERPT 10.21   *Continued*

f_0 changes. Enhanced neoglottic closure control might permit more rapid voicing onsets and offsets and a higher average SPL. The availability of a large air reservoir may allow both increased SPLs and/or the production of longer utterances. Finally, ability to modulate transneoglottic airflow via changes in intrathoracic pressure and upper vocal tract impedance might well allow a trade-off between increased SPL and increased utterance length.

The finding that some esophageal speakers are able to control f_0, SPL, and duration in a highly natural but somewhat inconsistent manner has significant clinical implications. In light of the data presented, it may be unjustifiable to dismiss patients when intelligible esophageal utterances are produced with relative fluency. Many laryngectomees may have the capability to go well beyond the point of merely functional esophageal speech. With intensive esophageal therapy emphasis on f_0, SPL, and duration, certain esophageal speakers may approximate suprasegmental normalcy more completely, more rapidly, and more consistently.

From "Acoustical Characteristics of Intended Syllabic Stress in Excellent Esophageal Speakers," by M. McHenry, A. Reich, and F. Minifie, 1982, *Journal of Speech and Hearing Research, 25,* pp. 564–573. Copyright 1982 by the American Speech-Language-Hearing Association. Reprinted with permission.

Implications for Future Research

As we mentioned earlier, no one research article can answer all of the relevant questions on a given topic. In fact, a particular research article may even raise more questions than it answers. Scientific progress depends on the cumulative efforts of a number of investigators and each of their efforts points toward new avenues of research. The Discussion section usually enumerates some of the questions for future research that occur to the author during the course of the investigation.

Future research may be suggested in a number of different areas, including, but not limited to, improvement of internal validity by refinement of the design and execution of the research, extension of external validity, further clarification of the relationship of results to previous research, additional empirical confirmation of theory, and elaboration of practical applications.

Suggestions for future research are often directed toward improvement of the internal validity of the research by refinement of the methods employed. For instance, the author may discuss limitations imposed on his or her conclusions by aspects of the method of investigation (i.e., threats to internal validity). The author may also incorporate suggestions for future research to overcome these limitations. These suggestions may be in the form of general comments or of specific delineations of procedural steps to be taken in a new study. Indeed, the author may already have such an investigation underway at publication time and readers may anticipate its subsequent publication. The suggestions offered may include replication with larger samples, use of more homogeneous or heterogeneous groups of subjects depending on the nature of the study, refinements in design or measurement techniques, or improvements in materials or instrumentation. Of course, if too many such suggestions are made, readers may wonder why the study was ever published in the first place. But a few suggestions for improvement are usually warranted because no study can ever be perfectly designed to avoid all of the possible pitfalls of research.

Suggestions for future research may also be directed toward external validity. The author may be concerned with extending the generalizability of results to other populations, settings, measures, or treatments. Procedures that are successful with adults may not necessarily work with children; replication with children would be needed to verify the generality of the procedure. By the same token, results obtained with one type of communicative disorder may not necessarily be obtained with another. Results may be limited to a particular setting and a systematic replication may be needed to extend generalization to another setting. Research suggestions aimed at extending external validity are often coupled with caveats discussed in practical implications and readers may be urged to await further research before attempting to generalize results to other subjects, settings, measures, or treatments.

Future research may also be suggested as a result of comparison of the results of a particular study to those of previous research. If there are disagreements between the results of a study and previous research, more research may be suggested to resolve the differences. The different results may be due to sampling or procedural differences that could be overcome by procedural comparisons, replications with different samples, or by control studies designed to evaluate the reliability and validity of different procedures with different samples. Agreement of previous research with the results of a particular study may also prompt suggestions for future research as such agreement may indicate that researchers have been pursuing a fruitful approach to the study of the particular phenomenon.

Suggested future research may also be related to the theoretical implications of the results. More research may be needed to firm up the empirical grounding of a theory supported by the results of a particular investigation. On the other hand, further research may be needed to account for discrepancies between the results of a study and existing theory. If a new or modified theory is advanced to explain the results, the new theory or modifications may contain predictions of behavior or phenomena that would need to be confirmed empirically by future research. Changes in type of subjects, research materials, instrumentation, or procedures might be necessary to test the predictions of the new theory.

As mentioned previously, the practical implications of a particular research study may not be immediately apparent or feasible and, therefore, further research may be suggested before practical applications can be accomplished. Such suggestions may include standardization of tests on larger samples, gathering of normative data on different populations, development of more efficient or less expensive (i.e., more clinically feasible) methods, or refinements in procedure to improve reliability and validity. Sometimes a procedure may be strongly advocated as useful with a well-defined, closely circumscribed clinical population, but caution is necessary regarding application to other populations until future research confirms the applicability of the measure or technique.

The next five excerpts present examples from Discussion sections that illustrate a variety of thoughtful suggestions for future research. The excerpts concern many of the different kinds of suggestions previously outlined.

Excerpt 10.22 is from a study of the effects of vocal pitch level on vowel spectral noise and perceived vowel roughness. The authors raised several questions based on their data and outlined a systematic series of research questions for future investigations. Although most of their questions concern methodological issues relative to subject selection and speech sample characteristics, note the practical application mentioned in the last paragraph regarding research aimed at producing more natural sounding synthetic speech.

EXCERPT 10.22

The data presented in this report raise several other questions. First, it is of interest to learn whether vowel samples from nonsingers would exhibit similar trends to those produced by singers. This study employed singers because of their ease in producing vowel samples that were acceptable for the analysis. It seems possible, however, that those singers may have developed a degree of laryngeal control not typical among nonsingers. Thus, it may not be reasonable to assume that the trends reported here would hold for all nonsingers.

Second, it seems pertinent to ask whether samples of vowels other than /ɑ/ would exhibit similar SNL and roughness-rating data. Some variation in those measurements has been shown across vowels in other studies (e.g., Coleman, 1969; Emanuel & Sansone, 1969; Lively & Emanuel, 1970); it seems reasonable to suspect, then, that SNL and perceived roughness characteristics of other vowels produced at different pitches might vary from productions of /ɑ/.

A third question concerns the relationship of SNL to jitter when vowel pitch is changed. Results of the present study indicated a highly linear relationship between pitch and SNL for vowel samples produced

by singers. One other investigation (Orlikoff & Baken, 1990), however, revealed a nonlinear relationship between pitch and jitter for vowel samples produced by vocally untrained subjects. Although these contrasting findings may exist because different subject populations were employed in the two studies, it also seems possible that SNL and jitter measurements may respond differently to changes in vowel pitch. Thus, a need exists to further our understanding of the relationship of vowel SNL to jitter, particularly when vowel pitch is changed.

Last, it would be of interest to know if synthetic vowel samples produced at different pitch levels would evidence the same SNL and perceived-roughness trends as samples produced by humans. Information of this type contributes to the synthesis of more natural-sounding speech.

From "Pitch Effects on Vowel Roughness and Spectral Noise for Subjects in Four Musical Voice Classifications," by R. A. Newman, and F. W. Emanuel, 1991, *Journal of Speech and Hearing Research, 34,* pp. 753–760. Copyright 1991 by the American Speech-Language-Hearing Association. Reprinted with permission.

Excerpt 10.23, taken from an article on quick incidental learning (QUIL) of words by children with and without specific language impairment, begins with a summary of the two major contributions of the findings of the investigation. The authors then pointed out that a great deal is still unknown about the process of QUIL and outlined several directions for future investigations, including studies of the effects of learner aptitude, contextual effects, and changes in children's performance over time.

EXCERPT 10.23   Conclusions

The results of this study contribute to our understanding of children's quick and incidental learning of words in at least two ways. First, the results provide a developmental perspective of QUIL as a function of age and learner aptitude. Like preschool chil-

dren, normally developing school-age children are able to pick up a remarkable number of words incidentally from oral contexts. Between the ages of 6 and 8 years, this ability gradually increases, although the magnitude of the gain is less dramatic when com-

Continued

EXCERPT 10.23   Conclusions   *Continued*

pared to the gain made during the preschool years. For children with SLI, this ability to incidentally learn words from an oral context is greatly reduced. Group differences in QUIL suggest at least two tracks for vocabulary development, one fast and one slow. Children following the fast track find vocabulary acquisition a serendipitous product of interacting with their environment. For children on the slow track, word acquisition is not so effortless.

A second contribution of this study is documentation of QUIL as a function of word type. For both normally developing children and those with SLI, quick and incidental word learning remains affected by word type throughout the early school years, with patterns of gain reflecting an object label advantage. This object label advantage, much like the home court advantage in collegiate sports, appears to cut across factors such as age and level of functioning, at least for children up to the age of 8 years.

There is still a great deal unknown about how children incidentally learn words from context and how this ability relates to the overall process of building a lexicon. Future investigations of QUIL should extend in a number of directions. One direction involves studying the processes by which children's representation of a new word changes over time, from the point of initial mapping to the state of full understanding and productive use. As pointed out by Rice (1990), what remains unclear in studies of quick and incidental learning and those of fast mapping, is the range of referents to which a child is prepared to extend a newly acquired word. Perhaps new word mappings are limited by perceptual similarities or other salient cues. Another possibility is that the initial phase of word learning is inherently conservative, with the initial mapping involving a one-to-one association with the observed referent and the phonological string of the

novel word. Further exploration of how children's meanings of new words change over time may help operationalize terms such as "initial mapping," "partial learning," and "incomplete knowledge," as well as illuminate the causal role different linguistic and nonlinguistic factors play in the short- and long-term storage of words.

The results of this study also highlight the need to examine further issues of learner aptitude as they relate to the on-line acquisition of words and the overall process of lexical expansion. Clearly, the ability to learn words incidentally from an oral context is not uniform across children. If incidental learning turns out to be the primary means by which lexical repertoires are built, children who demonstrate poor quick and incidental learning abilities are at risk for long-term lexical limitations as well as concomitant problems with reading and academic achievement.

Finally, the study of QUIL as a function of context (oral vs. print) should be pursued. Given the differences between the media of print and oral communication, it would not be surprising if certain contextual factors were found more critical for learning vocabulary from one context as compared to the other. However, we speculate that some processes of word acquisition cut across contextual boundaries, and it will be only through careful consideration of both media that a comprehensive understanding of vocabulary development will be achieved.

Excerpt 10.24, taken from the same study of syllabic stress with esophageal speakers that was used in Excerpt 10.21, illustrates several suggestions for research to extend the external validity of the study. Suggestions are made for studying other measures (e.g., variability within sentences, perceptual verification of stress magnitude) and comparing them

EXCERPT 10.24

The present study is limited by a number of factors. Three male and two female esophageal speakers with matched normals comprise a relatively small sample. Furthermore, large-sample perceptual evaluation of stress was not performed. For the purpose of this descriptive study of acoustical characteristics associated with intended syllabic stress, experimenter and trained-phonetician verification was considered adequate. The fact that significant stress main effects and nonsignificant group × stress interactions were found supports the notion that, for the most part, these esophageal speakers produced intended stress in a manner comparable to their matched normals. This, however, does not address the issue of how frequently or to what degree stress was realized. The necessity of excluding 14% of the esophageal but none of the normal productions implies that even excellent esophageal speakers lack consistent volitional control of the mechanisms underlying stress production. Large-sample perceptual verification of stress magnitude currently is underway in our laboratory. The results of the perceived stress-magnitude study will be correlated with dynamic as well as static acoustical characteristics known to be associated with syllable stress. We anticipated that certain dynamic aspects of prosodic patterning, such as rate of f_0 and SPL change within and between syllables, will correlate more highly with perceived stress magnitude than would the more static features investigated in the present study.

In addition, although the subjects did not seem to produce exaggerated contrasts between stimulus pairs, it is unlikely that the utterances are truly representative of ongoing conversational speech. Most subjects uttered each stimulus sentence as a single phrase. This eliminated the need for rapid air injections and releases that might tax their ability to produce longer, appropriately phrased utterances. Since each stimulus sentence was produced only once, within-sentence, intraspeaker variability data are unavailable. Within-sentence f_0, SPL, and durational variability data would provide information regarding the consistency with which esophageal speakers are able to manipulate these acoustical parameters to signal stress.

The need for further research regarding esophageal prosody is apparent. It will be interesting to investigate the ability of fair to good esophageal speakers to manipulate the acoustical characteristics associated with stress. Trading effects, such as signaling contrasts with durational rather than f_0 or SPL changes, may be evident. Research concerning the linguistic aspects of speech after laryngectomy, including studies of contrastive stress and intonation, would appear to be of great interest. Work addressing these questions currently is underway (Weinberg, Note 1).

From "Acoustical Characteristics of Intended Syllabic Stress in Excellent Esophageal Speakers," by M. McHenry, A. Reich, and F. Minifie, 1982, *Journal of Speech and Hearing Research, 25,* pp. 564–573. Copyright 1982 by the American Speech-Language-Hearing Association. Reprinted with permission.

to the measures reported in this study. Also, this study included only excellent esophageal speakers and the suggestion is made to study the abilities of fair to good speakers as well.

Excerpt 10.25 from a study of hearing-impaired speakers' intelligibility, includes two specific suggestions for future research. The first suggestion concerns examination of criterion validity of scaling measures in relation to word-identification tests of intelligibility and acoustical characteristics of speech. The second suggestion concerns extension of the external validity of the results to other populations with impaired intelligibility and to other measures (i.e., dimensions of speech that are scaled).

EXCERPT 10.25

Because the results of this study demonstrate the continuum of our hearing-impaired adults' speech intelligibility to be prothetic, we conclude that direct magnitude estimation has more construct validity than interval scaling for assessing this dimension. Future research should address the criterion validity of direct magnitude estimation by examining its functional relation to word identification tests of speech intelligibility and to acoustical parameters of speech (Monsen, 1978) found to be good predictors of intelligibility.

It is important to test the generalizability of these results to the speech intelligibility of hearing-impaired children, to other populations such as dysarthrics and esophageal speakers with impaired intelligibility, and to other dimensions of speech that are commonly scaled. For example, an interesting parallel is apparent between our results for speech intelligibility and the findings of Berry and Silverman (1972) regarding the inequality of intervals on the *Lewis-Sherman Scale of Stuttering Severity*. They used direct magnitude estimation to judge the widths between adjacent samples of stuttering previously scaled along a 9-point interval scale of stuttering severity and found smaller interval widths at the lower end than at the upper portion of the scale. This finding agrees well with Stevens's (1974) prediction for prothetic continua. Because a number of dimensions like stuttering severity, speech intelligibility, articulatory defectiveness, vocal qualities, etc., are commonly assessed with interval scaling in clinical and research work, it seems imperative that these dimensions be explored to determine whether they constitute metathetic or prothetic continua. A serious reconsideration of the widespread use of interval scaling may be necessary if a number of these continua are found to be prothetic.

As Stevens (1974) has stated:

> The human being, despite his great versatility, has a limited capacity to effect linear partitions on prothetic continua. He does quite well, to be sure, if the continuum happens to be metathetic, but, since most scaling problems involve prothetic continua, it seems that category and other forms of partition scaling generally ought to be avoided for the purposes of scaling. (p. 374)

From "Construct Validity of Direct Magnitude Estimation and Interval Scaling of Speech Intelligibility: Evidence from a Study of the Hearing Impaired," by N. Schiavetti, D. E. Metz, and R. W. Sitler, 1981, *Journal of Speech and Hearing Research, 24,* pp. 441–445. Copyright 1981 by the American Speech-Language-Hearing Association. Reprinted with permission.

Excerpt 10.26 is from a study of progressive hearing loss in children in relation to hearing-aid use and other etiological factors. This is a complicated area of research with many potential independent variables (etiological factors) that can cause deterioration in hearing in addition to the effect of high sound levels of hearing-aid output. The paragraphs excerpted indicate a number of variables that need further research in attempts to delineate the nature of progressive hearing loss in children. The first paragraph, taken from the beginning of the discussion, indicates the importance of following the time course of hearing-aid use and the progression of hearing loss, and the next two paragraphs, taken from the end of the discussion, indicate a number of variables that must be considered in clinical case studies and in future research studies. Excerpt 10.26 indicates the difficulty of generalization in this area without more research on a variety of potential independent variables and their interactions in causing progressive hearing loss in children.

EXCERPT 10.26

The potential of powerful hearing aids causing further hearing loss in hearing-impaired children cannot be discounted. However, an incentive to look beyond the hearing aid is provided by the large number of possible etiological factors associated with progressive hearing loss. Unfortunately, specific etiology in the individual case is often unknown. Scrutiny of factors such as the time relations between hearing aid application and the period of progression, therefore, become extremely significant.

. . . .

If progressive hearing loss is verified and not attributed to hearing aid use, immediate attention should be paid to all other possible factors. Careful questioning of illness, virus, allergy, noise exposure, medication, and family history is in order, and it should be verified that a physician is following the child. The gain and SSPL of auditory trainers, if used in the educational setting, need to be ascertained. In this connection, the Academy of Rehabilitative Audiology recommended to the Food and Drug Administration in 1976 that caution be exercised when SSPLs of over 132 dB are used in auditory trainers; but this level may be too high, according to Rintelman (1975).

Research is needed not only on the effects of gain and SSPL but also on the effects of steady stimulation from inherent noise in the hearing aid. Similarly, research is needed on temporary shifts with hearing aid use and their relation to permanent damage. We also need research on etiological factors in progressive hearing loss; for example, given a known causative agent, what is the rate, extent, and pattern of progression that might be expected once a change in hearing is seen. Finally, much greater emphasis should be placed on obtaining informative case history data. Although reflecting the present state of knowledge with respect to hearing impairment in children, any study such as this one is restricted in its comprehensiveness by the lack of adequate etiological information.

From "Progressive Hearing Loss in Children: Hearing Aids and Other Factors," by K. M. Reilly, E. Owens, D. Uken, A. C. McClatchie, and R. Clarke, 1981, *Journal of Speech and Hearing Disorders, 46,* pp. 328–334. Copyright 1981 by the American Speech-Language-Hearing Association. Reprinted with permission.

EVALUATION CHECKLIST

Instructions: The four-category scale at the end of this checklist may be used to rate the *Discussion* section of an article. The *Evaluation Items* help identify those topics that should be considered in arriving at the rating. Comments on these topics, entered as *Evaluation Notes,* should serve as the basis for the overall rating.

Evaluation Items   *Evaluation Notes*

1. Discussion was clearly related to research problem.

2. Limitations of the method were discussed.

3. Conclusions were drawn directly and fairly from results.

4. Reasonable explanations were given for unusual, atypical, or discrepant results.

5. There was thorough and objective discussion of agreements and disagreements of previous research.

6. The section related results to various theoretical explanations.

7. Implications for clinical practice were stated fairly and objectively.

8. Theoretical or clinical speculations were identified and justified.

9. Suggestions for future research were identified.

10. General comments.

Overall Rating (Discussion):   _____   _____   _____   _____
                                      Poor   Fair   Good   Excellent

Evaluation of the Complete Research Article: Three Examples

Overview

In Part II it was necessary to present a somewhat disjointed view of the evaluation process by showing examples of different parts of a research article instead of an integrated evaluation of a complete piece of research. In addition, we provided students with the link between each example in Part II and the principles discussed in Part I. In Part III we provide opportunities to synthesize the evaluation of three complete pieces of research and to find the links between these examples and the principles that were discussed in Part I.

We have reprinted three articles in Part III: one in audiology, one in speech disorders, and one in language disorders. In addition, we have put together the checklists from Chapters 7, 8, 9, and 10 as one reprintable checklist for students to use to guide them in the complete evaluation of each article as an integrating exercise. It then becomes the student's responsibility to draw upon the principles in Part I and the examples in Part II and synthesize these resources for the completion of the integrated evaluation.

We chose articles that we believe will illustrate many points discussed in the previous chapters. In general, the articles are examples of good research, but we expect students to make both positive comments and constructive criticisms for the improvement of future research. No single research study is expected to compensate for all possible threats to internal and external validity, given the practical problems of conducting research. Any published paper can profit from suggestions for improvement. The articles we have chosen make important contributions to our knowledge of communicative disorders and are used here to illustrate the process of evaluation: the weighing of positive and negative aspects of the research in order to arrive at a reasonable judgment about the overall adequacy of an article.

EVALUATION CHECKLIST—INTRODUCTION

Instructions: The four-category scale at the end of this checklist may be used to rate the Introduction section of an article. The *Evaluation Items* help identify those topics that should be considered in arriving at the rating. Comments on these topics entered as *Evaluation Notes* should serve as the basis for the overall rating.

Evaluation Items   *Evaluation Notes*

1. Title identified target population and variables under study.

2. Purpose, procedures, important findings, and implications were summarized in the abstract.

3. A clear statement of the general problem was given.

4. There was a logical and convincing rationale.

5. There was a current, thorough, and accurate review of literature.

6. The purpose, questions, or hypotheses were logical extensions of the rationale.

7. The introduction was clearly written and well organized.

8. General comments.

Overall Rating (Introduction):   _____   _____   _____   _____

                                      Poor   Fair   Good   Excellent

EVALUATION CHECKLIST—METHOD

Instructions: The four-category scale at the end of each part of the *Method* section checklist may be used to rate these parts of an article. The *Evaluation Items* help identify those topics that should be considered in arriving at the ratings. Comments on these topics, entered as *Evaluation Notes,* should serve as the basis for the ratings. An additional scale is provided to allow for an overall rating of the Method section.

Evaluation Items (Subjects)	*Evaluation Notes*

1. Sample size was adequate.

2. Subject selection and exclusion criteria were adequate and clearly defined.

3. Subjects were randomly selected and randomly assigned.

4. Overall or pair matching was employed.

5. Differential selection of subjects posed no threat to internal validity.

6. Regression effect controlled for subjects were selected on basis of extreme scores.

7. Interaction of subject selection and treatment posed no threat to external validity.

8. General comments.

Overall Rating (Subjects):

_____	_____	_____	_____
Poor	Fair	Good	Excellent

Evaluation Items (Materials)	*Evaluation Notes*

1. Instrumentation (hardware and behavioral) was appropriate.

2. Calibration procedures were described and were adequate.

3. Evidence presented on reliability and validity of hardware and behavioral instrumentation.

4. Experimenter and human observer bias was controlled.

5. Test environment was described and was adequate.

6. Instructions were described and were adequate.

7. There were adequate selection and measurement of independent (classification, predictor) variables.

8. There were adequate selection and measurement of dependent (criterion, predicted) variables.

9. General comments.

Overall Rating (Materials):   _____   _____   _____   _____

                                   Poor   Fair   Good   Excellent

Evaluation Items (Procedures)   *Evaluation Notes*

1. Research design was appropriate to purpose of study.

2. Procedures reduced threats to internal validity arising from:

   (a) history

   (b) maturation

   (c) pretesting

   (d) mortality

   (e) interaction of above

3. Procedures reduced threats to external validity arising from:

   (a) reactive arrangements

   (b) reactive effects of pretesting

   (c) subject selection

   (d) multiple treatments

4. General comments.

Overall Rating (Procedures):

_____	_____	_____	_____
Poor	Fair	Good	Excellent

Overall Rating (Method):

_____	_____	_____	_____
Poor	Fair	Good	Excellent

EVALUATION CHECKLIST—RESULTS

Instructions: The four-category scale at the end of this checklist may be used to rate the *Results* section of an article. The *Evaluation Items* help identify those topics that should be considered in arriving at the rating. Comments on these topics, entered as *Evaluation Notes,* should serve as the basis for the overall rating.

Evaluation Items

Evaluation Notes

1. Results were clearly related to research problem.

2. Tables and figures were integrated with text.

3. Summary statistics were used appropriately.

4. Organization of data was clear.

5. Statistical analysis was appropriate to:

    (a) level of measurement

    (b) number of observations

    (c) type of sample

    (d) shape of distribution

6. There was appropriate use of correlational and inferential analysis.

7. There was clear presentation of significant and nonsignificant correlations.

8. There was clear presentation of significant and nonsignificant differences.

9. General comments.

Overall Rating (Results):

_____	_____	_____	_____
Poor	Fair	Good	Excellent

EVALUATION CHECKLIST—DISCUSSION

Instructions: The four-category scale at the end of this checklist may be used to rate the *Discussion* section of an article. The *Evaluation Items* help identify those topics that should be considered in arriving at the rating. Comments on these topics, entered as *Evaluation Notes,* should serve as the basis for the overall rating.

Evaluation Items   *Evaluation Notes*

1. Discussion was clearly related to research problem.

2. Limitations of the method were discussed.

3. Conclusions were drawn directly and fairly from results.

4. Reasonable explanations were given for unusual, atypical, or discrepant results.

5. There was thorough and objective discussion of agreements and disagreements of previous research.

6. The section related results to various theoretical explanations.

7. Implications for clinical practice were stated fairly and objectively.

8. Theoretical or clinical speculations were identified and justified.

9. Suggestions for future research were identified.

10. General comments.

Overall Rating (Discussion):   _____   _____   _____   _____

                                     Poor   Fair   Good   Excellent

Example Article for Evaluation in Audiology

Masking of Speech in Young and Elderly Listeners with Hearing Loss

PAMELA E. SOUZA
CHRISTOPHER W. TURNER
Communication Sciences and Disorders
Syracuse University
Syracuse, NY

This study examined the contributions of various properties of background noise to the speech recognition difficulties experienced by young and elderly listeners with hearing loss. Three groups of subjects participated: young listeners with normal hearing, young listeners with sensorineural hearing loss, and elderly listeners with sensorineural hearing loss. Sensitivity thresholds up to 4000 Hz of the young and elderly groups of listeners with hearing loss were closely matched, and a high-pass masking noise was added to minimize the contributions of high-frequency (above 4000 Hz) thresholds, which were not closely matched. Speech recognition scores for monosyllables were obtained in the high-pass noise alone and in three noise backgrounds. The latter consisted of high-pass noise plus one of three maskers: speech-spectrum noise, speech-spectrum noise temporally modulated by the envelope of multi-talker babble, and multi-talker babble. For all conditions, the groups with hearing impairment consistently scored lower than the group with normal hearing. Although there was a trend toward poorer speech-recognition scores as the masker condition more closely resembled the speech babble, the effect of masker condition was not statistically significant.

Reprinted with permission from *Journal of Speech and Hearing Research, 37,* pp. 655–661, June 1994.

There was no interaction between group and condition, implying that listeners with normal hearing and listeners with hearing loss are affected similarly by the type of background noise when the long-term spectrum of the masker is held constant. A significant effect of age was not observed. In addition, masked thresholds for pure tones in the presence of the speech-spectrum masker were not different for the young and elderly listeners with hearing loss. These results suggest that, for both steady-state and modulated background noises, difficulties in speech recognition for monosyllables are due primarily, and perhaps exclusively, to the presence of sensorineural hearing loss itself, and not to age-specific factors.

KEY WORDS: speech recognition, masking, modulated noise, aging

---

The fact that background noise presents a special problem for listeners with sensorineural hearing impairment has been known for some time (e.g., Cooper & Cutts, 1971; Ross, Huntington, Newby, & Dixon, 1965). Recent research has suggested that elderly listeners have poorer speech recognition in difficult listening situations when compared to young listeners with similar hearing losses (e.g., Dubno, Dirks, & Morgan, 1984; Gelfand, Ross, & Miller, 1988; Helfer & Wilber, 1990); however, the relative contributions of threshold elevation versus age on speech understanding in noise are not yet clear.

Recent research has typically employed one of several methods to examine possible aging effects separately from the sensitivity loss that occurs with presbycusis. One frequently used approach is to recruit subjects with normal hearing for both the elderly and young groups. However, this approach presents difficulties because of the limited availability of elderly persons (over 60 years) with normal hearing. Additionally, even if "normal hearing" is defined as pure tone thresholds of 20 dB HL or better for the speech frequencies, there may still be a significant difference in hearing status between a group of elderly subjects with hearing thresholds of 20 dB HL and a group of younger subjects with hearing thresholds of 0 dB HL, although both groups fall within "normal" limits. Finally, normal hearing thresholds in elderly listeners may not ensure a lack of cochlear damage, because it has been shown that structural damage can exist in the aged auditory system that does not have a measurable effect on pure tone thresholds (e.g., Schuknecht & Woellner, 1955). A second experimental approach takes decreased hearing sensitivity into account by comparing older and younger groups with hearing loss, which are matched as closely as possible for audiometric thresholds. Although this method provides some practical difficulties because of the need to match thresholds closely, it offers a means to more closely control the effect of hearing sensitivity independent of possible aging effects. Alternatively, some researchers have attempted to eliminate the effect of hearing loss from that of aging by use of statistical methods. However, caution should be used when employing statistical controls because they may bias results if applied inappropriately (Martin, Ellsworth, & Cranford, 1991).

Even when researchers have attempted to control for hearing loss, the effect of aging per se on speech understanding remains in dispute. A number of studies have concluded that the primary factor in the speech recognition difficulties of elderly listeners with hearing loss is threshold elevation (e.g., Humes & Christopherson, 1991; Humes, Nelson, & Pisoni, 1991; Humes & Roberts, 1990; Nabelek, 1988; Takahashi & Bacon, 1992; Van

Rooij & Plomp, 1989, 1990, 1992). However, the variance in speech understanding does not appear to be completely accounted for by pure tone thresholds (Dubno, Dirks, & Morgan, 1984; Helfer & Huntley, 1991; Helfer & Wilber, 1990; Humes & Roberts, 1990), particularly for listeners over 75 years of age (Humes & Christopherson, 1991).

It is possible that the range of findings regarding the effect of age per se on speech understanding in noise is due to differences in test paradigm. Gordon-Salant (1987) suggested that an adaptive test paradigm rather than a fixed-level condition was necessary to show an effect of aging on speech understanding. Using an adaptive strategy, Dubno et al. (1984) did note an effect of age on speech recognition threshold in noise for listeners with normal hearing and hearing impairment despite equivalent performance in quiet and concluded that the decrease in performance in noise for the older listening groups could not be a result of threshold sensitivity differences. Although listener groups were not precisely matched for mean audiometric threshold, correlations with pure tone thresholds did not suggest a predictive relationship. However, poorer results (i.e., increased signal-to-noise ratio) for an adaptive task can result strictly from elevated high-frequency thresholds (Humes, 1991).

When comparing the speech-masking effects of different types of noise backgrounds, some investigators have reported a greater masking effect upon speech recognition from steady-state noise as opposed to single-talker competing speech (e.g., Carhart, Tillman, & Greetis, 1969; Festen & Plomp, 1990). However, this does not appear to hold true for multi-talker maskers, which can produce as much (Gordon-Salant & Wightman, 1983) or more interference (Danhauer & Leppler, 1979) than steady-state noise. Modulated maskers may interfere with the perception of the natural envelope cues in speech. On the other hand, it seems likely that a steady-state noise masker could produce more speech interference than a single-talker masker or some types of amplitude-modulated noise if large "quiet spots" are present in the modulated maskers. As more talkers are added, the quiet spots disappear and the speech masking effect of the modulated signal would increase. In a recent study, Takahashi and Bacon (1992) measured speech understanding of nonsense sentences as a function of signal-to-noise ratio in an unmodulated background noise and a background noise with a modulation frequency of 8 Hz and a modulation depth of 100%. They observed higher speech recognition scores for the modulated than for the unmodulated masking noise condition, even though the modulated-noise masker was presented at a slightly higher long-term level (1.7 dB) than the steady-state noise. This might have been due to the fact that 100% amplitude modulation of the noise produced large "quiet spots" that listeners used to advantage (Takahashi & Bacon, 1992).

Bronkhorst and Plomp (1992) measured speech-reception thresholds (SRTs) in a modulated noise background for listeners with normal hearing and hearing loss. The background noise was modulated by speech envelopes from one, two, four, or six interfering talkers and equated for long-term sound pressure level and average spectra. For both listeners with normal hearing and hearing impairment, SRT in noise improved as the number of talkers decreased. For all test conditions, the listeners with hearing loss performed significantly worse than the listeners with normal hearing, with the largest difference between the two groups occurring for a small number of talkers. The experimenters suggested that the listeners with hearing loss might be less able to take advantage of the masker modulations. Poorer performance for listeners with hearing loss in a modulated masker was also noted by Hygge, Ronnberg, Larsby, and Arlinger (1992), who interpreted this effect as a result of the poorer temporal resolution of the subjects with hearing loss.

A number of other studies have suggested that listeners with sensorineural hearing loss have poorer temporal resolution than listeners with normal hearing (Bacon & Gleitman, 1992; Bacon & Viemeister, 1985; Fitzgibbons & Wightman, 1982; Tyler, Summerfield, Wood, & Fernandes, 1982), although it appears that the loss of high-frequency sensitivity alone can lead to such results (Bacon & Gleitman, 1992; Bacon & Viemeister, 1985; Festen & Plomp, 1990; Humes, 1990; Humes & Christopherson, 1991). Poor temporal resolution has been implicated as a factor in the reduced speech reception abilities of some elderly persons. Huff (1988) demonstrated an association between reduced temporal processing abilities and speech understanding in noise for elderly listeners independent of the presence of sensorineural hearing loss. Humes and Christopherson (1991) measured performance on several psychoacoustic tasks (including temporal processing) as well as speech identification and found no differences in performance between young listeners with a masker-simulated hearing loss and elderly listeners (65–75 years) with hearing loss, implicating audibility as the primary factor in speech-recognition deficits for that age group. A group of persons with hearing loss aged 76–86 years performed significantly worse than a group aged 65–75 years with similar audiometric thresholds, suggesting deficits beyond those caused by audibility alone. Both groups of elderly listeners with hearing loss performed significantly worse than the young groups with normal hearing and simulated hearing loss on tasks that involved detection of a change in temporal sequence, suggesting that aging, in addition to audibility, may be a significant factor in these types of psychoacoustic tasks.

The present study was designed to examine further the effect of masker modulation in young and elderly subjects, with special care taken to control peripheral threshold effects. Sensitivity thresholds for young and elderly listeners with hearing loss were carefully equated. In addition, because it has been noted that nerve fibers with a high characteristic frequency are capable of coding lower frequency phonemic information (Delgutte, 1980; Kiang & Moxon, 1974; Van Tasell & Turner, 1984), and because our subjects were not closely matched for audiometric thresholds above 4000 Hz, we controlled for the possibility of confounding contributions from the basal end of the cochlea by adding a high-pass masker in all conditions. We also considered the possibility that an aging effect on speech recognition in noise, if it exists, might be related to excess amount of masking. A masked-threshold measure was therefore included to examine this possibility.

The specific questions addressed were: (a) As the background noise becomes more similar to speech in terms of temporal and/or spectral variation, with long-term spectral characteristics and average level held constant, is there a decrease in speech understanding for listeners with sensorineural hearing loss? (b) In view of the poorer temporal abilities that appear to exist in some elderly subjects (e.g., Huff, 1988), do elderly listeners with sensorineural hearing loss have greater difficulty in speech understanding than carefully matched young listeners as the modulations of the background noise become more similar to those of speech? (c) Do elderly listeners have higher-than-normal masked thresholds in a steady-state noise, and, if so, might these differences contribute to potential aging effects for speech recognition in noise?

> USE THE EVALUATION CHECKLIST TO GUIDE YOUR EVALUATION
> OF THE INTRODUCTION

Method

Subjects

Subjects were recruited into three groups. Ten young adult listeners (3 men and 7 women, age 22–35 years, mean age 29.8) with mild-to-moderate sensorineural hearing loss, 10 elderly adult listeners (2 men and 8 women, age 64–77 years, mean age 68.8) with mild-to-moderate sensorineural hearing loss, and 10 young adult listeners (1 man and 9 women, age 20–40 years, mean age 25.0) with normal hearing participated in the experiment. For group comparisons, the young listeners with hearing loss (YHI) and the elderly listeners with hearing loss (EHI) were matched for group mean audiometric thresholds to within 3 dB at 250, 500, 1000, 2000, 3000, and 4000 Hz. The listeners with normal hearing (NH) served as a control group and had pure tone thresholds of 10 dB HL (re ANSI, 1989) or better at 250, 500, 1000, 2000, 3000, and 4000 Hz. Mean audiometric thresholds are shown in Figure 1.

Only one ear of each subject was tested, and in the subjects with hearing loss the ear that most closely matched the desired group mean was chosen; however, in most cases audiometric thresholds were similar in both ears for a given subject. All subjects had normal static admittance and middle ear pressures and were native English speakers. All of the older subjects with hearing loss reported gradual onset of hearing loss relatively late in life; because no other underlying cause was present, these hearing losses were presumed to be age-related. The young subjects with hearing loss reported a variety of onset times of hearing impairment; all of these subjects reported the cause of their hearing loss as unknown, with the exception of one viral onset and two noise exposure histories.

Speech Stimuli

Our purpose was to investigate aging effects due to more peripheral, rather than central, factors, and to minimize cognitive demands on the listener. Therefore, we used monosyllabic words to reduce the possibility of syntactic cues. Four 50-word lists of Northwestern University Auditory Test No. 6 (NU6) (Tillman & Carhart, 1966), words spoken by a female talker and recorded on a compact disc (Audiology Section, VA Medical Center, 1989), were used as the speech stimuli. Each word was presented in the carrier phrase "Say the word - - - - - -." All test stimuli were presented simultaneously with a masker consisting of white noise high-pass filtered at 4000 Hz to minimize the contributions to speech recognition of the basal end of the cochlea, where sensitivity thresholds were not matched between the YHI and EHI groups. The high-pass noise was presented at a level of 60 dB SPL. Due to the low-pass roll-off of the headphones, this was actually a bandpass noise

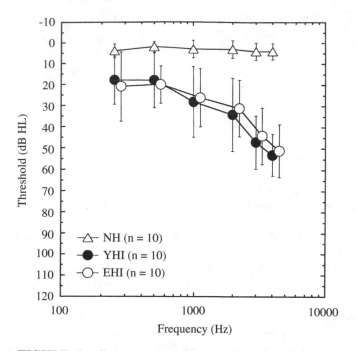

FIGURE 1   Group mean audiometric thresholds for young subjects with normal hearing (NH), young subjects with hearing loss (YHI), and elderly subjects with hearing loss (EHI). Error bars represent ± one standard deviation from the mean.

(–3 dB bandwidth 4–10 kHz). Speech items were presented in the high-pass noise only and in three different background conditions consisting of the high-pass noise plus one of three masking noises (described below). Speech was presented at 80 dB SPL, with each background noise presented at a long-term average level of 75 dB SPL for a signal-to-noise ratio of +5 dB.

Background Noises

The 12-talker babble from the Speech Perception in Noise (SPIN) test (Kalikow, Stevens, & Elliott, 1977) was used as background noise for the babble condition. The babble was the most speechlike of the three maskers, since it contained detailed temporal and spectral variations similar to "real speech."

To create the speech-spectrum masking noise, the output from a tape recording of the SPIN test 12-talker babble was routed to a spectrum analyzer (Hewlett-Packard 3571A), and the resulting frequency spectrum was used as a model to set the configuration of a spectrum shaper (Orban 672A). The output of a white noise generator (MDF 8156) was then passed through the spectrum shaper to create the speech-spectrum noise. One-third octave frequency spectra for the multi-talker babble and speech-spectrum noise were within ±2 dB from 125 to 4000 Hz and within ±5 dB from 5000 to 8000 Hz. The speech-spectrum noise was recorded on a 30-min audio tape. A sample of the speech-spectrum noise was also digitized for use in creation of the babble-modulated noise.

The final noise masker, referred to here as babble-modulated noise, was designed to have a temporal envelope similar to that of the multi-talker babble, but without the specific short-term spectral and temporal details of actual speech. A 6.5 sec sample of the SPIN test 12-talker babble was low-pass filtered at 30 Hz to yield essentially a flat-spectrum noise below this cutoff frequency. This signal was then full-wave rectified and multiplied by the speech-spectrum noise. Although this procedure is not identical to the traditional method of creating speech envelope noise, which rectifies the speech signal before low-pass filtering, our method did produce a masker having temporal envelope characteristics similar to those of the natural babble. Three-msec rise and fall times were added to the resulting signal, and it was played repeatedly for recording on a 30-min audio tape. One-third octave frequency spectra for the babble-modulated noise and the speech-spectrum noise were within ±2 dB from 125 to 8000 Hz.

Representative time waveforms for the three masking noises are shown in Figure 2.

Speech Recognition Procedures

Each subject participated in two test sessions, conducted approximately one week apart. A session consisted of one 50-word list presented in each of the four conditions (high-pass noise only [HP only], speech-spectrum noise plus high-pass noise [SSN+HP], babble-modulated noise plus high-pass noise [BMN+HP], babble plus high-pass noise [B+ HP]). Each subject was individually seated in a double-walled sound booth, with speech and background noise mixed and presented monaurally through a Beyer DT48 headphone. No word list was presented in the same condition twice, and for the second session the order of the conditions was reversed from that of the first session, to ensure that if fatigue influenced subjects' scores for the later presented conditions, this influence would not affect final results averaged over the two sessions.

Masked-Threshold Procedures

To investigate the contributions of masked thresholds to speech recognition in noise, masked pure tone thresholds at 125, 250, 500, 1000, 1500, 2000, 3000, and 4000 Hz were measured for each subject using an adaptive four-alternative forced-choice procedure to obtain an estimate of the 71%-correct level of detection (Levitt, 1971). The masker was the speech-spectrum noise described above presented at 75 dB SPL. The same high-pass noise as used in the four speech-recognition conditions was also presented during the masked-threshold task.

USE THE EVALUATION CHECKLIST TO GUIDE YOUR EVALUATION
OF THE METHOD

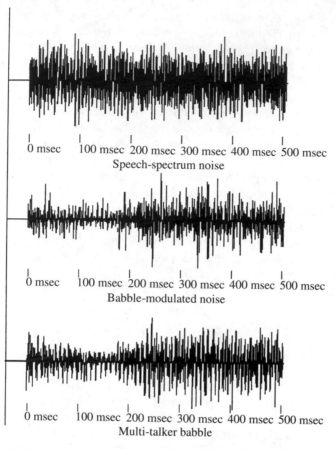

0 msec   100 msec 200 msec 300 msec 400 msec 500 msec
Speech-spectrum noise

0 msec   100 msec 200 msec 300 msec 400 msec 500 msec
Babble-modulated noise

0 msec   100 msec 200 msec 300 msec 400 msec 500 msec
Multi-talker babble

FIGURE 2   500-msec segments of the time waveforms for the three background noises. Top panel shows speech-spectrum noise; middle panel shows babble-modulated noise; bottom panel shows multi-talker babble.

Results

Speech Recognition

Speech recognition scores for the three subject groups are plotted in Figure 3. Error bars represent plus and minus one standard deviation about the mean. Before statistical analysis, percent correct scores were converted to rationalized arcsine values (Studebaker, 1985). An initial comparison of the group means in the HP-only condition was performed via a one-way analysis of variance (ANOVA); it indicated a significant effect of group,

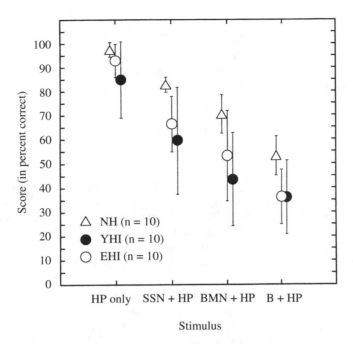

FIGURE 3 **Group mean speech recognition scores expressed in percent correct for subjects with normal hearing (NH), young subjects with hearing loss (YHI), and elderly subjects with hearing loss (EHI) for the four background conditions (high-pass noise only [HP only], speech-spectrum noise plus high-pass noise [SSN+HP], babble-modulated noise plus high-pass noise [BMN+HP], babble plus high-pass noise [B+HP]).**

F (2, 27) = 3.528, p <.05. A repeated-measure analysis of covariance was then performed on the scores obtained in noise. The score in the HP-only condition was used as the covariate to prevent between-group differences in this condition from influencing results for the speech-masking noise conditions. Results of this analysis indicated that the main effect of group (NH, YHI, EHI) was significant, F (2, 26) = 7.178, p <.005. Although the group mean speech-recognition results show a trend towards decreasing speech-recognition scores for all groups of subjects as the temporal and/or spectral variations in the masking noise became more speechlike, the effect of background condition (SSN+HP, BMN+HP, B+HP) was not found to be significant, F (2, 52) = 0.644, p = .529. The interaction between group and condition was also not significant, F (4, 52) = 0.777, p = .545, suggesting that all groups were similarly affected by the speechlike background noise types.

We were particularly interested in the presence or absence of an aging effect for these listening conditions. Fisher's Least Significant Difference post hoc tests with Type I error rate set at a maximum of .05 were performed to explore differences in the group effect, and results indicated significant effects for the young group with hearing impairment versus the group with normal hearing, as well as for the elderly group with hearing impairment versus the group with normal hearing. There was no significant difference between the young versus elderly groups with hearing impairment.

Masked Threshold

Mean masked thresholds (in dB SPL) for the three subject groups are shown in Figure 4. For all test frequencies, the groups with hearing loss had higher masked thresholds than the group with normal hearing. This effect was more pronounced at frequencies above 2000 Hz, where there was a greater difference in quiet thresholds between the listeners with hearing loss and the listeners with normal hearing (Trees & Turner, 1986). Because our primary question concerned possible differences between the young and elderly listeners with hearing loss, the listeners with normal hearing were excluded from further analysis. A two-factor repeated measures ANOVA was performed on the sets of masked thresholds for the two groups with hearing loss to examine possible aging effects. The within-subject effect of frequency (125, 250, 500, 1000, 1500, 2000, 3000, 4000) was significant, $F (7, 126) = 18.277$, $p < .0005$, as expected. The main effect of group (young listeners with hearing loss, elderly listeners with hearing loss) was not significant, $F (1, 18) = 0.097$, $p = .759$. These results are in agreement with those of Klein, Mills, and Adkins (1990), who found that elderly listeners with hearing loss did not show an excessive amount of masking when compared to younger listeners with hearing loss.

USE THE EVALUATION CHECKLIST TO GUIDE YOUR EVALUATION
OF THE RESULTS

Discussion

Although results showed a trend towards poorer speech-recognition scores as the temporal and/or spectral variations of the masking noise became more speechlike, with long-term masker level and spectral content held constant, this was not found to be significant. This effect is seen equivalently in listeners with normal hearing and listeners with hearing impairment, as demonstrated by the lack of interaction between condition and subject group. Although we found no improvement of speech recognition in a modulated versus a steady-state background noise, other research has noted an improvement in speech recognition (Takahashi & Bacon, 1992) or in speech-reception threshold (Bronkhorst & Plomp, 1992; Festen & Plomp, 1990) in a modulated background. However, the studies noted differ in the depth of modulation used. Use of 100% modulation depth, or single-talker backgrounds, is likely to result in larger "quiet spots" in which speech sounds can be more eas-

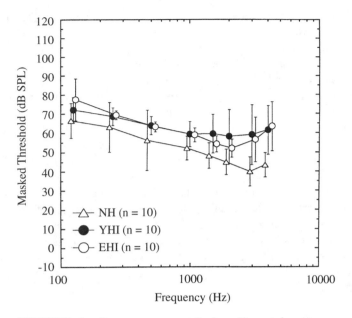

FIGURE 4   **Group mean masked audiometric thresholds for subjects with normal hearing (NH), young subjects with hearing loss (YHI), and elderly subjects with hearing loss (EHI). Masker was 75 dB SPL speech-spectrum noise. Error bars represent ± one standard deviation from the mean.**

ily detected, in contrast to the modulated noise used in the present research, in which virtually no "quiet spots" existed. In addition, each of the above studies used sentences (either meaningful or "nonsense" sentences) as the speech material. It seems likely that modulation of the masker may not be as helpful in the case of single words, where the length of the test material is shorter relative to the "quiet spots." In contrast, the presence of masker modulation may be more beneficial in the case of sentences, where greater redundancy of information is present.

The present study's results do not lend support to an age effect, at least for these types of speech stimuli and background maskers. There was no statistically significant difference in speech recognition scores between the young and elderly listeners with hearing loss across listening condition, nor was there an interaction between group (age) and noise condition. This lack of an aging effect is in agreement with the results of Takahashi and Bacon (1992). In our study, we took special care to match group mean hearing thresholds as well as to use a high-pass noise to equate contributions from the basal end of the cochlea between groups. This may have been responsible for the lack of an age effect found in our study. In summary, the poorer speech recognition in noise observed in our elderly subjects appears to be a simple consequence of the presence of sensorineural hearing loss.

Several additional factors may have influenced our findings, in view of previous studies of aging effects on speech recognition. Given that Gordon-Salant (1987) suggested that certain demands (such as an adaptive task) must be placed on the listener to reveal differences in speech recognition due to aging, it is possible that our speech-identification task was not sufficiently demanding. A second issue involves the age of our elderly listeners. Humes and Christopherson (1991) noted poorer performance on a filtered-speech identification task by a group of listeners aged 76–86 years as compared to a group of listeners aged 65–75 years with equivalent hearing loss. This suggests that where present an aging effect on speech recognition may be influenced by the age of the listener; a subject aged 85 years may perform more poorly on some tasks than a subject aged 65 years. Perhaps our elderly listeners were not "old enough" to show a significant effect of aging. Finally, our speech materials did not allow listeners to make use of syntactic cues, leaving open the possibility that aging effects in speech recognition may still exist in more "central" locations of the auditory system, and might be revealed when using speech materials that allow the listener to take advantage of contextual information. These factors may be resolved with further study.

USE THE EVALUATION CHECKLIST TO GUIDE YOUR EVALUATION
OF THE DISCUSSION

Acknowledgments

This research was supported in part by NIH grant #DC00377. We also thank Sid Bacon for helpful comments concerning our modulated noise.

References

American National Standards Institute. (1989). *Specification for Audiometers* (ANSI S3.6-1989). New York: ANSI.

Audiology Section, VA Medical Center, Long Beach, California. (1989). *Speech recognition and identification materials, Disc 1* (Compact Audio Disc). Washington, DC: Rehabilitation Research and Development Service.

Bacon, S. P., & Gleitman, R. M. (1992). Modulation detection in subjects with relatively flat hearing losses. *Journal of Speech and Hearing Research, 35,* 642–453.

Bacon, S. P., & Viemeister, N. F. (1985). Temporal modulation function in normal-hearing and hearing-impaired listeners. *Audiology, 24,* 115–134.

Bronkhorst, A. W., & Plomp, R. (1992). Effect of multiple speech-like maskers on binaural speech recognition in normal and impaired hearing. *Journal of the Acoustical Society of America, 92,* 3132–3139.

Carhart, R., Tillman, T. W., & Greetis, E. S. (1969). Perceptual masking in multiple sound background. *Journal of the Acoustical Society of America, 45,* 694–703.

Cooper, J. C., & Cutts, B. P. (1971). Speech discrimination in noise. *Journal of Speech and Hearing Research, 14,* 332–337.

Danhauer, J. L., & Leppler, J.G. (1979). Effects of four noise competitors on the California Consonant Test. *Journal of Speech and Hearing Disorders, 44*, 354–362.

Delgutte, B. (1980). Representation of speech-like sounds in the discharge patterns of auditory-nerve fibers. *Journal of the Acoustical Society of America, 68*, 843–857.

Dubno, J. R., Dirks, D. D., & Morgan, D. E. (1984). Effects of age and mild hearing loss on speech recognition in noise. *Journal of the Acoustical Society of America, 76*, 87–1144.

Festen, J. M., & Plomp, R. (1990). Effects of fluctuating noise and interfering speech on the speech-reception threshold for impaired and normal hearing. *Journal of the Acoustical Society of America, 88*, 1725–1736.

Fitzgibbons, P. J., & Wightman, F. L (1982). Gap detection in normal and hearing-impaired listeners. *Journal of the Acoustical Society of America, 72*, 761–765.

Gelfand, S. A., Ross, L., & Miller, S. (1988). Sentence reception in noise from one versus two sources: Effects of aging and hearing loss. *Journal of the Acoustical Society of America, 83*, 248–256.

Gordon-Salant, S. M. (1987). Age-related differences in speech recognition performance as a function of test format and paradigm. *Ear and Hearing, 8*, 277–282.

Gordon-Salant, S. M., & Wightman, F. L (1983). Speech competition effects on synthetic stop-vowel perception by normal and hearing-impaired listeners. *Journal of the Acoustical Society of America, 73*, 1756–1765.

Helfer, K. S., & Huntley, R. A. (1991). Aging and consonant errors in reverberation and noise. *Journal of the Acoustical Society of America, 90*, 1786–1796.

Helfer, K. S., & Wilber, L. A. (1990). Hearing loss, aging, and speech perception in reverberation and noise. *Journal of Speech and Hearing Research, 33*, 149–155.

Huff, S. J. (1988). *Temporal processing and speech intelligibility as a function of age*. Unpublished doctoral dissertation, University of Washington, Seattle.

Humes, L. E. (1990). Masking of tone bursts by modulated noise in normal, noise-masked normal, and hearing-impaired listeners. *Journal of Speech and Hearing Research, 33*, 3–8.

Humes, L. E. (1991). Understanding the speech-understanding problems of the hearing impaired. *Journal of the American Academy of Audiology, 2*, 59–69.

Humes, L. E., & Christopherson L. (1991). Speech identification difficulties of hearing-impaired elderly persons: The contributions of auditory processing deficits. *Journal of Speech and Hearing Research, 34*, 686–693.

Humes, L. E., Nelson, K. J., & Pisoni, D. B. (1991). Recognition of synthetic speech by hearing-impaired elderly listeners. *Journal of Speech and Hearing Research, 34*, 1180–1184.

Humes, L. E., & Roberts, L. (1990). Speech-recognition difficulties of the hearing-impaired elderly: The contributions of audibility. *Journal of Speech and Hearing Research, 33*, 726–735.

Hygge, S., Ronnberg, J., Larsby, B., & Arlinger, S. (1992). Normal-hearing and hearing-impaired subjects' ability to just follow conversation in competing speech, reversed speech and noise backgrounds. *Journal of Speech and Hearing Research, 35*, 208–215.

Kalikow, D. N., Stevens, K. N., & Elliott, L. L. (1977). Development of a test of speech intelligibility in noise using sentence materials with controlled word predictability. *Journal of the Acoustical Society of America, 61*, 1337–1351.

Kiang, N. Y. S., & Moxon, E. C. (1974). Tails of tuning curves of auditory-nerve fibers. *Journal of the Acoustical Society of America, 55*, 620–630.

Klein, A. J., Mills, J. H., & Adkins, W. Y. (1990). Upward spread of masking, hearing loss, and speech recognition in young and elderly listeners. *Journal of the Acoustical Society of America, 87*, 1266–1271.

Levitt, H. (1971). Transformed up-down methods in psychoacoustics. *Journal of the Acoustical Society of America, 49*, 476–477.

Martin, D., Ellsworth, R., & Cranford, J. (1991). Limitations of analysis of covariance designs in aging research. *Ear and Hearing, 12*, 85–86.

Nabelek, A. K. (1988). Identification of vowels in quiet, noise, and reverberation: Relationships with age and hearing loss. *Journal of the Acoustical Society of America, 84*, 476–484.

Ross, M., Huntington, D., Newby, H. A., & Dixon, R. (1965). Speech discrimination of hearing-impaired individuals in noise. *Journal of Auditory Research, 5,* 47–72.

Schuknecht, H. F., & Woellner, R. C. (1955, February). An experimental and clinical study of deafness from lesions of the cochlear nerve. *Journal of Laryngology and Otology, 75*–97.

Studebaker, G. A. (1985). A "rationalized" arcsine transform. *Journal of Speech and Hearing Research, 12,* 455–462.

Takahashl, G. A., & Bacon, S. P. (1992). Modulation detection, modulation masking, and speech understanding in noise in the elderly. *Journal of Speech and Hearing Research, 35,* 1410–1421.

Tillman, T. W., & Carhart, R. (1966). *An expanded test for speech discrimination utilizing CNC monosyllabic words: Northwestern University Auditory Test No. 6.* Brooks Air Force Base, TX: USAF School of Aerospace Medicine.

Trees, D. E., & Turner, C. W. (1986). Spread of masking in normal subjects and in subjects with high-frequency hearing loss. *Audiology, 25,* 70–83.

Tyler, R. S., Summerfield, Q., Wood, E. J., & Fernandes, M. A. (1982). Psychoacoustic and phonetic temporal processing in normal and hearing-impaired listeners. *Journal of the Acoustical Society of America, 72,* 740–752.

VanRooij, J. C. G. M., & Plomp, R. (1989). Auditive and cognitive factors in speech perception by elderly listeners. I: Development of test battery. *Journal of the Acoustical Society of America, 86,* 1294–1309.

VanRooij, J. C. G. M., & Plomp, R. (1990). Auditive and cognitive factors in speech perception by elderly listeners. II: Multivariate analyses. *Journal of the Acoustical Society of America, 88,* 2611–2624.

VanRooij, J. C. G. M., & Plomp, R. (1992). Auditive and cognitive factors in speech perception by elderly listeners. III: Additional data and final discussion. *Journal of the Acoustical Society of America, 91,* 1028–1033.

VanTasell, D. J., & Turner, C. W. (1984). Speech recognition in a special case of low-frequency hearing loss. *Journal of the Acoustical Society of America, 75,* 1207–1212.

Received April 12, 1993
Accepted December 21, 1993

Contact author: Paula E. Souza, PhD, Syracuse University, Communication Sciences and Disorders, 805 South Crouse Avenue,Syracuse, NY 13244. E-mail: souzapam@mailbox.syr.edu

Example Article for Evaluation in Speech Disorders

Effects of Temporal Alterations on Speech Intelligibility in Parkinsonian Dysarthria

VICKI L. HAMMEN
Audiology and Speech Sciences
Purdue University
West Lafayette, IN

KATHRYN M. YORKSTON
Department of Rehabilitation Medicine
University of Washington, Seattle

FRED D. MINIFIE
Department of Speech and Hearing Sciences
University of Washington, Seattle

The effect of two types of temporal alterations, paced and synthetic, on the intelligibility of parkinsonian dysarthric speech was investigated. Six speakers with idiopathic Parkinson's disease served as subjects. Paced temporal alterations were created by slowing each speaker to 60% of his/her habitual speaking rate. The synthetic alterations were created by modifying the habitual rate speech samples using digital signal processing. Three types of synthetic alterations were examined: Pause Altered, Speech Duration Altered, and Pause and Speech Duration Altered. The 60% of habitual speaking rate condition was more intelligible than the synthetic conditions. In addition, none of the

Reprinted with permission from *Journal of Speech and Hearing Research, 37,* pp. 244–253, April 1994.

synthetic alterations were found to be more intelligible than samples produced at habitual speaking rates. The results suggest that simple alterations of speech signals do not explain the differences in intelligibility that have been observed when parkinsonian dysarthric speakers reduce speaking rates. Reasons for the failure of synthetic alterations to increase speech intelligibility scores are discussed.

KEY WORDS: Parkinson's disease, dysarthria, speaking rate, acoustics

The temporal pattern of speech can be characterized by simple measures of duration of speech, number of pauses, and duration of pauses. These measures have been used to study how non-impaired individuals modify their speaking rates. Results indicate that as speaking rate is adjusted, the number and/or duration of pauses is primarily responsible for the observed changes in overall speech tempo (Goldman-Eisler, 1968; Lane & Grosjean, 1973; Minifie, 1973). Reviews by Miller (1981) and Gay (1981) present data indicating that the duration of consonant and vowel segments, as well as the spectral characteristics of these phonemes change as speaking rate is increased.

Alterations in the temporal pattern of speech are commonly associated with dysarthria. In their study of over 200 dysarthric speakers, Darley, Aronson, and Brown (1975) found that 80% had speaking rates that differed from normal. Patterns of temporal alteration vary with the type of dysarthria: most often speaking rates of dysarthric speakers are slower than those of non-impaired speakers, but rates may also be so rapid as to impair intelligibility. Treatment may then focus on techniques to slow overall speaking rate. Rate reduction techniques vary in their impact on the speech and pause components of the overall speech sample. Delayed auditory feedback (DAF) has been shown to increase both speech and pause duration when used to reduce the speaking rates of individuals with Parkinson's disease (Hanson and Metter, 1983). Hammen, Yorkston, and Beukelman (1989) reported that when small changes in overall rate were required, parkinsonian dysarthric speakers primarily altered speech duration. Increases in the pause duration occurred once substantial rate reductions were demanded.

These studies provide some insight into the type of temporal alterations that occur when parkinsonian speakers are asked to reduce speech rate. However, the differential effect of speech versus pause alterations on speech intelligibility has not been examined systematically. Canter and Van Lancker (1985) attempted to address this issue when they expanded speech samples obtained from one individual with Parkinson's disease using a computerized speech compressor/expander (Varispeech II). Intelligibility increased by 11% for the expanded version of the utterances.

Although few researchers have investigated the effects of temporal alterations on the speech intelligibility of dysarthric speakers, the impact of temporal changes on deaf speech has been examined by several authors (Maassen, 1986; Maassen & Povel, 1984; Osberger & Levitt, 1979). These researchers manipulated both the speech and pause characteristics of sentences read by deaf children. They also used digital processing techniques to create relative and absolute changes in phoneme and syllable duration. Maassen and Povel (1984), in an extension of Osberger and Levitt's (1979) work, found that none of the changes significantly improved speech intelligibility. The elimination of pauses, however, had a detrimental effect on speech intelligibility, leading the authors to conclude that the removal of pauses decreased listener processing time, thereby reducing intelligibility. Although Maassen (1986) found that intelligibility increased when pauses were inserted into sentences, a decelerated version of the sentences, created by an equal distribution of the increased length across the entire utterance, failed to improve intelligibility.

Relatively little attention has been directed toward understanding the differential effects of changes in pause and speech duration characteristics on the speech intelligibility of dysarthric speakers. One reason to examine temporal alterations in parkinsonian speech is that the patterning is distinctive and is considered a hallmark of the disorder. Such an investigation could provide insights regarding intervention and suggest factors that contribute to improved speech intelligibility when these individuals are asked to reduce speaking rates. In addition, identification of factors that contribute to improved speech intelligibility can facilitate the exploration of synthetic manipulations to bring it about (Bunnell, 1990).

The purpose of this study was to explore the impact of temporal alterations on the speech intelligibility of parkinsonian speakers. Speech was altered either through pacing or synthetically. In paced speech, parkinsonian speakers were asked to produce speech at rates slower than their habitual productions. In synthetically altered speech, recorded samples of habitual speech of these speakers were acoustically analyzed and manipulated to increase speech and/or pause duration. The questions addressed in this investigation were:

Does paced speech differ in intelligibility from habitual speech in parkinsonian dysarthria? Specifically, this research focused on whether speech intelligibility increased when parkinsonian individuals spoke at rates slower than their habitual rates. This question was asked in an effort to confirm results of previous work that suggested large intelligibility differences between speech produced at habitual and reduced rates (Yorkston, Hammen, Beukelman, & Traynor, 1990). Differences between habitual and paced speech also served as a benchmark against which to make other comparisons.

Does speech that is synthetically altered in pause and/or speech characteristics differ in intelligibility from habitual productions? This question was posed in an effort to obtain some insight into possible contributors to improved intelligibility. One theory suggests that changes in articulatory characteristics may not occur when speaking rates are reduced, but that increases in the number and duration of pauses provide listeners with more time to decode the distorted speech signal (Maasen, 1986; Maasen & Povel, 1984; Osberger & Levitt, 1979; Yorkston et al., 1988). An examination of the effects of speaking rate reduction through synthetically imposed alterations of pause and/or speech duration characteristics would provide insight into how these features affect the intelligibility of parkinsonian dysarthric speech.

Finally, does the intelligibility of paced speech differ from that of synthetically altered speech? A second theory proposes that reducing speaking rate provides dysarthric speakers with more time to achieve articulatory targets accurately (Hardy, 1983; Yorkston et al., 1988). Comparing the intelligibility of speech that has been synthetically altered with samples produced by a speaker at reduced rates would provide insight into the applicability of this theory and give us a better understanding of which factors contribute to improved speech intelligibility in the parkinsonian dysarthric population.

USE THE EVALUATION CHECKLIST TO GUIDE YOUR EVALUATION
OF THE INTRODUCTION

Methods

Subjects

The speakers with idiopathic Parkinson's disease who participated in this project were part of a larger study (Hammen, 1991). They met the following selection criteria: (a) hypokinetic dysarthria of sufficient severity for subjects or their families to report reduction in speech intelligibility; (b) 1 year or more post-diagnosis of Parkinson's disease; (c) no reported motoric side effects or on/off fluctuations from the antiparkinsonian medications they were currently taking; (d) adequate vision with corrective lenses to read from a computer screen; (e) no additional medical or neurological conditions, such as CVA, that could contribute to the observed speech disorder; and, (f) no history of hearing loss. Two speech-language pathologists experienced in differential diagnosis of dysarthria listened to audio-recorded samples of each subject's speech to confirm the presence of hypokinetic dysarthria utilizing the perceptual attributes identified by Darley and colleagues (1975) and Ludlow and Bassich (1983).

Subjects included 5 males and 1 female with a mean age of 70 years and a range of 56 to 77 years. The subjects' neurologist provided information about the date of diagnosis, severity of the Parkinson's disease, current medications, and any side effects (See Table 1). The time post-diagnosis averaged 12 years with a range from 7 to 17 years. Disease severity, rated on the scale developed by Hoehn and Yahr (1967), ranged from Stage III–V. The

TABLE 1   Subject characteristics

Subjects	Years of Age	Gender	Years Post Diagnosis	Severity*	Intelligibility at Habitual Rate**	Medications
S1	77	M	17	IV	92%	Sinemet Artane
S2	56	M	8	III	95%	Sinemet Symmetrel Bromocriptine
S3	71	M	7	III	97%	Sinemet Symmetrel
S4	73	M	13	V	77%	Sinemet Symmetrel Bromocriptine
S5	68	M	16	V	67%	Sinemet Artane Bromocriptine
S6	73	F	11	V	46%	Sinemet Artane

*Hoehn and Yahr Stage (1967).
**Sentence Test, *Computerized Assessment of Intelligibility of Dysarthric Speech* (1984).

mean sentence subtest score from three experienced listeners on the Computerized Assessment of Intelligibility of Dysarthric Speech (CAIDS) (Yorkston, Beukelman, & Traynor, 1984) was used to determine each subject's intelligibility score. Sentence intelligibility ranged from 46.4 to 96.5%, with 2 subjects greater than 80% intelligible and 3 less than 80% intelligible.

Speech Sample and Recording Equipment

A 132-word passage (See Appendix) was designed to include a number of features. A relatively long sentence length (from 20 to 26 words) was employed to encourage speakers to pause at least once when reading each sentence. The number of syllables in the sentences to be used for temporal alteration was relatively the same (from 28 to 31). Sentences were imbedded in a paragraph with a logical contextual flow to minimize misreading. Two sentences were included at the beginning of each computer screen so the speaker could adjust to the pacing rate prior to reading a sentence targeted for temporal alteration.

High-quality tape recordings of the reading passage were obtained in a quiet room on a reel-to-reel tape recorder (TEAC A3320). A Realistic electret microphone (33-1063) was positioned 10 cm from the speaker's lips at 90 degrees to the airstream using a lightweight, head-mounted apparatus throughout the recording session. Subjects were recorded one-half hour after taking antiparkinsonian medications and the entire recording session lasted no more than 2 hours. The session ended no later than one-half hour prior to their next scheduled medication dose. This was done to avoid any performance variations related to medication cycle.

Recording Tasks

Habitual speaking condition. The stimulus passage was displayed on the screen of an Apple IIe computer. Prior to the recording, the paragraph was read aloud to subjects in an effort to minimize reading errors. Subjects were asked to read exactly what appeared on the screen. No instructions regarding speaking rates were given. The duration of the passage was timed with a stop watch and habitual speaking rate (in syllables per minute) was calculated from each sample. Each subject was recorded first at habitual speaking rate and then at 60% of habitual using the procedure described below.

Paced speaking condition. Speaking rate was controlled using computerized pacing software, PACER (Beukelman, Yorkston, & Tice, 1988). This program allows a user to pace reading material at a specified syllable-per-minute rate. An algorithm in the program assigns a unit of time to each syllable in the text depending on the specified speaking rate. The durational patterning of the cursor movement through the passage is determined by the number of syllables in a word and number of junctures (i.e., commas, periods). Thus, multisyllabic words were assigned a longer duration than monosyllabic words and syntactic junctions (specified by commas or periods) were assigned one unit of time. A specific speaking rate was selected, a portion of the passage was displayed on the screen, and an underline moved through the passage indicating to the speaker the rate at which the passage was to be read. Subjects were instructed to keep up with the underlining cursor but not to get ahead of it. Previous investigations have shown that this method of speaking rate reduction reliably reduces oral reading rate of hypokinetic dysarthric speakers

(Beukelman, Yorkston, & Dowden, 1986; Hammen et al., 1989; Yorkston et al., 1990). The 60% of habitual speaking rate was used in the current study as the target paced speaking rate because the results of previous studies suggest that the greatest increases in speech intelligibility occurred at this rate.

Signal Processing

The Interactive Laboratory System (ILS-PC, version 6.0) installed on an IBM-AT compatible computer was used to process the acoustic signals in order to generate listening tapes. Five listening conditions were generated: two unaltered conditions (habitual and paced) and three synthetic temporal alteration conditions (pause altered, speech duration altered, and speech duration & pause altered). A flowchart of the signal processing appears in Figure 1.

Unmodified speaking conditions. Previous reports of synthetic alteration of deaf speech (Maasen & Povel, 1984) suggested that the resynthesis process required to create

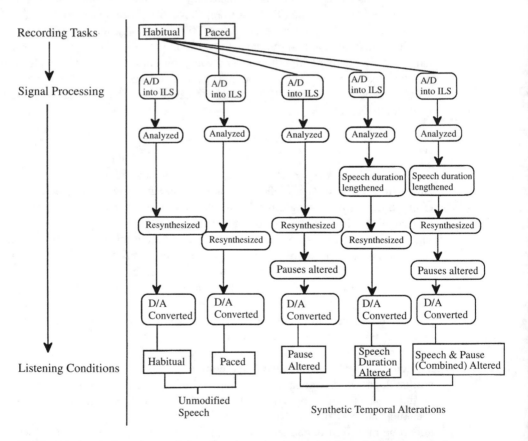

FIGURE 1 A flowchart of the signal processing steps by which the speech samples used for the intelligibility task were created.

some alterations can degrade the speech signal. Therefore, the signals for the unmodified speaking conditions (habitual and paced) were processed in a manner similar to those that were synthetically altered in order to insure consistency across samples. The unmodified speaking conditions were not subjected to additional temporal alteration. Habitual and paced speaking samples were low-pass filtered at 5000 Hz, amplified, and analog-to-digital (A/D) converted using a 10 kHz sampling rate into a sample data file. Input signal energy remained within 10 V peak-to-peak as monitored on an oscilloscope.

Synthetic temporal alterations. Samples from the habitual speaking condition were altered such that the duration of the synthetic conditions was essentially equal to the duration obtained during the paced condition. The habitual speech samples were altered in the following ways:

Pause altered. Existing pauses were lengthened and pauses were inserted within sentences at predetermined, syntactically appropriate locations in order to achieve the target duration. Several rules were consistently applied. No more than three pauses were lengthened or inserted within each sentence. The increase in duration was divided equally among the three pauses. Pauses that a speaker inserted in his or her habitual production were lengthened first. If more than three pauses occurred in the habitual sample, the pauses closest to the predetermined pause locations were lengthened. At least two words had to occur between pauses or a predetermined pause would have been used. The effect of this and other alterations to the habitual samples appears in Figure 2, showing amplitude by time plots for all conditions. The pause characteristics were added and/or increased by transferring the section of the sentence just prior to a pause to a second file following resynthesis. Because some pauses were inserted within a continuous acoustic signal, the signal surrounding a pause was modified with a special program, RAMP, that provided gradual onset and offset of the signal into and out of the silence that represented a pause.

Speech duration altered. Other researchers have changed the relative and absolute duration of phonemes in addition to overall lengthening of the speech signal to study the effects on intelligibility of changing speech duration (Maassen, 1986; Maassen & Povel, 1984; Osberger & Levitt, 1979). Pilot work showed that consistent identification of all segment boundaries in an utterance across all subjects was not possible. Therefore, as a first attempt to investigate the effect of several types of temporal alterations on speech intelligibility, lengthening of the entire speech portion of the sample was selected. Pauses that occurred in the habitual speaking rate sample were removed because we wished to examine the effect only of altering speech duration. Therefore, increases in speech duration were created by lengthening the speech portion of utterance until the duration was equivalent to the 60% of habitual speaking rate sample for each subject.

Alteration of the speech duration characteristics was completed after the sampled data file had been subjected to linear predictive coding (LPC) analysis. A hamming window and pre-emphasis were applied. Twelve coefficients were used in the analysis. The output of the LPC procedure was a series of analysis frames that represented 5.0 msec windows of the original sample. Lengthening of the samples was accomplished through the use of a specially designed program (CHANGE) that lengthens a speech sample by replicating analysis frames and repeating this process following an interval of a specified number of frames. The samples were lengthened such that the number of frames in the speech duration altered file was equal to the number of frames in the paced speaking condition file.

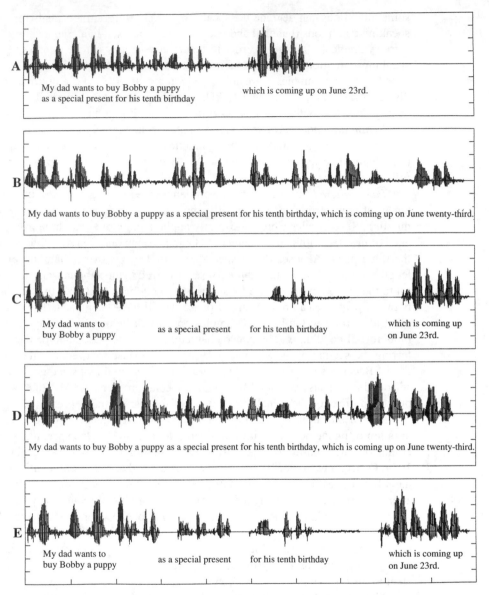

FIGURE 2 **Amplitude by time plots provide examples of the effect of temporal alteration on the habitual rate samples. (A) habitual rate, (B) paced, (C) pause-altered, (D) speech-duration altered, (E) speech-duration & pause-altered.**

For example, if the paced condition file consisted of 2208 analysis frames, and the habitual sample 1182 frames, then 1026 analysis frames were added to the habitual rate file using the CHANGE program. The increase was accomplished by submitting the analysis file to the CHANGE program twice for this example. The first pass had two frames between each replication, which resulted in a file that contained 1772 frames. The second pass had 4 analysis frames between replications to add the remaining 436 frames. Although the CHANGE program does not result in a shift of the fundamental frequency (pitch) characteristics of the original speech samples, the slope of the intonational, as well as formant frequency contour would be affected. Once the CHANGE program was run, the sample was resynthesized within ILS-PC using the SNS (synthesize sampled data) command which incorporates a routine that has a smoothing effect on the signal. The lengthened speech segments were transferred to a second data file to reduce the length of any pauses that had occurred in the habitual rate sample to 100 msec or less (See Figure 2). A hundred milliseconds was used since it represented a duration less than that used by other researchers as a criterion for identifying pauses in a speech signal (Maassen & Povel, 1984).

Pause and speech duration altered. The overall increase in sample duration was equally divided between increases in pause duration and speech duration. These combined alterations were completed by first using the CHANGE program to lengthen the entire speech sample, resynthesizing the analysis file, and then altering the pause characteristics. As in the pause-altered condition, no more than three pauses were lengthened or added to each of the experimental sentences. Pauses occurring in the habitual sample were lengthened during the speech duration process. However, if more pause time was required after the lengthening procedure to achieve the target duration, the added pause time was inserted at the same locations used for the pause-altered condition (See Figure 2).

Intelligibility Measures

Research design. A 5×5 Latin square (Listeners x Sentences) was created for each subject, with the five conditions counterbalanced under the rows and columns of the square (Edwards, 1985). An example of a 5×5 Latin Square appears in Table 2. In this design the levels of two sources of error that the experimenter wishes to control are assigned to the columns and rows of the square. The treatment conditions are then assigned to the square once per row and column. The advantage of this design is that a reduced number of listeners are required to obtain measures of intelligibility. Because each listener is presented a different sentence for each condition, the problem of listener familiarity confounding the intelligibility measure is avoided. This design eliminates determining the reliability of the listeners using correlation methods. Therefore, relative homogeneity of the variables assigned to the rows and columns (i.e., listeners and sentences) is assumed. Additional information regarding this design may be found in Winer (1971) or Snidecor and Cochran (1967).

Generation of listening tapes. A total of 150 sentence files was created during the signal processing phase of the project (5 sentences $\times$ 5 conditions [2 unmodified and 3 synthetic temporal alterations] $\times$ 6 speakers). A Latin square design was employed to create the listening sequence for the audio tapes from which speech intelligibility was scored.

TABLE 2   Example of a 5 × 5 (Judges × Sentences) Latin square. The treatments are represented by the letters (A, B, C, D, E) within the square.

JUDGES

	1	2	3	4	5
1	B	A	E	C	D
2	A	B	C	D	E
3	E	C	D	B	A
4	D	E	A	A	C
5	C	D	B	E	B

(SENTENCES — row labels 1–5)

A = Habitual Rate
B = 60% of Habitual Rate
C = Pausal Alteration
D = Speech Duration Alteration
E = Combined Alteration

Each listener listened to a different sentence for each condition, thereby controlling for listener familiarity with the speech samples.

Tasks. Five different listeners were required for each dysarthric speaker, so a total of 30 undergraduate students served as inexperienced listeners. Listeners reported no hearing problems and had English as their primary language. They participated in the following tasks.

Practice tasks. Two practice tapes served to familiarize listeners with the orthographic transcription task and speaker characteristics. These tapes contained five sentences (Yorkston et al., 1984) produced by parkinsonian speakers with hypokinetic dysarthria who were not subjects in the current study. Intelligibility measures for these speakers were obtained from three experienced listeners using the procedures outlined in the CAIDS manual. These listeners had from 1 to 3 years of experience scoring sentence CAIDS tests. The speaker used for practice task #1 was 94.8% intelligible, and the speaker for practice task #2 was 78.3% intelligible.

The inexperienced listeners listened to the audio tapes individually in a quiet room under circumaural headphones (Superex, APS II). Listeners were instructed to adjust the volume control during the first sentence so they could easily hear the sentences. Volume was not readjusted during the remainder of the task. Listeners were asked to write down what they understood from the practice tapes. They were instructed to listen to the whole sentence once, then listen to it a second time and write down what they thought the speaker said. Each sentence was presented a third time for listeners to modify what they had written. Listeners were not allowed to listen to a sentence more than three times. These procedures differ from the CAIDS procedure in that listeners were allowed to listen to a sentence three rather than two times. This deviation from standard scoring was done so that the practice tasks were the same as the experimental task. Pilot studies indicated that listeners required three passes at the sentence to fully understand non-dysarthric speech. Listeners were provided with the list of sentences read by the speaker and asked to review their responses after completing the first practice tape. The second practice task was completed in the same manner.

Because listeners listened to a different sentence for each experimental condition and were considered biased once they had been exposed to a sentence produced by a given speaker, the Latin square design assumes relative homogeneity among the listeners. This issue was examined by comparing listeners' performance on the practice tasks with the mean scores from three experienced listeners. Eighty-three percent (25/30) of the listeners were within +/–5% or better of the mean intelligibility score from experienced listeners on the first practice task. Scores for this task ranged from 76.6 to 98.4%. The second speaker was less intelligible than the first so a +/–10% range was used for comparison. Ninety percent (27/30) of the listeners were within +/–10% or better of the mean of the experienced listeners on the second practice task. These data suggest that the majority of the listeners' scores after practice were equivalent to or higher than those of experienced listeners; therefore, relative homogeneity among the listeners could be assumed.

Experimental task. Listeners completed the experimental listening task after the two practice tapes. They received the same instructions as in the practice tasks. They were informed that the sentences would be longer than the practice sentences, and the speaker may be more or less intelligible than those heard during the practice tasks. The listeners were again instructed to adjust the volume during the first sentence so that it was at a comfortable listening level for them. The percentage of words correctly transcribed served as the measure of speech intelligibility for each sentence. The entire listening task, two practice tapes and one experimental tape, required approximately 30 minutes to complete.

USE THE EVALUATION CHECKLIST TO GUIDE YOUR EVALUATION
OF THE METHOD

Results and Discussion

Prior to presenting the results of the intelligibility tasks, confirmation of the parkinsonian speakers' ability to achieve the paced speaking rate target accurately is warranted. Table 3 contains each subject's habitual speaking rate, the target speaking rate at which speech was paced (60% of habitual speaking rate), actual paced speaking rate that subjects achieved,

TABLE 3   Habitual speaking rates, targeted paced speaking rates (60% of habitual), actual paced rate achieved, and the percentage difference between the target and actual speaking rates for the 6 subjects. All speech rates are reported in syllables per min.

Subject	Habitual Speaking Rate	Target Paced Rate	Actual Paced Rate	Difference from Target
S1	188	113	118	+4.4%
S2	269	161	163	+1.2%
S3	258	155	161	+3.8%
S4	305	183	196	+7.1%
S5	195	117	115	−1.7%
S6	392	235	237	+0.8%
Mean	268	161	165	+2.6%

*Mean habitual speaking rate for 6 control subjects was 216 syll/min (sd = 37.9).

and the percentage difference between target and actual paced speaking rate. Five of 6 subjects were within +/–5% of the targeted speaking rate during the paced condition. The remaining subject, S4, was within 7% of the targeted rate. These results confirm the effectiveness of the Pacer technique in controlling speaking rate and are consistent with other reports in the literature (Yorkston et al., 1990).

The mean intelligibility scores for each condition appear in Table 4. It should be noted that data for only 5 subjects appear in this table. The intelligibility scores for S1 across all conditions ranged from 96 to 99%, creating a ceiling effect. Therefore, the data for that subject were eliminated from further analysis. Because the Latin square design used five different listeners and sentences for each condition the data have been averaged across the five listeners/sentences for each subject and condition. The mean intelligibility scores across subjects for the unmodified speaking conditions were 47% for the habitual condi-

TABLE 4   Mean percentage intelligibility for the two unmodified speech conditions (habitual and paced), and the three synthetic alterations (pause-altered, speech-duration-altered, and speech- & pause-altered). Data for each subject have been averaged across five listeners.

Subject	Unmodified Speech		Synthetic Alterations		
	Habitual	Paced	Pause-Altered	Speech-Altered	Speech- & Pause-Altered
S2	83	88	84	81	91
S3	81	83	80	50	70
S4	54	67	48	54	57
S5	14	26	26	21	14
S6	3	16	6	4	5
Mean	47.0	56.0	48.8	42.0	47.4

tion and 56% for the paced condition. The synthetic conditions of pause-altered, speech-duration-altered, and pause- and speech-duration-altered were, in order, 48.8%, 42%, and 47.4% intelligible.

A mixed model analysis of variance was performed so that a priori single contrasts could test the comparisons of interest. An arcsine transformation was completed prior to performance of all statistical tests because the intelligibility scores were in the form of percentages. Since a Latin square design was used the Subject × Condition interaction term served as the denominator in the contrast analysis. The results of the single contrast analyses appear in Table 5.

The first question of interest was: Does paced speech differ in intelligibility from habitual speech in parkinsonian dysarthria? A review of Table 4 indicates that all subjects' scores increased under the paced condition. In addition, the contrast between the habitual and paced conditions (see Table 4) indicated that the paced condition was significantly more intelligible than the habitual condition [$F (1,16) = 4.94, p < .042$].

Although statistically significant, the difference between the means for the two conditions is not as large as has been reported in other studies, and is not consistent across subjects. The hypokinetic dysarthrics studied by Yorkston and colleagues (1990) showed an average increase in speech intelligibility of 26% when speaking rates were reduced to 60% of habitual. No subject in the current study demonstrated more than a 13% difference. One factor that may contribute to the differences in findings between the current investigation and those of previous studies is the habitual intelligibility level of some of our subjects. The subjects in the Yorkston et al. study were all below 80% intelligible, allowing for a greater potential difference between the two conditions. Because these subjects were selected as part of a larger study, they also demonstrated a range of speaking rates. The increase in intelligibility during the paced condition may have been larger if only subjects with excessively fast speaking rates had been included. Data from the current study support earlier findings of increased speech intelligibility with reduced speaking rates despite differences in the magnitude of the effects.

The second research question addressed was: Does speech that is synthetically altered differ in intelligibility from habitual productions? The contrast between the habitual condition and all synthetic temporal alterations (Table 5) failed to reach statistical significance [$F (1,16) = 0.09, p < .770$]. Therefore, synthetic alterations were not found to be more intelligible than habitual speech. Several possible causes for the lack of significant differences between the intelligibility of speech samples produced at habitual speaking rates and the synthetically altered samples can be identified. First, the intent of this study was to

TABLE 5   Results of the a priori single contrast analysis

Source	Mean Square	df	F	p value
Paced versus habitual	0.319	1,16	4.91	0.042
Habitual versus all synthetic temporal alterations	0.014	1,16	0.22	0.645
Paced versus all synthetic temporal alterations	0.590	1,16	9.06	0.008

examine the relative contribution of pause and speech duration changes on speech intelligibility. The duration alterations used were simple, global changes that allowed for considerable experimental control. These alterations, however, did not replicate the more complex types of alterations that occur when speakers change overall speech rate. Gay (1981) showed that increases in speaking rate are not the result of simple linear compression of the speech signal. Therefore, it is likely that reductions in speaking rate are not accomplished by simple expansion of the speech signal.

Aspects of the signal processing required to complete the experimental manipulations might have contributed to the failure of this contrast to reach significance. Low pass filtering of the signal during digitization may have eliminated some high frequency components that may have provided more information for the listeners. Errors in the LPC analysis necessary for creating some of the alterations may have resulted in a degraded speech signal following resynthesis. Recall that the synthetic alterations were based on the habitual speaking rate samples produced by the parkinsonian subjects. Changes in vocal quality resulting from impairment of the phonatory system could have made voicing decisions difficult during LPC analysis of the signal. No corrections of the analysis file were completed prior to resynthesis in order to retain consistency across all subjects. It is also likely that the accuracy of the LPC analysis would vary with habitual intelligibility level. Interestingly, S1's intelligibility remained quite high, producing a ceiling effect, despite filtering and LPC analysis. It is important to note that this subject's speech was highly intelligible at the outset. The impact of speech analysis and synthesis on the intelligibility of dysarthric speech needs to be examined in future investigations. Determining the effect of filtering and LPC analysis on speech samples of varying levels of intelligibility and speech characteristics (e.g., vocal quality, resonance) would be an important area for further research if these experimental methods are to be used with dysarthric populations.

Any reduction in articulatory precision that was present would have been replicated during the lengthening procedure required for both the speech-duration-altered and speech-duration and pause-altered conditions. Whereas at the segmental level, some changes in duration that may have had a positive effect on speech intelligibility were created during the lengthening process (i.e., longer stop closure duration, longer voice onset times). However, other spectral characteristics such as formant duration and slope were changed, but likely not improved. Reduced formant transition rate and lower onset frequency of F1 have been noted for parkinsonian speakers when producing syllable strings (Connor, Ludlow, & Schultz, 1989). An investigation by Di Benedetto (1989) suggests that changes in the frequency of formant (F1) onset and trajectory can affect perceived vowel height. The temporal relationship between consonants and vowels as discussed by Gay (1981) was not directly modified as the result of the alterations used in this study. These factors may have had an important role in the failure of the synthetic alteration conditions to be more intelligible than the habitual speech samples. Further research is needed to characterize the effect of the synthetic modifications used in this study on specific acoustic features of the speech signal.

Inserting pauses into a very rapid stream of speech may have served only to increase its perceived bizarreness. The decisions we made regarding placement and distribution of pauses, that is, while providing experimental control, may have created speech samples that sounded unusual. These findings suggest that although the use of synthetic alterations provides the examiner with a highly controlled method to examine features theorized to affect speech intelligibility, caution must be exercised when altering the speech of dysarthric individuals by computerized methods. This is especially true when synthesis of the speech signal is required.

The final question of interest was: Does the intelligibility of paced speech differ from that of synthetically altered speech? As evident in Table 5, the results from the orthogonal contrasts show significant differences between the paced condition and all synthetic alteration conditions [F (1,16) = 9.06, p < .008], indicating that the paced condition was more intelligible. The finding that improvements in intelligibility were detectable, regardless of any additional distortion due to the resynthesis process, speaks to the robustness of the effect of speaking rate reduction with parkinsonian dysarthric individuals. This is not to suggest that paced rate control is more effective than other strategies in increasing the intelligibility of dysarthric individuals.

One intent of this investigation was to identify factors that contribute to the improvement in speech intelligibility with reduced speaking rates. However, the failure of any of the synthetic alterations to be as intelligible as the paced condition does not allow these factors to be determined. Although they provide experimental control, the alterations employed in this study may not reflect the actual temporal alterations used when speaking rate is reduced. In addition, the method used to decrease speech rate may also affect the type of temporal alteration that occurs. One might expect that use of a rate control strategy in which the subject was asked to slow down rather than follow an external pacer may result in different temporal alterations of the speech signal. It has been theorized that reduced speaking rates may allow the speaker to more accurately achieve articulatory targets. The computerized alterations used in this study did not directly test this theory. The failure of the synthetic alteration conditions to be as intelligible as the paced condition may suggest that in addition to any overall changes in the temporal domain, improvements at the segmental level are responsible for the increased intelligibility.

In conclusion, the findings of the current study indicate that temporal alterations as created by the paced condition result in speech that is significantly more intelligible than habitual speech or samples that were synthetically altered. This suggests that the type of synthetic, computerized alteration strategies used in the present study (simple expansion of the speech signal, addition of pauses, or both) did not explain the differences in intelligibility that have been observed when parkinsonian dysarthric individuals reduce speaking rates through use of the PACER program. This failure may be due to several factors. Although the use of synthetic alterations provides the researcher with a highly controlled method to empirically examine features theorized to affect speech intelligibility, caution must be exercised when synthetically altering the speech of hypokinetic dysarthric individuals. It must be remembered that only one method of expansion was used in this study (overall temporal changes). Different forms of computer expansion (such as increases in the duration of the steady-state portions of the signal, or proportional changes in consonant and vowel duration) may have resulted in more intelligible samples for some subjects.

The results of this investigation do not clearly indicate the type of changes occurring during the paced condition that were responsible for the improvements in speech intelligibility. Because we failed to find an improvement in intelligibility with the synthetic temporal alterations, one may suspect that one result of speaking rate reduction is an alteration in the segmental characteristics of the speech sample. This study does not contain data to explore this possibility. One way to examine this question would be to increase the rate of speech samples obtained using the Pacer program. The techniques employed in this study to decrease speech rates could be used in reverse, to accelerate the speech samples. If the intelligibility of the accelerated samples remains similar to the original Paced speech samples, one could argue that tempo alone was not the basis of improved intelligibility.

Secondly, a detailed acoustic examination of the temporal features of speech produced at habitual and reduced speaking rates as generated by a variety of strategies would provide insight into potential features contributing to increased intelligibility when decreased speech rates are used with individuals with parkinsonian dysarthria. Such work would allow future research in this area to model the computerized alterations after documented temporal-segmental changes that occur as the result of speaking rate reduction.

USE THE TWO EVALUATION CHECKLISTS TO GUIDE YOUR EVALUATION
OF THE RESULTS AND DISCUSSION

Acknowledgments

This work was supported in part by Grant #H133B80081 from the National Institute of Disability and Rehabilitation Research, Department of Education, Washington D.C., and a graduate student scholarship from the American Speech-Language-Hearing Foundation to the first author. Grateful thanks to Ed Belcher who wrote some of the programs used in this study. The authors would also like to thank Carol Stoel-Gammon, Harry Cooker, Marjorie Anderson and Michael McClean for their input regarding this research. James Hillenbrand and three anonymous reviewers provided helpful suggestions during the preparation of this manuscript.

References

Beukelman, D. R., Yorkston, K. M., & Dowden, P. D. (1986). *Impact of speaking rate reduction on respiratory patterns of dysarthric speakers.* Paper presented at the annual convention of the American Speech-Language-Hearing Association, Detroit, MI.

Beukelman, D. R., Yorkston, K. M., & Tice, B. (1988). *Pacer/Tally.* Tucson: Communication Skill Builders.

Bunnell, H. T. (1990). Determinants of intelligibility in dysarthric speech. *Journal of Rehabilitation Research and Development, 28,* 372.

Canter, G. J. (1965). Speech characteristics of patients with Parkinson's disease: III. Articulation, diadochokinesis, and overall adequacy. *Journal of Speech and Hearing Disorders, 30,* 217–224.

Canter, G. J., & Van Lancker, D. R. (1985). Disturbances of the temporal organization of speech following bilateral thalamic surgery in a patient with Parkinson's disease. *Journal of Communication Disorders, 18,* 329–349.

Connor, N. P., Ludlow, C. L., & Schultz, G. M. (1989). Stop consonant production in isolated and repeated syllables in Parkinson's disease. *Neuropsychologia, 27,* 829–838.

Darley, F, L., Aronson, A. E., & Brown, J. R. (1975). *Motor speech disorders.* Philadelphia: Saunders.

Di Benedetto, M. (1989). Frequency and time variations of the first formant: Properties relevant to the perception of vowel height. *Journal of the Acoustical Society of America, 86,* 67–77.

Edwards, A. L. (1985). *Experimental design in psychological research.* New York: Harper & Row.

Goldman-Eisler, F. (1968). *Psycholinguistics: Experiments in spontaneous speech.* New York: Academic Press.

Hammen, V. L. (1991). Effects of speaking rate reduction in parkinsonian dysarthria. (Doctoral dissertation, University of Washington, 1990). *Dissertation Abstracts International, 51,* 4304.

Hammen V. L., Yorkston K. M., & Beukelman, D. R. (1989). Pausal and speech duration characteristics as a function of speaking rate in normal and dysarthric individuals. In K. M. Yorkston & D. R. Beukelman (Eds.), *Recent Advances in Clinical Dysarthria* (pp. 213–224). Austin: Pro-Ed.

Hanson, W. R., & Metter, E. J. (1983). DAF speech rate modification in Parkinson's disease: A report of two cases. In W. R. Berry (Ed.), *Clinical dysarthria* (pp. 231–252). Austin: Pro-Ed.

Hardy, J. (1983). *Cerebral palsy.* Englewood Cliffs, NJ: Prentice-Hall.

Hoehn, M. M., & Yahr, M. D. (1967). Parkinsonism: Onset, progression and mortality. *Neurology, 17,* 427–442.

Kent, R. D., & Rosenbek, J. C. (1982). Prosodic disturbance and neurologic lesion. *Brain and Language, 15,* 259–291.

Lane, H., & Grosjean, F. (1973). Perception of reading rate by listeners and speakers. *Journal of Experimental Psychology, 97,* 141–147.

Ludlow, C. L., & Bassich, C. J. (1983). The results of acoustic and perceptual assessment of two types of dysarthria. In W. R. Berry (Ed.), *Clinical dysarthria* (pp. 121–154). Austin: Pro-Ed.

Massen, B. (1986). Marking word boundaries to improve the intelligibility of the speech of the deaf. *Journal of Speech and Hearing Research, 29,* 227–230.

Massen, B., & Povel, D. J. (1984). The effect of correcting temporal structure on the intelligibility of the deaf. *Speech Communication, 3,* 123–135.

Minifie, F. D. (1973). Speech acoustics. In F. D. Minifie, T. J. Hixon, & F. Williams (Eds.), *Normal Aspects of Speech, Hearing and Language* (pp. 235–284). Englewood Cliffs: Prentice-Hall.

Osberger, M. J., & Levitt, H. (1979). The effect of timing errors on the intelligibility of deaf children's speech. *Journal of the Acoustical Society of America, 66,* 1316–1324.

Osberger, M. J., & McGarr, N. S. (1982) Speech production characteristics of the hearing impaired. In N. Lass (Ed.), *Speech and Language: Advances in basic research and practice* (pp. 221–283). New York: Academic Press.

Parkhurst, B. G., & Levitt, H. (1978). The effect of selected prosodic errors on the intelligibility of deaf speech. *Journal of Communication Disorders, 11,* 249–256.

Snidecor, G. W., & Cochran, W. G. (1967). *Statistical methods.* Ames: The Iowa State University Press.

Weismer, G. (1984). Articulatory characteristics of parkinsonian dysarthria: Segmental and phrase-level timing, spirantization, and glottal-supraglottal coordination. In M. R. McNeil, J. C. Rosenbek, & A. E. Aronson (Eds), *The dysarthrias* (pp, 101–130) Austin: Pro-Ed.

Winer, B. J. (1971). *Statistical Principles in Experimental Design.* New York: McGraw-Hill.

Yorkston, K. M., Beukelman, D. R., & Bell, K. R. (1988). *Clinical Management of Dysarthric Speakers.* Austin: Pro-Ed.

Yorkston, K. M., Beukelman, D. R., & Traynor, C. (1984). *Computerized Assessment of Intelligibility of Dysarthric Speech.* Austin: Pro-Ed.

Yorkston, K. M., Hammen, V. L., Beukelman, D. R., & Traynor, C. (1990). The effect of rate control on the intelligibility and naturalness of dysarthric speech. *Journal of Speech and Hearing Disorders, 55,* 550–560.

Received January 28, 1992
Accepted August 30, 1993

Contact author: Vicki L. Hammen, PhD, Audiology and Speech Sciences, 1353 Heavilon Hall, Purdue University, West Lafayette, IN 47907.

Appendix

The Passage Read by the Dysarthric Speakers *(The Experimental Sentences Are in Italics)*

What is the best gift a boy can be given? *My dad wants to buy Bobby a puppy as a special present for his tenth birthday, which is coming up on June twenty-third. We have looked at many beautiful dogs, with shiny coats, happy expressions and the biggest feet you have ever seen. I pointed out that keeping the gift a secret will be much harder than choosing a sheepdog from the ones we have encountered.* The plan is to wrap the pet in a box. *I wonder how much noise the dog will make in the package while we join our voices in song and light the candles on the cake.* It will be good fun to watch my brother taking on the responsibility of feeding and walking his new pet.

Example Article for
Evaluation in Language Disorders

Plural Acquisition in Children
with Specific Language Impairment

JANNA B. OETTING
Louisiana State University
Baton Rouge

MABEL L. RICE
University of Kansas
Lawrence

A plural elicitation task and a nominal compounding task were administered to a group of children with SLI and two groups of normally developing children, an age-equivalent group (CA) and a language equivalent group (MLU). Across tasks, differences between the CA and SLI groups were significant, but differences between the MLU and SLI groups were not. These findings suggest that by 5 years of age, children with SLI demonstrate a productive and differentiated plural system. However, unlike the normally developing children, the pluralization skills of the children with SLI were affected by input frequency, with nouns that are frequently pluralized in everyday conversation more readily inflected than ones that are infrequently pluralized. Three explanations within a model of linguistic normalcy are proposed to account for the frequency effect. These include (a) delayed independence of rule use, (b) linguistic vulnerability, and (c) a faulty lexicon.

KEY WORDS: specific language impairment, plural acquisition, morphology, number marking

Reprinted with permission from *Journal of Speech and Hearing Research, 36,* 1236–1248, December 1993.

Children with specific language impairment (SLI) frequently demonstrate difficulty learning particular aspects of morphology. This claim is based on findings from a collection of English-speaking investigations (cf. Johnston, 1988; Leonard, 1989), with cross-linguistic validation from studies involving German, Hebrew, and Italian (Clahsen, 1989; Leonard, Sabbadini, Leonard, & Volterra, 1987; Rom & Leonard, 1990). Traditionally, the linguistic problems of children with SLI have been viewed as the product of either a delayed or deviant language mechanism. Argument over which interpretation best defines SLI started over 30 years ago with Menyuk's (1964) claims of deviancy, and a number of issues inherent to the debate remain unresolved.

Recently, notions of language delay and language deviancy have been set within theoretically motivated frameworks of linguistics and language acquisition (e.g., Clahsen, 1989; Connell, 1986; Crago, Gopnik, Guilfoyle, & Allen, 1991; Leonard, 1989; Loeb & Leonard, 1991). Examining SLI within a theoretical model of normal acquisition is appealing because of the conceptual framework it provides for looking at various patterns of linguistic weakness or strength. In this paper we examine the plural morphology of children with SLI using a current learnability model of inflectional development, that of the dual mechanism account. This model was initially proposed by Pinker (1984) and further developed by Pinker and his colleagues to explain children's acquisition of past tense (Marcus et al., 1992; Pinker, 1991; Pinker & Prince, 1991; Prasada & Pinker, in press). The model is of interest because it generates specific predictions for input frequency effects and word formation processes. Thus, it is possible to conduct an analysis of the inflectional systems of children with SLI at the level of acquisition mechanisms.

Plural acquisition is of particular interest because current accounts of SLI predict plurals to be either missing, as in the case of the Missing Feature hypothesis (Crago et al., 1991; Gopnik, 1990a, 1990b; Gopnik & Crago, 1991), or delayed in acquisition, as suggested by the Surface account (Leonard, 1989; Leonard, Bertolini, Caselli, McGregor, & Sabbadini, 1992). However, in a recent study, we found the spontaneous plural use of children with SLI to be comparable to that of language-equivalent, normally developing children (Rice & Oetting, 1993). The number of subjects in that study was relatively large in comparison to previous studies of SLI morphology (50 children with SLI and 58 MLU-equivalent children). In addition, a rigorous set of criteria was used to identify the two groups of subjects. The results of this study extend the findings from our previous work with data collected from two elicitation tasks. In the following session, Pinker's dual mechanism model is discussed in terms of its usefulness for testing the claims of the Missing Feature hypothesis and the Surface account.

Dual Mechanism Model of Plural Development

The dual mechanism model is an enhanced version of the traditional rule versus rote approach to inflectional morphology. Like the traditional model, regular and irregular inflections rules are learned through different modes of acquisition. Differences between Pinker's model and the traditional approach include a more specified regular rule component and a rote component that is embedded within an associative memory network.

Within the dual mechanism model, the learning of regular inflectional rules is paradigmatic. As depicted in Figure 1, children first construct a small number of word-specific paradigms for a given feature, such as number (e.g., *ball-balls, eye-eyes, shoe-shoes*). After a small set of word-specific paradigms is generated, a general morphological paradigm develops. Once established, a child should be able to inflect an infinite number of unique word stems. Also, the development of a general paradigm should generate consistent use of regular suffixes in obligatory contexts and overregularization (e.g., *foots*). A critical feature of the dual mechanism model is that a general paradigmatic rule should render inflectional use that is independent of input frequency (cf. Marcus et al., 1992). In other words, a child should not have to hear the inflected form of a word before spontaneously producing it.

In contrast, irregular forms are learned through rote learning devices within an associative memory network. Following the connectionist framework of Rumelhart and McClelland (1987), the acquisition of irregular forms is heavily dependent on input frequency. This means that irregular forms are learned individually after repeated exposure, with frequently produced irregular forms more likely to be learned by children than ones that are rarely produced. Thus, one would not expect a child to produce an irregular form before hearing the form in the input.

Research involving children's acquisition of regular plural supports Pinker's model. For example, children typically undergo a qualitative change in their plural use, in which limited use is replaced with frequent use and overregularization. The time span between initial plural production and this qualitative shift has ranged between 1 and 4 months in children who have been studied longitudinally (Cazden, 1968; Mervis & Johnson, 1991). The early age at which regular plural use becomes productive also has been documented in a number of studies involving nonce forms (Anisfeld & Tucker, 1968; Berko, 1958; Hecht, 1983).

It should be noted that an alternative model to plural development is one of connectionism, in which the learning of both regular and irregular plurals is explained within one

Word Specific Paradigms for English Plural	
Singular	Plural
ball	balls
eye	eyes
shoe	shoes
General Paradigm for English Plural	
Singular	Plural
--	-s

FIGURE 1 **Development of Pinker's regular rule component**

general associative memory network (e.g., Marchman & Bates, 1991; Plunkett & Marchman, in press; Seidenberg & Daugherty, 1992). However, one finding that a single mechanism approach has yet to explain is why regular and irregular nouns relate to word formation processes differently.[1] For example, in English, when regular nouns are compounded, the singular form of the noun must be used (e.g., *rat-eater* but not *rats-eater*). In contrast, when irregular nouns are compounded, either the singular or plural form is grammatical (e.g., *mice-eater, mouse-eater*). This pattern of word formation also occurs in German (Clahsen, Rothweiler, Woest, & Marcus, 1993). Within the dual mechanism model, differences in compounding are explained; regular and irregular plurals are learned through separate mechanisms, and these subsystems relate to word formation processes differently.

Within theories of lexical morphology, differences between regular and irregular plurals are well-recognized. For example, Kiparsky (1982, 1983) developed a set of level-ordering constraints for inflectional and derivational morphology that assumes a psycholinguistic distinction between regular and irregular plural forms. According to Kiparsky's model, morphology involves three distinct levels of application (See Figure 2). At Level 1, irregular inflections are formed along with primary affixes (e.g., *-ian, -ous, -ion*). At Level 2, secondary affixes of derivational morphology (e.g., *-er, -ism, -ness*) and nominal compounding are generated. At Level 3, regular inflection that characteristically shows neither semantic idiosyncrasy nor stem deformation is applied.

According to Kiparsky's model, rule application proceeds through the three levels such that rules at a later level may not be applied prior to those at a previous level. This constraint is referred to as the Elsewhere Condition. Given that regular plural marking (Level 3) occurs after nominal compounding (Level 2), regular plurals inside of noun compounds are ungrammatical. Take *mouse* and *rat* as examples. They are similar in meaning, yet one is irregular and the other regular. The irregular noun, *mouse,* is pluralized to mice at Level 1. In contrast, at Level 1 *rat* remains *rat,* because regular plural marking does not occur until Level 3. At Level 2, *mice* and *rat* can be compounded to *mice-eater* and *rat-eater.* The Elsewhere Condition states that regular plural suffixation (Level 3) cannot be applied prior to the more specific rule of compounding (Level 2). As predicted, *rats-eater* is ungrammatical. If the word rat is not compounded, Level 3 rules are not blocked by the Elsewhere Condition and the regular plural suffix can be felicitously applied (e.g., *rats*).[2]

Acquisition research by Gordon (1985) involving children's nominal compounds supports the dual mechanism hypothesis. In Gordon's study, children between the ages of

---

[1]The purpose of this study was not to test the differences between a connectionist and symbolic approach to morphology. To the extent that a single associative mechanism can account for differences between regular and irregular word formation processes, the results of this study are not necessarily incompatible with a unitary architecture for inflectional development.

[2]As pointed out by an anonymous reviewer, some compounds involving irregular plurals may be ungrammatical to some adult speakers (e.g., men-hater vs. man-hater). The ungrammatical nature of these compounds does not violate Kiparsky's model, because either the singular or plural form of irregulars may enter into the word formation process. We speculate that preferences for some irregular compounds over others occur for reasons such as Amoff's Blocking principle or Wexler's Uniqueness principle, that fall outside of Kiparsky's model (cf. Ullman & Pinker, 1990). Readers are also referred to Allen (1978) and Siegel (1977) for additional discussion of level-ordering constraints and Gordon, Alegre, and Jackson (1993) for the results of a study on syntactic recursion in children's compounding.

Level	Properties	Examples	
		Irregular	Regular
		Mouse	Rat
Level 1	Irregular Inflection Derivational, irregular, semantically idosyncratic host deforming, stress shift vowel reduction, unproductive	Mice	Rat
Level 2	Compounds Derivational non-deforming (more) semantically predictable productive	Mice-eater	Rat-eater
Level 3	Regular inflection non-deforming semantically predictable		Rats

FIGURE 2   Kiparsky's model of word formation

3 and 5 overwhelmingly used the singular form when producing regular noun compounds, even though the probes involved plural stimuli. As predicted by Kiparsky's and Pinker's models, the children's irregular compounds included the plural form.

The dual mechanism model provides a useful framework for examining the plural morphology of children with SLI. If these children acquire a normal plural system, their plural use should reflect a dual mechanism, one in which regular plurals are generated by a rule and irregular plurals are individually memorized. One consequence of a dual system is the ability to generate a diverse set of regular plurals, regardless of whether the inflected forms of the words are heard in the input. Thus, the duality of a plural system can be tested by examining the productivity of regular inflection. Another consequence of a dual system is differential treatment of regular and irregular plurals when completing various word formation processes, such as noun compounding. If children with SLI exploit a dual system, they should compound regular and irregular plurals differently.

Alternatively, if children with SLI present a deviant plural system, atypical plural use may surface. For example, in the case of the Missing Feature account, the inflectional rules of individuals with SLI are thought to be impaired, and it is hypothesized that inflected forms are learned through the lexicon (Gopnik & Crago, 1991). Within the dual mechanism model, this would mean that children with SLI learn both regular and irregular plurals within a single associative network. In other words, whereas children following normal developmental patterns have access to a dual mechanism, an abstract rule for regular plurals and an associative memory network for irregulars, children with SLI only have access to the latter. Two predictions emerge from this deviant account. First, if children with SLI have access only to a single, lexically driven system, their ability to pluralize a diverse set of novel noun stems should be extremely limited. Specifically, children with

SLI should be able to generate plural forms for frequently pluralized nouns, but inflection of forms that are rarely pluralized in the input should be nearly impossible. Also, overregularizations and pluralization of nonce forms should be extremely difficult because they must be rule-generated. Even if one granted the associative system the use of analogical processes, only word stems that were similar to previously learned inflected forms, in either semantic or phonological content, could be productively pluralized. Work on normally developing individuals suggests that morphological productivity via analogy is weak (MacWhinney, 1978). Thus, if normally developing individuals have difficulty using analogy to produce productive forms, it seems counterintuitive that children with SLI might present such an ability. Therefore, if the plural system of children with SLI is driven by the lexicon, their ability to pluralize a diverse set of nouns should be significantly reduced.

A second prediction of the Missing Feature account concerns the organization and storage of the plural system of children with SLI. If these children have access only to a single plural mechanism, storage of regular and irregular plurals should be isomorphic. Consequently, their productions of regular noun compounds should be the same as those involving irregular nouns. The reason for this is that a single plural mechanism would generate both regular and irregular plurals at Level 1 of Kiparsky's (1982) model. Noun compounding, because it occurs at Level 2, must include the lexical derivations that were allowed at Level 1. Therefore, both regular and irregular plurals would be available for nominal compounding. In other words, *rats-eater* and *mice-eater* would be equally felicitous to a child with SLI.

This study was designed to examine the plural systems of children with SLI by means of two experimental tasks. The first task examined the children's ability to pluralize a diverse set of noun forms. Four types of nouns were included in the task: frequently pluralized regular nouns, infrequently pluralized regular nouns, irregular nouns, and nonce forms. The second task involved a noun compounding activity.

> USE THE EVALUATION CHECKLIST TO GUIDE YOUR EVALUATION
> OF THE INTRODUCTION

Method

Subjects

The subjects of this study included a total of 55 children. Eighteen of the subjects were identified as SLI (henceforth SLI group) and the other 37 were classified as developing language appropriately.[3] Nineteen of the latter group were equivalent to the subjects in the SLI group on the basis of age (henceforth CA group) and the other 18 were equivalent on

---

[3]Initially 57 subjects completed the study. However, 2 of the SLI subjects were dizygotic twins. To meet the ANOVA assumption of independent observations, 1 twin and the corresponding control subject were randomly excluded from the analyses. See Oetting (1992) for further details concerning the unique behaviors of the twins.

the basis of MLU (henceforth MLU group). All of the subjects were drawn from native English-speaking homes and were enrolled in one of several area preschool or day care programs in eastern and central Kansas. The participating programs served predominately Caucasian middle-class children, with the exclusion of two programs that served families of low socio-economic status.

The following criteria were used to identify subjects in the SLI group: (a) diagnosed as language-impaired by a certified speech-language pathologist and enrolled in a pre-school program for language-impaired children; (b) presented normal nonverbal intelligence, as evidenced by an age deviation score of 85 or above on the Columbia Mental Maturity Scale (Burgemeister, Blum, & Lorge, 1972); (c) presented normal hearing, according to a hearing screening conducted within 6 months of the study; (d) scored one or more standard deviations below the mean on the Peabody Picture Vocabulary Test—Revised (Dunn & Dunn, 1981); (e) produced an MLU one or more standard deviations below the mean expected for age as reported by Miller (1981, p. 27); (f) lacked mastery of three or more grammatical morphemes appropriate for age; and (g) produced final /s/ and /z/ with at least 90% accuracy when asked to produce 13 nonmorphophonemic monosyllabic words, 3 of which involved a final /s/ consonant cluster (e.g., fox). Measures of MLU and morpheme use were based on analyses of a language sample that was at least 100 utterances.

The 18 subjects in the SLI group ranged in age from 55 to 68 months ($M = 60.33$; $SD = 4.29$). Nine of the subjects were males, and 9 were females. All of these subjects met the aforementioned criteria, except for Subject 17 whose MLU of 4.43, although low, was within one standard deviation of the mean for his age (for a child 55 months of age, an average MLU of 5.12, $SD = 1.08$, is expected [Miller, 1981. p. 27]). Given that MLU can be a highly variable index of overall language development when it exceeds the 4.00 range (cf. Rondal, Ghiotto, Bredart, & Bachelet, 1987), additional analysis involving Lee's (1974) developmental sentence score (DSS) procedures were conducted. The subject's overall DSS score was 5.2. This score is below the 10th percentile expected for his age. In addition, this subject demonstrated limited use of 8 of the 14 morphemes expected for his age. Both the reduced DSS score and limited use of morphology confirmed this subject's SLI classification.

The Goldman-Fristoe Test of Articulation (GFTA) (Goldman & Fristoe, 1986) was also administered to measure each subject's general phonological development. The GFTA percentile ranks of the subjects in the SLI group ranged from 01 to 62. In general, the subjects' errors consisted of initial cluster reduction, sound distortions, and sound substitutions of late emerging sounds. Although the SLI phonological systems were limited, none of the children's errors involved word final omission of /s/ and /z/. Also, the phonological abilities of the children did not significantly reduce the accuracy of language sample transcription; 96% of their complete utterances were intelligible. Subject profiles for the SLI group are listed in Table 1.

Both groups of normally developing children presented normal hearing according to teacher report, scored within or above +/– one standard deviation but not exceeding two standard deviations above the mean on the Peabody Picture Vocabulary Test—Revised, demonstrated an age-appropriate MLU, and completed the /s/ and /z/ articulation probe with at least 90% accuracy. The 19 CA children ranged in age from 57 to 67 months ($M = 60.58$; $SD = 3.86$). Six were males and 13 were females. The ages of the 18 MLU children ranged from 30 to 40 months ($M = 35.44$; $SD = 3.27$). The MLU group consisted of 9 males and 9 females. Subject profiles for the CA and MLU groups are listed in Tables 2 and 3.

The MLU of each child in the language-equivalent group was within .24 morphemes of the MLU of 1 child in the SLI group. It should be noted that the use of MLU to place children in the SLI and MLU groups involves the subjects' ability to spontaneously produce plural forms. Given that the focus of this study is on children's plural marking, it is important to establish that the grouping variable does not inadvertently capture the variance of interest in the dependent variable. In other words, one would want to ensure that the grouping criterion is not dependent upon the subjects' plural use. In order to test this, each subject's MLU in words (MLU-W) was calculated. Similar group means were observed in this analysis (SLI = 3.29; MLU = 3.21). Also, the correlation between MLU and MLU-W was high for both groups(SLI, $r = .91$; MLU, $r = .93$). Thus, it does not appear that the grouping variable of MLU is significantly influenced by morphological affixation for either group of children.

Elicitation Task

The stimuli included 36 nouns and 12 nonce forms (See Table 4). Twenty-four of the nouns were common regular count nouns, 12 of which were documented to be frequently pluralized in everyday language, and 12 infrequently pluralized. A number of criteria were used to select the 12 frequently pluralized nouns. They had to be (a) of the variable regular type (e.g.,

TABLE 1   Individual subject profiles: SLI group

ID	Sex	Age	Columbia[a]	PPVT[b]	GFTA[c]	ARTIC PROBE[d]	MLU
01	M	65	103	75	24	100	3.70
02	M	59	111	79	12	100	3.12
03	M	59	115	84	3	100	3.61
04	F	58	100	79	6	92	3.41
05	M	63	85	72	1	92	3.92
07	M	59	99	61	66	100	3.76
09	F	57	93	81	38	100	3.21
11	F	66	99	85	17	100	4.06
12	F	57	99	76	14	100	3.36
13	M	59	86	69	4	100	3.30
14	F	68	95	83	13	100	2.82
15	F	58	115	75	52	100	3.16
16	M	68	96	65	26	100	3.88
17	M	55	108	73	62	100	4.43
18	F	65	102	82	4	100	3.36
19	M	57	100	79	12	100	3.48
20	F	56	89	83	7	100	3.32
21	F	57	90	73	4	100	3.19
M		60.33	99.17	76.33	20.27	99.11	3.50

[a]Colombia Mental Maturity Scale, age deviation score reported; [b]Peabody Picture Vocabulary Test—Revised, standardized score reported; [c]Goldman Fristoe Test of Articulation, percentile rank reported; [d]Articulation Probe, percentage correct reported.

dogs, cats), (b) easy to depict via line drawings, (c) produced by preschool children in the singular and plural form as documented by Hall, Nagey, and Linn (1984), and (d) used frequently by adults in the plural form in a number of different genres as documented by Francis and Kucera (1982). Similar criteria were used to select the infrequently pluralized nouns, but the plural forms of these nouns had to be infrequently pluralized by adults and not produced in the plural form by children. For both groups of regular nouns, the singular form was monosyllabic, and allomorphic variations of the plural suffix were counterbalanced.

Nonce forms and irregular noun stems were included to elicit novel applications of the regular plural affix. For the nonce stimuli, 12 monosyllabic words were created following the procedures of Anisfeld and Tucker (1968). The 12 irregular nouns consisted of 6 variable nouns and 6 invariable nouns. Again, allomorphic variations were counterbalanced for both the nonce and irregular forms. Although the irregular nouns, in correct usage, do not carry the plural suffix, they were classified according to potential allomorphs based on their final consonant.

For each of the 48 items, line drawings were created in the singular and multiple form. For the nonce items, line drawings of made-up creatures were developed. Each line drawing was approximately 2¼ inches by 2¼ inches. Line drawings were created using MacDraw software and a Macintosh personal computer. The line drawings were presented on an 8 × 6-inch piece of white paper. The singular forms of the 48 line drawings were bound into five 8 × 6-inch books. The order of presentation was fixed to permit counterbalancing. To reduce priming effects of the high-frequency regular plurals on the other stimuli, noun type and allomorph

TABLE 2   Subject profiles: CA group

ID	Sex	Age	Columbia[a]	PPVT[b]	ARTIC GFTA[c]	PROBE[d]
61	M	62	113	114	99	100
62	F	57	105	107	99	100
63	F	62	101	98	99	92
64	F	63	101	118	99	100
65	F	58	111	129	57	100
66	F	57	106	107	89	100
67	M	58	100	109	90	100
68	F	55	120	112	99	100
69	F	65	101	104	99	92
70	F	59	105	118	88	100
71	M	67	103	104	99	100
72	F	58	123	131	89	100
74	M	65	93	91	99	100
75	F	57	100	97	99	100
76	M	57	111	101	83	100
77	F	66	111	120	99	100
78	F	62	94	99	77	100
79	F	66	106	128	99	100
80	M	57	102	94	76	100
M		60.58	105.58	109.53	91.47	99.16

[a]Columbia Mental Maturity Scale, age deviation score reported; [b]Peabody Picture Vocabulary Test—Revised, standardized score reported; [c]Goldman Fristoe Test of Articulation, percentile rank reported; [d]Articulation Probe, percentage correct reported.

TABLE 3   Subject profiles: MLU group

ID	Sex	Age	PPVT[a]	GFTA[b]	ARTIC PROBE[c]	MLU
31	M	36	93	94	92	3.77
32	F	30	97	37	92	3.12
33	M	33	117	65	92	3.57
34	F	34	116	99	100	3.38
35	F	38	108	99	100	3.90
37	F	39	100	98	100	3.86
39	M	39	100	98	100	3.33
41	F	40	125	99	100	3.82
42	M	35	115	72	92	3.31
43	M	30	108	83	100	3.42
44	M	36	102	91	100	2.89
45	F	33	112	99	100	3.13
46	M	32	109	97	92	3.95
47	F	40	96	99	100	4.33
48	F	36	113	99	100	3.26
49	M	38	93	87	100	3.40
50	F	32	117	99	100	3.43
51	M	37	94	93	100	3.24
M		35.44	106.11	89.33	97.78	3.50

[a]Peabody Picture Vocabulary Test—Revised, standardized score reported; [b]Goldman Fristoe Test of Articulation, percentile rank reported; [c]Articulation Probe, percentage correct reported.

TABLE 4   Stimuli

Allomorph	Frequently Pluralized Nouns	Infrequently Pluralized Nouns	Nonce Forms	Irregular Nouns[a]
−z	door	lid	dob	child
−z	hand	moon	duug	man
−z	girl	sun	keem	glue
−z	dog	stove	med	corn
−s	heart	clock	heek	foot
−s	hat	belt	tat	tooth
−s	cup	sack	tuup	milk
−s	coat	mat	bith	meat
−əz	horse	nose	baz	dice[b]
−əz	glass	church	gij	goose
−əz	box	couch	dooch	juice
−əz	bridge	brush	tees	cheese

[a]Irregular items are classified by allomorph according to potential for a regular plural affix, given the final consonant of the stem. [b]Irregular items taking the −z allomorph were extremely difficult to find. Irregular like *ice* were not easily depicted in the singular and plural. *Dice* was chosen as an invariable irregular. Although *dice* is variable (i.e., *die/dice*), *die* is infrequent and not used by children or by adults talking with children as confirmed by Hall, Nagey, and Linn (1984) and Francis and Kucera (1982).

ending were counterbalanced. A similar set of books was created for the multiple forms of the line drawings and the subjects were given the books of the multiple line drawings.

Directions for the task involved telling a subject that both the examiner and subject were to tell each other what they had in their books. The examiner then opened her booklet and said, "I have a X. Look in your book. What do you have?" and if needed, "You have many. . . . You have lots of. . . ."

Nominal Compounding Task

Fourteen nouns were included in the nominal compounding task (See Table 5). Seven of the items were regular with the others being irregular. A line drawing of each noun was created in the singular and multiple form. First, each subject was asked to name the 14 plural pictures. These responses were used to prompt for the nominal compounds. For example, if a subject produced mouses for the picture of mice, teeth for the picture of teeth and doggies for the picture of dogs, the examiner used mouses, teeth, and doggies when prompting for the subject's production of a noun compound.

To introduce the nominal compounding task, the examiner presented a puppet to the subject and stated that the puppet liked to eat different things. Using mass nouns, the examiner modelled nominal compounds involving the derived noun eater. For example, the examiner said, "My puppet loves to eat things. If he likes to eat dirt, I would call him a dirt-eater. Can you say that? Call him a dirt-eater." Six mass nouns were used for training the subject to spontaneously produce nominal compounds involving X-eater (e.g., money-eater, popcorn-eater). Following training, the subject was asked to produce nominal compounds that involved the 14 experimental items. Upon completion of this task, the subjects were asked to produce the singular form of the experimental items to verify that they had at their disposal both the singular and plural form of the nouns when compounding. This was especially critical for children's irregular plural compounds (e.g., *teeth-eater*). If subjects could not produce the singular form of teeth after producing *teeth-eater*, they were judged as not having both forms readily available for the compounding task.

Reliability

Ten percent of the data (two audiorecordings of each task per group) was transcribed and coded by a second person. Reliability was calculated by dividing the total number of agreements by the total number of opportunities for agreement. Interrater reliability was 98% (282/288) for the elicitation task and 98% (248/252) for the compound task. Across

TABLE 5   Noun compound stimuli

Regular nouns	Irregular nouns
ball	tooth
rat	mouse
eye	foot
doll	man
horse	fish
dog	deer
duck	goose

tasks, disagreement concerned the presence of the plural marker. Of the 10 disagreements, four involved *-s,* four involved *-z,* and two involved *-əz.*

USE THE EVALUATION CHECKLIST TO GUIDE YOUR EVALUATION
OF THE METHOD

Results

Preliminary Analysis

A preliminary analysis between the SLI and MLU group consisted of a comparison of regular and irregular plural use in spontaneous language production. Percentage of correct use for each subject was calculated and averaged for each group. Data for this comparison were taken from the language samples that were collected to measure MLU. All three groups of children demonstrated consistent marking of regular plurals in obligatory contexts (SLI = 90%; MLU = 94%; CA = 98%). The average number of obligatory contexts of regular plurals was 7.3 for the SLI group, 9.0 for the MLU group, and 12.5 for the CA group. In addition, the number of children from each group who produced at least one overregularized plural (e.g., *foots*) was: SLI 6, MLU 3, CA 0. For irregular plurals, 10 SLI children, 12 MLU children, and 14 CA children produced an irregular form. These included: *people, feet, women,* and *teeth.* The overall high level of plural use in obligatory contexts and the presence of overregularization errors in the SLI, as well as the control groups, replicate the basic findings of Rice and Oetting (1993).

Elicitation Task

Regular nouns. A three-way mixed ANOVA was run with group as a between-subject factor (three levels: SLI, MLU, CA), and noun type (two levels: frequently and infrequently pluralized) and allomorphic ending (three levels: *-s, -z, -əz*) as fully-crossed within-subject factors. Table 6 presents means and standard deviations of the individual cells. A significant two-way interaction (Group × Noun) was present ($F_{(2,52)} = 3.47$, $p < .05$). This interaction is displayed in Figure 3.

Two follow-up ANOVAs indicated that there were group differences at both levels of noun type (frequently pluralized nouns: $F_{(2,52)} = 8.31$, $p < .05$; infrequently pluralized nouns: $F_{2,52)} = 11.80$, $p < .05$). Three planned comparisons at each level of noun type were conducted to further examine the differences between the three groups. Follow-up analyses employed Fisher's Least Significance Difference method. For the frequently pluralized nouns, the CA group pluralized more items than either the SLI group ($t_{(27.3)} = 4.04, p < .05$) or the MLU group ($t_{(27)} = 3.38, p < .05$). Similarly, for the infrequently pluralized nouns, the difference between the CA group and either of the other two groups was significant (CA vs. SLI: $t_{(23.9)} = 4.92, p < .05$; CA vs. MLU: $t_{(24.8)} = 3.82, p < .05$). There were no significant differences between the SLI and MLU group at either levels of noun type.

TABLE 6   Regular plural affixation: group means and standard deviations[a]

	Frequently pluralized nouns[b]		
	−s	−z	−əz
CA	4.00 (.00)	3.95 (.23)	3.37 (1.07)
MLU	3.78 (.43)	3.50 (1.10)	2.11 (1.37)
SLI	3.66 (.49)	3.72 (.57)	1.50 (1.69)
	Infrequently Pluralized Nouns[b]		
	−s	−z	−əz
CA	4.00 (.00)	3.95 (.23)	3.32 (1.20)
MLU	3.50 (.86)	3.50 (1.04)	1.72 (1.32)
SLI	3.17 (.99)	3.17 (1.15)	1.39 (1.71)
	Irregular Nouns		
	−s	−z	−əz
CA	2.89 (1.05)	2.63 (.96)	1.79 (1.18)
MLU	3.00 (1.14)	2.89 (1.02)	1.11 (1.18)
SLI	2.27 (1.07)	2.56 (.98)	.55 (1.19)
	Nonce Forms		
	−s	−z	−əz
CA	3.79 (.42)	3.84 (.38)	1.21 (1.18)
MLU	2.61 (1.38)	2.89 (1.23)	.61 (1.15)
SLI	2.22 (1.45)	2.83 (1.47)	.22 (.55)

[a]Total correct is 4; [b]Arcsine transformations were conducted on the data before the analyses were completed given a left skew.

In addition, planned paired t tests were completed on the transformed data to further examine the two-way interaction. For both the CA and MLU groups, differences in noun type were not significant. For the SLI group, significant differences were found ($t_{(17)} = 3.86$, $p = .001$), with more frequently inflected items pluralized than infrequently inflected items. The effect size of this difference was .91 (.80 or above is considered large by conventional definition).

Main effects for group, noun type, and allomorphic ending also were significant. Main effects for group and noun type were considered in the two-way interaction. Figure 4 illustrates the main effect of allomorphic ending with group and noun type collapsed. Three paired t tests were completed on the combined scores. Significant differences were present between the -s and -$əz$ items ($t_{(54)} = 8.04$, $p < .05$) and the -z and -$əz$ items ($t_{(54)} = 7.69$, $p < .05$). No difference was found between the -s and -z items. Thus, the effect is largely attributable to the low performance on the -$əz$ ending.

Irregular nouns. A two-way mixed ANOVA (Group x Allomorphic ending) was used to analyze these data. Although the primary interest was application of the regular plural suffix to novel stems, correct irregular plural production also must be considered when interpreting the irregular items. Recall that seven of the irregular nouns were invariable (e.g., milk) and could not be coded for correctness, having a total of five items for possible correct irregular use. As it turned out, the number of correct irregular plural forms produced by each group varied: CA = 12; SLI = 5; MLU = 2. This complicates matters because the opportunity to overregularize the irregulars was different for each group. Because there is no clearly preferred way to address this complication, analyses for the

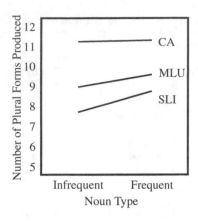

FIGURE 3
Regular nouns: Group × Noun
Interaction. Total correct is 12.

irregular nouns were conducted twice, with and without inclusion of the correct forms. Tests of significance did vary somewhat, so both analyses are reported here.

When correct irregular forms were excluded, the main effects for group ($F_{(2,52)} = 3.33$, $p < .05$) and allomorphic ending ($F_{(2,51)} = 32.58$, $p < .05$) were significant. There were group differences between the SLI group and either of the other two ND groups (SLI vs. CA: $t_{(52)} = -2.42$, $p < .05$; SLI vs. MLU: $t_{(52)} = -1.99$, $p < .05$). To examine the main effect for allomorph, group scores were collapsed and three paired t tests were conducted. Items taking the -əz allomorph were found to be significantly more difficult than items taking either the -s or -z (-s vs. -əz: $t_{(54)} = 7.61$, $p < .05$ and -z vs. -əz: $t_{(54)} = 7.31$, $p < .05$). There was no significant difference between -s and -z productions.

When correct irregular plural productions were included in the analyses, group differences were still significant ($F_{(2,52)} = 4.60$, $p < .05$), with the CA group pluralizing more items than the SLI group ($t_{(52)} = 3.30$, $p < .05$). However, unlike the earlier analysis, the difference between the SLI and MLU group was no longer significant. All other analyses concerning allomorphic effects did not change.

Nonce forms. A two-way mixed ANOVA (Group × Allomorphic ending) was used to analyze these data. Main effects for group ($F_{(2,52)} = 9.27$, $p < .05$) and allomorph ($F_{2,51} = 103.84$, $p < .05$) were significant. Significant group differences were between the CA group and the other two groups (CA vs. SLI group: $t_{(24.5)} = 4.44$. $p < .05$ and CA vs. MLU: $t_{(24.2)} = 3.45$, $p < .05$). As depicted in Figure 4, items taking the -əz allomorph were significantly more difficult than items taking either of the other two allomorphic endings (-s vs. -əz: $t_{(54)} = 123.71$, $p < .05$ and -z vs. -əz: $t_{(54)} = 14.43$, $p < .05$). There was also a difference between items taking -s and items taking -z ($t_{(54)} = -2.22$, $p < .05$).

Compounding Task

Each subject was asked to pluralize and compound 14 nouns. However, the categorization of each response was dependent upon how the children chose to initially pluralize the sin-

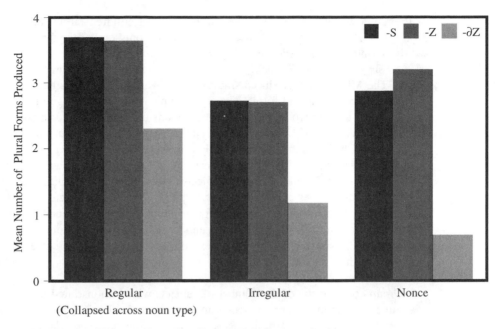

FIGURE 4 **Allomorph main effects. Total correct is 4.**

gular noun forms. If a subject pluralized the word *dog* as *dogs,* the compound of this item would be classified as involving a regular plural. If a subject pluralized the word *foot* as *foots,* the compound would be classified as involving an overregularization. If a subject pluralized the word foot as feet, the compound would be classified as involving an irregular plural. Therefore, seven of the nouns could be categorized as compounds involving regular pluralization and seven could be categorized as compounds involving overregularized plural forms. Of these latter seven, a subject may have produced the correct irregular plural form for five of them (i.e., *men, feet, mice, teeth, geese* but not *deer* and *fish*).

In the event that a subject could not provide a plural form for an item (i.e., only repeated the base stem) or could not compound the item for some reason, the data point for that item could not be used in the analysis. In addition, the number of subjects who completed the nominal compounding task varied across the three groups. Therefore, not only did the total number of data points per subject vary, but the total number of subjects in each group was different. Table 7 presents the number of subjects per group who completed the nominal compounding task as well as a breakdown of each group's responses. Both the frequency of each response type by group and the percentage of each response type out of each group's total number of responses are presented. Four of the SLI and 6 of the MLU children were unable to complete the task. Failure was determined if a child could not produce a noun compound after 10 to 15 training trials. A typical failed response of the MLU children was either to refuse to attempt a compound or to produce only one of the target words (e.g., *popcorn* or *eater*). The SLI children rarely refused compound production. However, their responses involved either only one of the target words or both words but in the wrong order (e.g., *popcorn, eater popcorn* or *eat popcorn*).

As shown in Table 7, each group pluralized a similar percentage of regular plural nouns. The MLU group produced slightly more overregularizations but did not produce any correct irregular plural forms. The SLI group's higher percentage of bare stems was primarily due to their production of irregular nouns in the singular form rather than over-regularizing like the MLU group or correctly producing the irregular plural form like the CA group. Of the items that were correctly produced in the irregular plural form, *foot* and *tooth* were most common. However, *mouse* and *man* were also produced as irregular plurals by the SLI and CA children; only subjects in the CA group pluralized goose correctly.

The first three types of response patterns presented in Table 7 were of particular interest. All three groups rarely produced a regular plural form in compounds even though the stimuli involved multiple plural referents, and the examiner used the plural form to prompt each response. A similar pattern was observed for the nouns that were overregularized. In contrast, for the irregulars, the majority of the nominal compounds included the plural form (e.g., *geese-eater*).

Group comparisons of the number of subjects who demonstrated the correct pattern of regular and irregular noun compounding were examined using the test of significance between two proportions (Bruning & Kintz, 1977). Subjects were classified as correctly compounding the regular nouns if they used the singular form in all, or all but one, of their productions. As indicated in Table 8, the difference between the proportions of SLI and CA children who used the singular form in compounds was significant (SLI vs. CA: $z = 2.12$),

TABLE 7   Summary of subjects' nominal compounding responses by group[a]

	SLI ($n = 14$)	MLU ($n = 12$)	CA ($n = 19$)
Correctly produced the regular plural affix	91 (46%)	77 (46%)	131 (49%)
Correctly overregularized the regular plural affix	52 (27%)	54 (32%)	56 (21%)
Correctly produced the irregular plural form	10 (5%)	0	47 (18%)
Provided the bare stem or an ambiguous response[b]	36 (18%)	20 (12%)	29(11%)
Could not compound	1 (1%)	5 (3%)	0
Provided the correct irregular plural form but could not produce the singular form of the irregular	6 (3%)	8 (5%)	3 (1%)
Excluded because of examiner error[c]	0	4 (2%)	0
Total Responses	196	168	266

[a]Frequencies of response types are presented in the table. Percentage of each response type from each group's total number of responses is included in the parentheses. [b]All responses were bare stems except for two. One subject pluralized rat as mouse and another would only use mouse to compound the word rat. Both of these were included in this response category. [c]All errors involved a child's overregularization that the examiner incorrectly provided as a bare stem during the compounding task.

but the difference between the SLI and MLU groups was not (SLI vs. MLU: $z = .75$) as $z > +/-1.96$ is needed for significance. Group differences were not observed when compounds involving overregularizations were examined (SLI vs. CA: $z = 1.18$; SLI vs. MLU: $z = .11$). As expected, for the irregular compounds the majority of SLI and CA children used the plural form. The difference between the proportion of SLI and CA children who followed this pattern was not significant (SLI = 88%; CA = 94% $z = .60$).

USE THE EVALUATION CHECKLIST TO GUIDE YOUR EVALUATION
OF THE RESULTS

Discussion

The dual mechanism model (Pinker, 1984) was used as a framework for investigating the plural acquisition of children with SLI. The productivity and dual nature of their plural mechanism were examined. In this study, children with SLI demonstrated an ability to produce rule-generated plurals as readily as children in the language-equivalent normative comparison group. Specifically, both the SLI and MLU groups were able to productively pluralize frequently and infrequently pluralized regular nouns and nonce forms. Moreover, across these productivity analyses, differences between the SLI and MLU groups were not significant. Although the CA and MLU groups produced more overregularizations of the irregular noun items than the SLI group, the difference between the SLI and MLU groups was not significant when correct irregular plurals were included in the overregularization count. On the noun compounding task, all three groups compounded regular nouns differently than irregulars. Following a dual mechanism account, these observed patterns of plural use indicate that by 5 years of age children with SLI have arrived at a productive and differentiated plural marking system that is sufficiently robust to guide word formation processes.

One finding that is somewhat discrepant with a normative dual mechanism model is the apparent effect of input frequency on regular plural marking for children with SLI. These children performed better with nouns that are frequently pluralized in everyday conversation as compared to those that are infrequently pluralized. According to the dual mechanism model, once a general paradigmatic rule is established, rule use should be independent of input frequency. Although both groups of normally developing children demonstrated frequency independence, the SLI group did not. A number of explanations may account for this finding. However, one interpretation that does not seem adequate is that of the Missing Feature hypothesis (Crago et al., 1991; Gopnik & Crago, 1991), as it claims that children with SLI are missing an abstract regular plural rule. In this study, the children with SLI clearly demonstrated rule-governed behavior on the pluralization task. Moreover, differential treatment of regular and irregular plural forms during noun compound productions would not have been possible if the SLI children had not possessed a dual plural mechanism.

TABLE 8   Number of subjects who used the singular form inside compounds

Regular noun compounds	
Group	Number of subjects
CA	19/19 (100%)[a]
MLU	10/12 (83%)
SLI	11/14 (79%)[a]
Overregularized noun compounds	
Group	Number of subjects
CA	19/19 (100%)
MLU	11/12 (92%)
SLI	13/14 (93%)

[a]Significant group differences

Another interpretation that does not seem appropriate is one of a general delay in plural rule establishment. The average MLU of the SLI subjects was 3.50; the range was 2.82 to 4.43. Work by Lahey, Liebergott, Chesnick, Menyuk, and Adams (1992) suggests that it is not until after the 3.00 to 3.50 MLU range that some normally developing children achieve plural mastery, as measured by 80% use across two consecutive sessions (p. 389). If the SLI subjects of this study demonstrated a pronounced delay in the establishment of a general paradigmatic plural rule, they should have demonstrated significantly less productive and less accurate plural use than the language-equivalent group. This finding was not observed. Given that some of the subjects' MLUs were greater than 4.00, it is possible that a difference between the SLI and MLU groups was present, but only for children at the less advanced MLU levels. We checked this possibility by comparing the productivity scores of the 6 least-advanced SLI children to their language-equivalent counterparts. An MLU of 3.30 or less was used to identify the less-advanced children. Group differences were not present. In fact, the less-advanced SLI children demonstrated greater pluralization skills than the MLU group.

If plural acquisition of children with SLI is not atypical, and establishment of a regular plural rule is not delayed relative to general language level, then what accounts for the apparent frequency effect? Three explanations seem plausible. These include (a) delayed independence of rule use, (b) rule vulnerability, and (c) a faulty lexicon. Each of these will be briefly discussed (See Oetting, 1992, for elaboration).

A possible explanation of the frequency effect is that part of normal plural development involves a paradigmatic rule that is initially affected by input frequency. During this early period, the more often a word is pluralized the easier it is for the system to generate the inflection. If this is the case, children with SLI present a normal regular plural component, but it takes longer for the system to become independent of frequency effects. Whereas a child with a normally developing language mechanism achieves frequency independence very quickly after a general rule has been established, the plural system of a child with SLI remains frequency-dependent until much later stages of linguistic development. Given this scenario, the ability of children with SLI to achieve rule use that is independent of input frequency may be interpreted as delayed. It should be pointed out that this account does not suggest, as in the case of the Surface account (Leonard, 1989; Leonard et al. in press), that it is the establishment of the plural rule that is delayed. Rather, the rule develops in pace with general linguistic maturation, but an aspect of rule use (i.e., frequency independence) takes longer to develop.

Another explanation may be that effects of input frequency surface anytime a linguistic task becomes difficult for an individual, in the sense that task difficulty requires greater allocation of resources. Young children's variable performance on plural marking across different tasks has been documented elsewhere (cf. Hecht, 1983; Winitz, Sanders, & Kort, 1981). In this study, the metalinguistic requirements of the elicitation task may have been relatively easy for the control children. The normally developing children's near-ceiling performance on the infrequently pluralized regular nouns suggest this to be the case. As such, input frequency effects could not significantly help their performance. On the other hand, the elicitation task may have presented additional sources of difficulty for children in the SLI group. There was some clinical suggestion of this possibility, in that children in the SLI group often required longer latency to formulate their responses and were more likely to revise their answer.

Additional support for this interpretation comes from differences in the group profiles of the MLU and SLI groups when spontaneous plural production is compared to elicited plural production. During spontaneous production, both groups of children produced the plural morpheme with a high percentage of accuracy (above 90%). However, during elicited production, the scores of the SLI group were consistently lower than the MLU group, although group differences were not significant. On this interpretation, the plural rule of SLI children, although represented in the expected way, may nevertheless be more vulnerable to task demands at the linguistic level targeted in this study.

A third explanation for the frequency effect may be that children with SLI have a regular plural rule, but access to the rule is always influenced by input frequency. Thus, the plural system of these children would still involve a dual mechanism, but the role of input frequency would affect both components of the system rather than just irregular plural development. If this explanation is correct, the cause of their persistent dependence on input frequency may be difficult to identify. Perhaps the difficulty involves inefficient access of the lexicon. Thinking back to Kiparsky's model of word formation, a lexeme must enter the different derivation levels to receive target inflections or derivations. If children with SLI are less able to access words that are rarely taken through the word formation process, then infrequently pluralized words would be more difficult for these children to inflect.

Alternatively, the plural rule of children with SLI may be affected by input frequency because of a poorly constructed lexicon. In current work on the dual mechanism model, Pinker and his colleagues are exploring whether inflected forms that are learned during the word-specific period of inflectional development occasionally stay in the lexicon as unanalyzed forms (cf. Pinker & Prince, 1991). Perhaps the lexicon of normally developing children undergoes efficient and frequent reorganization that helps the system rid itself of nonproductive inflected forms. In contrast, the lexical system of SLI children may not reorganize as readily, and nonproductive forms could remain in their lexicon. Although the storage of these nonproductive forms probably hinders the usefulness of a lexicon in the long run, access to these forms may have helped the children in the SLI group during the pluralization task. Thus, the SLI group's higher scores with the frequently pluralized items as compared to the infrequently pluralized forms may have been a product of inefficient lexical storage.

Additional support for this line of reasoning can be found in the regular and overregularized compound productions of the SLI group. Of the 21 ungrammatical compounds (e.g., *rats-eater*) the SLI group produced, 16 were with regular plural forms. Overregularized nouns were less likely to be compounded incorrectly (5 errors out of 52 opportunities). This pattern of findings may have occurred because the SLI children, at times, produced a regular noun compound with an unanalyzed plural form (e.g., *rats*). Ungrammatical compounds were less likely to be produced for the overregularized nouns because the plural forms of these items had to be rule-generated. As a result, they could not be accessed from the lexicon.

A possible test of an inefficient lexicon hypothesis would be to examine the plural systems of language-impaired children who do not demonstrate reduced vocabulary ability. As noted earlier, the SLI children of this study demonstrated a range of vocabulary impairment as measured by the PPVT-R (standard scores ranged between one and three standard deviations below the means expected). If input frequency does not affect the pluralization skills of impaired children who present a normally developing vocabulary, an inefficient lexicon hypothesis may provide a plausible explanation for the observed frequency effect.

To summarize, the findings of this study indicate that the plural system of 5-year-old children with SLI is constructed in a manner that is similar to that of normally developing children who demonstrate equivalent language abilities. Within the dual mechanism model, this means that their plural mechanism involves two subsystems, a paradigmatic component for representing a regular plural rule and an associative memory network for acquiring and storing irregular plural forms. Contrary to the Missing Feature account, the children in the SLI group demonstrated rule-governed behavior. Contrary to the Surface account, the predicted difficulty with plural rule establishment for children with SLI was not observed. Rather, a type of performance factor that affects children's ability to apply the plural suffix independent of input frequency may be operative at the level of lexical marking. In the case of children with SLI, they may take longer to relinquish a familiarity effect than children without SLI. Two alternative accounts, rule vulnerability and the use of a competent plural system in the presence of a faulty lexicon, should also be considered as plausible explanations of SLI children's plural omissions.

At the same time, the full complexity of plural marking entails consideration of number marking beyond the level of individual lexical items as assessed here. Elsewhere (Rice & Oetting, 1993) we argue that another way in which the plural uses of children with SLI differ from their language-equivalent control group is in the syntactic contexts in which omissions are likely. Within a full noun phrase, noun phrases with quantifiers (e.g., *two balls*) create more difficulties for children with SLI than for normally developing children. These errors were not interpretable as an effect of frequency for the lexical items involved. Considered together, the two studies suggest that although the underlying representation of regular plural affixation is intact for children with SLI, there are nevertheless some points of vulnerability for less frequently encountered lexical items and certain syntactic constructions. The findings of this study indicate that the probable sources of the vulnerability are outside the representation of plural morphology per se. Fruitful areas for further investigation include studies of older children with SLI to determine if the frequency effect at the lexical level persists, if plural marking remains influenced by certain syntactic contexts, and if there is an interactive effect of lexical and grammatical factors on SLI plural use.

USE THE EVALUATION CHECKLIST TO GUIDE YOUR EVALUATION
OF THE DISCUSSION

Acknowledgments

This manuscript summarizes the findings of the first author's doctoral dissertation, completed while she was a U.S. Department of Education Trainee at the University of Kansas #H029090046-90. As part of a larger project this study was also supported by NIDCD 1 R01 NS26129, awarded to the second author. Appreciation is extended to Pat Cleave, Soyeong Pae, and Colette Thomas for their assistance in subject recruitment, language sample elicitation and transcription, and reliability calculation. We are also grateful to the children, teachers, and parents of the following day care centers and preschools in Lawrence: Children's Learning Center, Community Child Care Services, Head Start, Hilltop Child Development Center, Stepping Stones, United Christian Development Center, Hutchinson Early Education Center, and the public school systems of Baldwin and Shawnee Mission, whose cooperation made this study possible.

References

Allen, M. (1978). *Morphological investigations.* Unpublished doctoral dissertation. University of Connecticut, Storrs, CT.

Anisfeld, M., & Tucker, G. (1968). English pluralization rules of six-year-old children. *Child Development, 38,* 1201–1217.

Berko, J. (1958). The child's learning of English morphology. *Word, 14,* 150–177.

Bruning, J., & Kintz, B. (1977). *Computational handbook of statistics.* Glenview, IL: Scott, Foresman, and Company.

Burgemeister, B., Blum, H., & Lorge, I. (1972). *The Columbia Mental Maturity Scale.* New York: Harcourt Brace Jovanovich.

Cazden, C. (1968). The acquisition of noun and verb inflections. *Child Development, 39,* 433–448.

Clahsen, H. (1989). The grammatical characterization of developmental dysphasia. *Linguistics, 27,* 897–920.

Clahsen, H., Rothweiler, M., Woest, A., & Marcus, G. (1993). Regular and irregular inflection in the acquisition of German noun plurals. *Cognition, 45,* 225–255.

Connell, P. (1986). Teaching subjecthood to language-disordered children. *Journal of Speech and Hearing Research, 29,* 481–493.

Crago, M., Gopnik, M., Guilfoyle, E., & Allen, S. (1991). *Familial aggregation of a developmental language disorder.* Paper presented at the annual conference of the American Speech-Language-Hearing Association, Atlanta, GA.

Dunn, A., & Dunn, A. (1981). *Peabody Picture Vocabulary Test—Revised.* Circle Pines, MN: American Guidance Service.

Francis, W., & Kucera, H. (1982). *Frequency analysis of English usage: Lexicon and grammar.* Boston, MA: Houghton Mifflin.

Goldman, R., & Fristoe, M. (1986). *Goldman-Fristoe Test of Articulation.* Circle Pines, MN: American Guidance Service.

Gopnik, M. (1990a). Feature blindness: A case study. *Language Acquisition, 1,* 139–164.

Gopnik, M. (1990b). Feature-blind grammar and dysphasia. *Nature, 334,* 715.

Gopnik, M., & Crago, M. (1991). Familial aggregation of a developmental language disorder. *Cognition, 39,* 1–50.

Gordon, P. (1985). Level-ordering in lexical development. *Cognition, 21,* 73–93.

Gordon, P., Alegre, M., & Jackson, T. (1993). *Finding the red rats eater: Lexical recursion in children's compounding.* Paper presented at the annual Stanford Child Language Research Forum, Stanford University, Stanford, CA.

Hall, W., Nagey, W., & Linn, R. (1984). *Spoken words: Effects of situation and social group on oral word usage and frequency.* Hillsdale, NJ: Lawrence Erlbaum Associates.

Hecht, B. (1983). *Situations and language: Children's use of plural allomorphs in familiar and unfamiliar settings.* Unpublished doctoral dissertation. Stanford University, Stanford, CA.

Johnston, J. (1988). The language disordered child. In N. Lass, L. McReynolds, J. Northern, & D. Yoder (Eds.), *Handbook of speech-pathology and audiology* (pp. 685–715). Toronto: B. C. Decker.

Kiparsky, P. (1982). From cyclic phonology to lexical phonology. In H. van der Hulst & N. Smith (Eds.), *The structure of phonological representations* (pp. 131–175). Dordrecht, Netherlands: Foris.

Kiparsky, P. (1983). Word-formation and the lexicon. In F. Ingemann (Ed.), *Proceedings of the 1982 Mid-America Linguistics Conference.* University of Kansas, Lawrence, KS.

Lahey, M., Liebergott, J., Chesnick, M., Menyuk, P., & Adams, J. (1992). Variability in the use of grammatical morphemes: Implications for understanding language impairment. *Applied Psycholinguistics, 13,* 373–398.

Lee, L. (1974). *Developmental sentence analysis.* Evanston, IL: Northwestern University Press.

Leonard, L. (1989). Language learnability and specific language impairment in children. *Applied Psycholinguistics, 10,* 179–202.

Leonard, L., Bertolini, U., Caselli, M., McGregor, K., & Sabbadini, L. (1992). Morphological deficits in children with specific language impairment: The status of features in the underlying grammar. *Language Acquisition, 2 (2),* 151–180.

Leonard, L., Sabbadini, L., Leonard, J., & Volterra, V. (1987). Specific language impairment in children: A cross-linguistic study. *Brain and Language, 32,* 233–252.

Loeb, D., & Leonard, L. (1991). Subject case marking and verb morphology in normally developing and specifically language-impaired children. *Journal of Speech and Hearing Research, 34,* 340–446.

MacWhinney, B. (1978). The acquisition of morphophonology. *Monographs of the Society for Research in Child Development, 43 (1–2).*

Marchman, V., & Bates, E. (1991). Vocabulary size and composition as predictors of morphological development. *Center for Research in Language Technical Report #9103.* University of California.

Marcus, G., Ullman, M., Pinker, S., Hollander, M., Rosen, T., & Xu, F. (1992). Overregularization in language acquisition. *Monographs of the Society for Research in Child Development, 57 (4).*

Menyuk, P. (1964). Comparison of grammar of children with functionally deviant and normal speech. *Journal of Speech and Hearing Research, 7,* 109–121.

Mervis, C., & Johnson, K. (1991). Acquisition of the plural morpheme: A case study. *Developmental Psychology, 27,* 222–235.

Miller, J. (1981). *Assessing language production in children.* Austin, TX: PROED.

Oetting, J. (1992). *Language-impaired and normally developing children's acquisition of English plural.* Unpublished doctoral dissertation. University of Kansas, Lawrence, KS.

Pinker, S. (1984). *Language learnability and language development.* Cambridge, MA: Harvard University Press.

Pinker, S. (1991). Rules of language. *Science, 253,* 530–535.

Pinker, S., & Prince, A. (1991). Regular and irregular morphology and the psychological status of rules of grammar. *Proceedings of the 1991 Meeting of the Berkeley Linguistics Society.* University of California, Berkeley.

Plunkett, K., & Marchman, V. (in press). From rote learning to system building: Acquiring verb morphology in children and connectionist nets. *Cognition.*

Prasada, S., & Pinker, S. (in press). Generalization of regular and irregular morphological patterns. *Language and Cognitive Processes.*

Rice, M., & Oetting, J. (1993). Morphological deficits of children with SLI: Evaluation of number marking and agreement. *Journal of Speech and Hearing Research, 36,* 1254–1262.

Rom, A., & Leonard, L. (1990). Interpreting deficits in grammatical morphology in specifically language-impaired children: Preliminary evidence from Hebrew. *Clinical Linguistics and Phonetics, 4,* 93–105.

Rondal J., Ghiotto, M., Bredart, S., & Bachelet, J. (1987). Age-relation, reliability, and grammatical validity of measures of utterance length. *Journal of Child Language, 14,* 433–446.

Rumelhart, D., & McClelland, J. (1987). Learning past tenses of English verbs: Implicit rules or parallel distributed processing? In B. MacWhinney (Ed.), *Mechanisms of language learning* (pp. 195–248). Hillsdale, NJ: Erlbaum.

Seidenberg, M., & Daugherty, K. (1992). Rules or connections? The past tense revisited. In *Proceedings of the Fourteenth Annual Conference of the Cognitive Science Society,* Hillsdale, NJ: Lawrence Erlbaum.

Siegel, D. (1977). *Topics in English morphology.* Unpublished doctoral dissertation. Massachusetts Institute of Technology, Cambridge, MA.

Ullman, M., & Pinker, S. (1990). *Why do some verbs not have a single past tense form?* The 15th Annual Boston Conference on Language Development, Boston College, Boston, MA.

Winitz, H., Sanders, R., & Kort, J. (1981). Comprehension and production of the /-əz/ plural allomorph. *Journal of Psycholinguistic Research, 10,* 159–271.

Received January 15,1993
Accepted July 7, 1993

Contact author: Janna B. Oetting, PhD, Department of Communication Sciences and Disorders, Louisiana State University, Baton Rouge, LA 70803–2606. e-mail: cdjanna @ lsuvm.sncc.lsu.edu

Author Index

Subject Index